Anthropology in Medical Education

Iveris L. Martinez • Dennis W. Wiedman
Editors

Anthropology in Medical Education

Sustaining Engagement and Impact

Springer

Editors
Iveris L. Martinez
Center for Successful Aging, College of Health and Human Services
California State University – Long Beach
Long Beach, CA, USA

Dennis W. Wiedman
Department Global and Sociocultural Studies, School of International and Public Affairs
Florida International University
Miami, FL, USA

ISBN 978-3-030-62276-3 ISBN 978-3-030-62277-0 (eBook)
https://doi.org/10.1007/978-3-030-62277-0

This Springer imprint is published by the registered company Springer Nature Switzerland AG.
The registered company address is: Gewerbestrasse 11, 6330 Cham, Switzerland

I dedicate this book to my children in hopes of inspiring them to make this a better world in whatever capacity they may. To my parents and sister for pushing me to always do my best. For Marcie who is my role model of resilience and my best friend.

—Iveris L. Martinez

This book and my chapters represent a lifetime of endeavors to improve health care for peoples of the world. Through these decades my children Crescent, Danielle, and Denison were always supportive in their many ways. I give thanks to my parents, Frances and John, and especially my wife Felicia, whose lives instilled in me the value of caring for others.

—Dennis W. Wiedman

Contents

About the Editors

Iveris L. Martinez, PhD, is Professor, Archstone Foundation Endowed Chair in Gerontology, and Director of the Center for Successful Aging at California State University, Long Beach. She was a founding faculty member of the Herbert Wertheim College of Medicine (HWCOM) at Florida International University where she served as chief of the Division of Medicine and Society and chaired the admissions committee for the college for 5 years. Between 2009 and 2018, she taught the first-year introductory course and other course content on health disparities, cultural competency, and social determinants of health at HWCOM, as well as led an annual interprofessional clinical workshop across the health sciences. An applied anthropologist, she has received funding from the National Institutes of Health, the Macarthur Foundation, and others for her community-based research on social and cultural factors influencing health, with an emphasis in aging, Latinos, and minority populations. Her current research interests include improving services for caregivers of persons with Alzheimer's, reducing social isolation in aging, as well as interprofessional efforts to create age-friendly communities. She previously served as the Chair of the Board of the Alliance for Aging, Inc., the local area agency on aging for Miami-Dade and Monroe Counties, and President of the Association for Anthropology, Gerontology, and the Life Course. She holds a joint Ph.D. in Anthropology and Population and Family Health Sciences (Public Health) from Johns Hopkins University.

Dennis W. Wiedman PhD, is Professor of Anthropology, Department of Global and Sociocultural Studies, Florida International University, Miami, Florida. He received his Ph.D. in Anthropology from the University of Oklahoma in 1979 where he trained in medical anthropology at the University of Oklahoma College of Medicine. Employment in the Department of Psychiatry at the University of Miami School of Medicine in the Office of Transcultural Education and Research grounded him in clinical anthropology as Director of a Department of Psychiatry community mental health unit. He is the Founding Director of the FIU Global Indigenous Forum with the mission to bring the indigenous voice to FIU, South

Florida, and the world. His research interests include Native American health, organizational culture, applying anthropology, and directing culture change. He specializes in social and cultural factors for the global pandemic of type II diabetes and metabolic syndrome. He teaches courses in medical anthropology, anthropological theory, and ethnohistorical research methods. During more than a decade in the FIU Provost Office, he was the Assistant to the Provost, University Accreditation Officer and first Director of Program Review. As lead strategic planner for the university's first major strategic plan he had a key role in planning and envisioning the new FIU Medical School incorporating medical anthropology principles and a community focus. He served on the Executive Board of the American Anthropological Association (AAA) in the practicing/professional seat, and was President of the National Association for the Practice of Anthropology (NAPA). Throughout these academic, applied, and practicing leadership experiences, he consistently published on organizational culture theory and analysis in leading journals and book chapters.

Chapter 1
Anthropological Engagement in Medical Education: An Introduction

Iveris L. Martinez and Dennis W. Wiedman

> *Medicine is a social science and politics is nothing else but medicine on a large scale. Medicine as a social science, as the science of human beings, has the obligation to point out problems and to attempt their theoretical solution; the politician, the practical anthropologist, must find the means for their actual solution. The physicians are the natural attorneys of the poor, and social problems fall to a large extent within their jurisdiction.*
>
> *Rudolf Virchow (1848–1849)* Die Medizinische Reform

It has long been recognized that the field of anthropology has much to contribute to medicine and medical education. Anthropologists by training and vocation possess an excellent skill set in cross-cultural communication and critical analysis that can contribute to greater understanding of the human condition, illness, and healing systems around the world, including the current hegemonic system of allopathic medicine. Since the 1890s, anthropologists have served in medical schools in an array of roles in teaching, curriculum development, administration, evaluation, research, and planning. Yet, for over a century, anthropologists teaching in medical schools have experienced uneven success and tangible frustrations. Careers of anthropologists in medicine have followed diverse tracks and have significantly transformed over time. Recent changes in medical education focusing on diversity, social determinants of health, and more humanistic patient centered care opens the door for anthropologists in medical schools. However, throughout history, sustaining anthropological engagement and impact within medical education has proved

I. L. Martinez (✉)
Center for Successful Aging, College of Health and Human Services, California State University – Long Beach, Long Beach, CA, USA
e-mail: iveris.martinez@csulb.edu

D. W. Wiedman
Department Global and Sociocultural Studies, School of International and Public Affairs, Florida International University, Miami, FL, USA
e-mail: wiedmand@fiu.edu

I. L. Martinez, D. W. Wiedman (eds.), *Anthropology in Medical Education*,
https://doi.org/10.1007/978-3-030-62277-0_1

challenging at times, albeit not impossible and oftentimes very rewarding. In fact, according to Hemmings, "Medical anthropology is still largely ignored in clinical settings and training, or considered at best peripheral" (2005: 92). This is not to say that anthropology has nothing to offer medical education, or that medicine could not benefit even greatly from engagement with anthropology, its to say that we need to find ways to do it better.

The purpose of this book is to reflect on how anthropologists have engaged in medical education, and to positively influence the future careers of anthropologists who are currently engaged, or considering a career in medical education. In doing so, we also seek to enhance the important role of anthropology in educating physicians throughout the world to improve patient care and population health. We describe various ways in which anthropologists have been and are currently engaged in training physicians in various countries, suggesting potential new directions for the field. Anthropologists working to prepare future physicians must not only be familiar with the culture of biomedicine, but also aware of the culture of medical education as well as the health systems in which medical students work. Chapters in this peer-reviewed book describe the past and current experiences of anthropologists in medical schools, the modes and magnitude of this engagement, and reflect on these experiences from diverse settings in medical education.

This edited volume emerged organically from a collaboration by us on the role of anthropological theory and methods in organizational culture, namely the establishment of a new medical school at an urban public university where we were both faculty. Using longitudinal cultural theme analysis we compared the 1996 University Strategic Plan calling for the establishing of the medical school compared to the 2015 medical school strategic plan written 9 years after the school opened its doors (Wiedman and Martinez 2017). Our conversation while collaborating on this journal article led us to at first a perfunctory exploration of the historical role of anthropologists in medical education, and later to a much more systemic and deeper exploration. Chapter 2 of this book details the role of anthropologists in US medical education from 1890 to the present.

From this research we realized that the recent history of anthropological involvement in medical education was not well documented and that the lessons we could learn from each other and past experiences were buried in the anthropological literature. The lessons of this historical research resonated with many of the experiences that we personally had. Wondering what the experience was of others currently teaching in medical education, we decided to convene symposia on the subject of "sustaining anthropological engagement in medical education" and put a call out to organizational networks for participants. The first symposium was held at the Society for Applied Anthropology meetings in Santa Fe, New Mexico on March 28, 2017. The second was held the following Fall at the annual conference of the American Anthropological Association held in Washington DC on December 1, 2017. A number of the chapters in this volume had their inception during these presentations and discussions.

Building upon the barriers to engagement both from the medical school culture and our diverse anthropological training, chapters focus on solutions to these barriers, identifying useful theoretical paradigms and successful strategies. We consider not only individual level issues, but institutional and organizational structures that allow for sustained engagement. Moreover, potential models or strategies for continued and significant impact in medical education are highlighted. A purpose of this book is to initiate dialogue while providing constructive solutions to make anthropological engagement in medical education more effective and sustainable. Each of the chapters address the context of the current emergence of interests in the social sciences in medicine in their respective locations, and consider whether the current resurgence is a sustainable trend. Ultimately, the goal is to consider how anthropologists can have a continued and significant impact in medical education. Applied medical anthropologists primarily emphasize improving health outcomes for populations, including changing health care delivery for the better. Strategically, one of the key ways to do this is to influence the training of physicians.

Several factors are opening up opportunities to anthropologists in the field of medical education. These include changes in accreditation standards for medical schools around the globe that require the incorporation of behavioral factors in understanding and addressing the social determinants of health, a recognition of the impact of diversity on health care, and the call for interprofessional approaches to improve patient outcomes. Furthermore, new opportunities for recent graduates of anthropology graduate programs are increasingly outside the traditional employment sectors of anthropology and more and more in applied settings, such as medical education and healthcare.

In order to better contribute to these efforts, anthropologists and anthropology students need to be prepared to effectively assume these roles in medical education. Therefore, this book should be of primary interest to doctoral students in anthropology, or other anthropologists who want to, or are thinking about going into medical education as a profession. It will also be useful to medical and applied anthropology programs actively seeking curriculum to train anthropologists to work within the medical profession as it provides numerous examples of how anthropology has and can contribute to the medical field. Additionally, this information has importance for the history of medicine and of anthropology. Finally, this book should be of interest to medical educators and deans of curriculum who are seeking to integrate anthropology into current pre-med and medical school curriculum to address the current focus on diversity, social determinants of health, and more humanistic patient centered care. Therefore, because writing for multiple audiences across different disciplines can pose challenges, we have done our best to keep the language jargon-free and speak to the interests and concerns of diverse readers.

While the experience of anthropologists in medical education has been documented in several articles and anthropology meeting proceedings, there are no recent books published on the various roles of anthropologists in medical school education. In 1982, Chrisman and Maretzki published an edited book titled *Clinically Applied Anthropology: Anthropologist in Health Science Settings* that took a broad look at the role of anthropologists in health science faculties and beyond the academic settings in these fields. This book was followed by Peggy Golde and Demitri B. Shimkin's *Clinical Anthropology: A New Approach to American Health*

Problems (1983) that highlighted the many facets of anthropologists in the clinical setting. Howard Stein's 1990 book, *American Medicine as Culture*, provided a psychological anthropology perspective on the culture of medicine with specific chapters on the socialization and process of becoming a physician including paradoxes of medical training. In 1996, John Rush published the book *Clinical Anthropology: An Application of Anthropological Concepts within Clinical Settings* with the aim to find common threads between social sciences and biomedical sciences to propose a model for clinical practice. More recently, in 2011, Good et al. published a volume Shattering Culture: American Medicine Responds to Cultural Diversity presenting ethnographic studies of health-care settings focused on one aspect of anthropological engagement in medical education—the recent preoccupation with cultural competence. Two recent issues of the *Journal of Culture, Medicine, and Psychiatry* published two special editions (Holmes et al. 2011) and (Carpenter-Song and Willen 2013) highlight some of the experiences of anthropologists teaching medical students, as well as some of their ethnographic research of medical education at the center of anthropological engagements with medicine since the 1980s. Most recently in *Practicing Anthropology*, Barnes et al. (2020), present the 2009 initiation of the masters degree in medical anthropology in the Boston University School of Medicine. They discuss how anthropology research paradigms are translated to clinical settings leading to their student's careers in community-based anthropology. However, until now there has not been a book that serves as an accessible resource for those in anthropology seeking to work in the training of physicians or to raise awareness among medical schools and medical educators of the long-standing history, constraints, and strategies for facilitating the integral knowledge and skills that anthropologists bring to educating future physicians.

About This Book

The volume provides throughout its chapters the history of anthropological involvement in medical education—a legacy that is not yet available in one easily accessible format that can be studied and built upon in current applied and research efforts. Chapters highlight the global health experience of the integration of anthropology in medical education in Canada, France, the United Kingdom, Japan, Mexico, Uganda, and the United States. The book is organized in four parts that capture some of the major contemporary themes of anthropology in medical education.

Medical School Culture

The first theme in the book is medical school culture. Every organization and profession has a culture with shared beliefs, practices, and material objects. Over historical time the culture of medicine and medical school culture patterned individual values and behaviors of faculty and students. First, Wiedman and Martinez outline the history of anthropological contributions in medical education in the United States since the 1890s. This chapter is intended to outline a history that until now has been inaccessible to anthropologists entering the field of medical education, or others such as medical educators seeking to understand how anthropology has and can positively influence medical education and the care of patients. While we do not claim this to be a comprehensive history, the intent is to give the reader a starting point to explore further this rich canon.

The next chapter, by Samuel Leze, provides a rich description of the colorful and deeply rooted rituals of medical school culture in France. Based on his teaching experience at the École Normale Supérieure de Lyon, France, Leze describes how a moral economy of care organizes medical education to humanize physicians. Historically, the beginnings of allopathic physician training began in the surgical theatres of France. Leze teaches that the dominating, authoritative, and paternalistic physician is no longer the best moral attitude to convey good care. From this portrayal of medical school organizational culture and folkore as a *rite-de-passage*, he shares how to teach contemporary medical education in France as a moral career with at least two turning points that are decisive and structuring in access to the profession of doctor, to medical training, and to clinical practice.

Junko Iida and Hiroshi Nishigori describe their joint efforts to develop and implement between anthropologists and medical doctors in Japan for conducting "collaborative clinical case conferences" as a means of helping physicians and medical students manage the uncertainty, or *moyamoya*, that often emerges in clinical practice. This uncertainty, where clinical decision-making is not as straightforward as clinicians would hope, they argue, is increasing due to the rise of chronic diseases in an aging society. In doing so, they examine the "new anthropology" that emerges from this collaboration. It is noteworthy that traditionally in medical anthropology such morphing and fusing of anthropology with medicine has not been considered as legitimate within the field of medical anthropology.

Furthermore, in this section, Lisa Dikomitis presents an analysis of how medical students "think about" the social sciences, including anthropology, in the United Kingdom. Dikomitis uses autoethnography and other ethnographic techniques implemented at two medical schools in which she has taught to examine medical students' views about social scientific learning content, especially anthropology, and the challenges and opportunities of integrating anthropology in medical education. In doing so she explores students enthusiasm and apprehension for anthropological content, as well as the "hidden curriculum" and other constraining factors. She also notes the relative "invisibility" and limited understanding of anthropology in medicine and outlines critical incidents that can facilitate the teaching of anthropology in medicine. Her chapter also provides a useful methodological example of how to use ethnography to understand the impact of anthropologists teaching in medicine.

Dennis Wiedman also uses an autoethnography approach to describe the training, research, and work experiences that prepared him for a leading role in planning the future of an entire university with a vision for a new medical school to train physicians focused on community care at Florida International University in

Miami, Florida. Reflecting on factors shaping anthropology and medicine over the past 50 years, the lessons learned are important for future students assessing applied, practicing and academic careers. More specifically, he discusses theories, methods, skills and perspectives useful for understanding medical school culture. He notes ways to maintain an anthropologist identity while taking leadership roles in institutions and professional organizations to facilitate the influence of anthropology and organizational culture change.

Beyond Cultural Competency

The second section titled "Beyond Cultural Competency" includes chapters that highlight contemporary contributions of anthropologists to issues of how to work with patients of diverse cultural backgrounds.

Mutale Chileshe reflects on 4 years of teaching behavioral sciences as part of an interdisciplinary team at the Copperbelt University School of Medicine in Zambia using participatory anthropology. Her role is particularly remarkable as the field of anthropology is virtually non-existent in Zambia given its links to colonization. Chileshe demonstrates how the utilization of unique and creative anthropological approaches and "participatory anthropology," including ethnography and fieldwork, can deeply impact student learning of the contextual factors of health.

William McKellin describes how anthropology played a significant role in elevating the patient's point of view during a period of curricular reform in the Canadian medical education system in the 1990s and 2000s. Both health care and medical education are publicly funded in Canada which stimulates medical curricula to reflect social responsibilities to their communities and patients. This wave of curriculum change was an opportunity to include anthropological perspectives and ethnographic methodologies in the MD program at the University of British Columbia through the development of new required, multi-disciplinary courses. These courses brought together medical anthropology, epidemiology, community health, and medical ethics. He guided students in conducting ethnography in communities and interviewing patients in their homes confronting the student's tension between epidemiological evidence and individual patient experiences.

Maya and Vega describe the long-standing history of anthropology in medical education in Mexico and explore anthropological instruction within medical education at the National Autonomous University of Mexico (UNAM). They focus on the curriculum's strengths, limitations, and potential directions for future growth. This undergraduate course of study leads to a Bachelor of Surgery medical degree. Medical anthropologists also contribute to graduate degrees in medical anthropology and certificate-granting workshops. Since the mid-1980s medical anthropology faculty in the medical school have influenced medical student curriculum to reflect an anthropological approach to patient care and population health, in particular with respect to the Indigenous population in rural regions. Reflexive analysis provides recommendations for integrating anthropology into pre-med and medical school curriculums.

Ethics and Humanities

Ethics and humanities programs are perhaps one of the places where anthropologists are most likely to work in medical schools today. The increase in health humanities programs in medical schools has created new meanings and opportunities for anthropologists in medical education. More than transmitting anthropological theories and methods to medical students, ethnographic understanding of how efforts to transform medical education itself are necessary for sustainable contributions to the human experience of illness.

Juliette McMullin and Sharon Rushing provide an ethnographic study of how anthropologists engaged in an interdisciplinary effort to develop a medical and health humanities program in a newly established school of medicine at the University of California, Riverside. They discuss the process of bringing together multiple paradigms and pedagogies of the humanities (arts and social sciences) with those of medical education. Most notable is their reflection on the institutional aspects of development across multiple administrative levels, academic calendars, faculty permissions, and institutional justifications for humanities content in medical curriculum. They note that co-constructing content that forwards humanistic knowledge in medical education requires continuous dialogical engagement and attentiveness to systems and practices that exclude perspectives from other disciplines.

Arlene Macdonald and Jerome Crowder explore the challenges anthropologists face integrating their critical perspectives in medical humanities programs. Based on their experience at the University of Texas Medical Branch, they describe the "many hats" they wore and strategies they adopted for legitimizing anthropological content within the biomedical context and make suggestions for facilitating the process of integration for future anthropologists entering the medical humanities. This chapter also delivers a brief history of the growth of medical humanities in medical schools since the 1970s, and the emerging tensions between contrasting views of traditional perspectives of biomedicine with its individualistic perspective of the 'humanist self' and broader understandings offered by anthropology and other critical fields.

Lee X. Blonder provides a comprehensive history of integrative and alternative medicine and how she as an anthropologist was able to make this a more significant part of medical education at the University of Kentucky College of Medicine. Her experience illuminates many of the presumptions inherent in biomedicine and provides a way to expose students to non-conventional healing modalities and traditions that challenge their views and enhance their educational experience. Ultimately her goal is to demonstrate how anthropologists can present options not offered in a "diagnose and dispense" model of healthcare in which prescription drugs are often the principal approach to prevention and treatment.

Addressing Socio-cultural Determinants of Health and Health Disparities

The last section of the book provides several examples of one of the most recent thematic formulations within medical education, how anthropologists are addressing socio-cultural determinants of health and health disparities.

Iveris Martinez (California State University, Long Beach) in the chapter "Anthropology in the Implementation of a New Medical School in South Florida" describes her role as founding faculty at the Herbert Wertheim College of Medicine, Florida International University in Miami where she played a key role in the content development and implementation of an innovative medical curriculum that addressed the needs and perspectives of this urban multicultural community. She describes how her anthropological and public health training and prior experiences led her to this unique opportunity as Chief of the Division of Medicine and Society, and Chair of the college's admission committee, among other roles. She reflects on the main challenges she faced as a medical school faculty member and shares some of the strategies she learned in the process to be more effective in her role as an administrator and medical teacher.

Robert Rubinstein and Sandra Lane describe how they developed and implemented anthropologically-based innovations in several health professional schools in Upstate New York using a community-based collaborative model. The authors have been engaged in this process of curriculum development and research since 1994. They highlight the role of anthropology in responding to the social determinants of health at the local level through community-based research. They stress relationship building as the foundation for creating change.

Mary Alice Scott, Ernesto Moralez, and John Andazola describe a family medicine curriculum they developed using a structural competency framework to address social determinants of health and health equity, focusing on the anthropological contributions to this curriculum. The Southern New Mexico Family Medicine Residency Program's mission is to "eliminate health disparities in New Mexico and train family physicians who will stay in the border region after graduation." The curriculum they developed as part of an interprofessional team of experts shifts community rotations from the traditional clinic environment to community-based experiences in local agencies and other settings that give residents a better appreciation of the social and structural barriers to health their patients face.

The book explores the various ways anthropologists are currently involved, as well as the barriers and opportunities for sustained involvement, in medical education. What are the potential roles for anthropologists in medicine? What can they accomplish within the field? And, how can the fields of anthropology and medicine facilitate ways for anthropologists to fulfill emerging roles in medical education? In this book, we focus on anthropological contributions to medical education, interactions with medical students, curriculum development, educational research and management, in contrast to focusing on anthropological research on biomedicine which encompasses the large part of medical anthropology publications. Through these chapters we aspire to propose better ways for sustained engagement of anthropology in medical education. It is our firm belief that anthropology has much to contribute to medical education. It is our hope that this volume will inform the future training of physicians and contribute to improvements in population health for generations to come.

Acknowledgments The chapters in this book greatly benefited from the perspectives of peer reviewers working in both medicine and anthropology who generously gave of their time and knowledge to improving the individual chapters in this volume: Amy Blue, PhD, Thomas Breslin, Ph.D, Noel Chrisman, PhD, Juan Cocum, PhD, Angela Jenks, PhD, Catherine Mas, PhD, Aimee Medeiros, PhD, Bryan Page, PhD, Amy Paul-Ward, PhD, and Bill Ventres, MD, MA. Students in Dennis Wiedman's medical anthropology courses at Florida International University greatly enhanced Chap. 2 by locating sources and writing essays on various medical education topics and careers of anthropologists. Special thanks goes to students Katlyn Cabrera, Victoria Davide, Lauren De La Torre, Jordan Evans, Maria Fernandez, Angelica Roger, and especially Joshua Falcon. We would also like to thank Stephen Schensul, Allan Burns, Alba Amaya-Burns, Robert Rubinstein, Sandra Lane, Juliet McMullin, Sharon Rushing, Jerome Crowder, Arlene McDonald and Edward Rohn for their engagement in the initial conversations that inspired this volume during the 2017 annual conferences of the Society for Applied Anthropology and the American Anthropological Association. Thank you to Carmen Estrada for her invaluable assistance proofreading and formatting the chapters in this volume.

References

Barnes, Linda L., Lance D. Laird, and Bayla Ostrach. 2020. From medical anthropology at a medical school to careers in community-based applied anthropology. *Practicing Anthropology* 42 (1): 36–42.

Carpenter-Song, Elizabeth, and Sarah S. Willen, eds. 2013. Special issue: Cultural competence in action: Multidisciplinary perspectives on four case studies. *Culture, Medicine and Psychiatry* 37 (2): 241–402.

Chrisman, Noel J., and Thomas W. Maretzki, eds. 1982. *Clinically applied anthropology: Anthropologists in health science settings*. Dordrecht: Springer.

Golde, Peggy, and Demitri B. Shimkin, eds. 1983. *Clinical anthropology: A new approach to American health problems?* Lanham, MD: University Press of America.

Good, Mary-Jo DelVecchio, Sarah S. Willen, Seth Donal Hannah, Ken Vickery, and Lawrence Taeseng Park, eds. 2011. *Shattering culture: American medicine responds to cultural diversity*. New York: Russell Sage Foundation.

Hemmings, Colin P. 2005. Rethinking medical anthropology: How anthropology is failing medicine. *Anthropology & Medicine* 12 (2): 91–103.

Holmes, Seth M., Angela C. Jenks, and Scott Stonington, eds. 2011. Special issue: Anthropologies of clinical training in the 21st century. *Culture, Medicine, and Psychiatry* 35 (2): 103–330.

Rush, John A. 1996. *Clinical anthropology: An application of anthropological concepts within clinical settings*. Westport, CT: Praeger.

Stein, Howard. 1990. *American medicine as culture*. Boulder: Westview Press.

Virchow, Rudolph. 1848–1849. *Die Meizinishe Reform. Eign Wochenschrift*, 10 July 1848–29 June 1849. Berlin: Druck & Verlag von G. Reimer.

Wiedman, Dennis, and Iveris L. Martinez. 2017. Organizational culture theme theory and analysis of strategic planning for a new medical school. *Human Organization* 76 (3): 264–274.

Iveris L. Martinez, PhD is Professor, Archstone Foundation Endowed Chair in Gerontology, and Director of the Center for Successful Aging at California State University, Long Beach. She was a founding faculty member of the Herbert Wertheim College of Medicine (HWCOM) at Florida International University where she served as chief of the Division of Medicine & Society and chaired the admissions committee for the college for five years. Between 2007 and 2018, she taught the first year introductory course and other course content on health disparities, cultural competency, and social determinants of health at HWCOM, as well as led an annual interprofessional clinical workshop across the health sciences. An applied anthropologist, she has received funding from the National Institutes of Health, the Macarthur Foundation, and others for her community-based research on social and cultural factors influencing health, with an emphasis in aging, Latinos, and minority populations. Her current research interests include improving services for caregivers of persons with Alzheimer's, reducing social isolation in aging, as well as interprofessional efforts to create age-friendly communities. She previously served as the Chair of the Board of the Alliance for Aging, Inc., the local area agency on aging for Miami-Dade and Monroe Counties, and President of the Association for Anthropology, Gerontology, and the Life Course. She holds a joint Ph.D. in Anthropology and Population & Family Health Sciences (Public Health) from Johns Hopkins University.

Dennis W. Wiedman, PhD, is Professor of Anthropology, Department of Global and Sociocultural Studies. Florida International University. Miami, Florida. He received his Ph.D. in Anthropology from the University of Oklahoma in 1979 where he trained in medical anthropology at the University of Oklahoma College of Medicine. Employment in the Department of Psychiatry at the University of Miami School of Medicine in the Office of Transcultural Education and Research grounded him in clinical anthropology as Director of a Department of Psychiatry community mental health unit. He is the Founding Director of the FIU Global Indigenous Forum with the mission to bring the Indigenous voice to FIU, South Florida, and the world. His research interests include Native American health, Type II diabetes, organizational culture, applying anthropology, and directing culture change. He specializes in social and cultural factors for the global pandemic of Type II diabetes and metabolic syndrome. He teaches courses in medical anthropology, anthropological theory, and ethnohistorical research methods. During more than a decade in the FIU Provost Office he was the University Accreditation Officer and first Director of Program Review. As lead strategic planner for the university's first major strategic plan he had a key role in planning and envisioning the new FIU Medical school incorporating medical anthropology principles and a community focus. He served on the Executive Board of the American Anthropological Association (AAA) in the practicing/professional seat, and was President of the National Association for the Practice of Anthropology (NAPA). Throughout these academic, applied, and practicing leadership experiences, he consistently published on organizational culture theory and analysis in leading journals and book chapters.

Part I
Medical School Culture

Chapter 2
Anthropologists in Medical Education in the United States: 1890s to the Present

Dennis W. Wiedman and Iveris L. Martinez

Introduction

For the past 130 years, anthropologists have worked in diverse roles in medical schools including teaching, curriculum development, research, planning and administration, as well as the management and development of community projects, with the goal of training practitioners and changing health outcomes. Additionally, anthropologists as observers, researchers, and critics of biomedicine, contributed to the understanding of health and illness in cross-cultural contexts since the turn of the twentieth century. As early as 1892, the English physician Havelock Ellis, known for his work on human sexuality, made the argument for the importance of anthropology in medical education in the medical journal "The Lancet," one of the most renowned medical journals. In fact, Ellis proposed the elimination of what he considered to be less important courses, such as pharmacopoeia and botany, as a way to accommodate the study of anthropology in medicine (Ellis 1892). He stated that anthropology and knowledge of "anthropometric cannons" would add to the scientific rigor of understanding and diagnosing disease through systematic observation. He states: "It is only accurate observation that counts." In addition to the role of anthropology in understanding comparative anatomy, Ellis cites the utility of anthropology for the study of insanity or "madness," criminality, and for practicing medicine abroad. This was a time when British imperialism was at its peak,

D. W. Wiedman (✉)
Department Global and Sociocultural Studies, School of International and Public Affairs, Florida International University, Miami, FL, USA
e-mail: wiedmand@fiu.edu

I. L. Martinez
Center for Successful Aging, College of Health and Human Services, California State University – Long Beach, Long Beach, CA, USA
e-mail: iveris.martinez@csulb.edu

I. L. Martinez, D. W. Wiedman (eds.), *Anthropology in Medical Education*,
https://doi.org/10.1007/978-3-030-62277-0_2

coinciding with the emergence of anthropology as a discipline. Ellis also lists an array of other nineteenth century physicians who had made advances to the field of comparative human anatomy not only in England, but in France, Italy, and Germany.

Among these physicians was Rudolf Virchow, a German pathologist, known for his advancements in the application of cell theory to understandings of disease and as the father of cellular pathology. Virchow is known as the father of social medicine for his studies of the social causes of disease, as well as his social activism. Critical medical anthropology considers the work of Virchow as the foundation of the political economy of health (Singer and Baer 1995). His study of the typhus epidemic between 1847 and 1848 in the Prussian Province of Upper Silesia is often cited as a foundational in understanding the social causes of disease disparities. As an outside expert appointed to report on the epidemic, he used observational methods which have been described as anthropological, to investigate the forces causing the epidemic. In his report he described the role of the Catholic Church, occupations, housing conditions and education as key contributing factors. He notes that while the disease, like others, has a biological basis, its spread is dictated by social factors, providing an epidemiological analysis of morbidity and mortality by demography, occupation and class (Taylor and Rieger 1984). He concluded that the typhoid epidemic was ultimately the result of poverty and underdevelopment. Therefore, instead of medical interventions, he recommends social reforms such universal education, industrial development, and agricultural reform. He famously stated in the journal he edited, *Medical Reform,* that "Medicine is a social science, and politics nothing but medicine on a grand scale" (Virchow 1848–1849).

Another major physician anthropologist at the turn of the twentieth century was William Halse Rivers. An English medical psychologist and anthropologist, Rivers is principally known for his two ethnographies in Melanesia and India. Trained at St. Bartholomew's hospital, he qualified to practice medicine at age of 22 in 1886. Appointed lecturer at the University of Cambridge in 1897, he became the first director of Britain's experimental psychology laboratory at the University of London. In 1898, Rivers joined the Cambridge expedition to the Torres Strait between Australia and New Guinea administering sensory functions tests to Melanesians which initiated his interest in anthropological methods. His 1902 ethnographic study of the Toda of southern India led to his major contributions to kinship and social organization (Rivers 1914). In the history of British social anthropology, he is considered a predecessor to Malinowski and Radcliffe-Brown (Barnard 2000: 179). A prolific scholar, his early experimental methods in psychology were his foundation for advances in ethnological methods as a science. His comparative analyses of color, visual acuity, neurasthenia and psychotherapeutics were well recognized in the field of psychology, while his genealogical methods for analysis of systems of social relationships is foundational in anthropology. In a series of FitzPatrick lectures in 1915, delivered before the Royal College of Physicians of London, and published in *Lancet*, he compared "Medicine, Magic, and Religion," as three social processes by which "mankind has come to regulate his behavior towards the world around him." Using historical, psychological, and sociological methods he presents a comparative perspective to understand processes of diagnosis, prognosis and beliefs of disease causation (Rivers 1916: 59). Throughout these years he continued to be engaged as a physician in hospitals and as psychologist to the Royal Air Force. In 1906, he presented the prestigious Croonian Lecture to the Royal College of Physicians. He served as President of the English Folklore Society (1920–1921). At the time of his death in 1922, he was President of the Royal Anthropological Institute (Haddon and Bartlett 1922; Bartlett 1923).

Considering these origins, the history of anthropology in medical education and the contributions of anthropologists in the training of physicians has not been published in one place. This history and contributions are often unknown to anthropologists entering the field of medical education, as well as physicians and medical school administrators. In this chapter we provide a history of anthropology in medical education in the United States from 1892 to the present based on published literature, as well as our experiences in the field of medicine. This chapter is by no means a review of the entire literature of anthropology in medical education, particularly after the mid-1980s when the involvement of anthropologists in the field exploded. A comprehensive history of anthropology and anthropologists in medical education is beyond the scope of a single chapter. Our goal in this chapter is to identify the phases, trends, and continuous themes of how anthropologists have engaged in the training of physicians, medical school curriculum, and management. We situate the contributions of anthropologists in the larger context of the political, economic, and technological developments of health care systems. Understanding historical changes in medical education reveals the roles and opportunities for anthropological perspectives and skills providing a foundation for the chapters in this book, which offer contemporary examples.

We begin this chapter by explaining our methodologies for locating and analyzing publications with an emphasis on those authored by anthropologists employed in medical schools. The chapter is organized into sections based on this analysis of the publications, weaving together historical approaches, theoretical models, and continuous themes. From the earliest publication in 1892 up to the 1960s portrays the contributions of physical anthropology to medicine. In the 1960s and 1970s a shift from physical anthropology to cultural anthropology began a rapid expansion of anthropologists in the practice of medicine. Overall, we identify two major approaches where anthropologists were valued in medical schools: community medicine and clinical anthropology. We also identify the roles and medical specialties where anthropologists tend to be employed within the structure of medical schools. During the 1970s and 1980s the major theoretical models referenced today were developed, refined, and incorporated into medicine and the other health professions. While the exact terms employed vary throughout this time period, from the frequency and proportion of the publications, three major themes can be discerned that continue to pattern anthropology's influence on medical school curriculum: the culture of medicine, cultural competency, and community medicine / social determinants of health. The conclusion section provides critical perspectives challenging future anthropologists, medical school faculty, and administrators on the multitude of possible roles for anthropologists in medical school education and administrative structures.

Methods

This chapter is based on an extensive literature review in the anthropological and medical literature on the role of anthropology in medical education in the United States. We have limited this history to the United States for several reasons. In our review of the literature, we have found very few English-language publications on the role of anthropology in medical education globally. This may be due in part to the way anthropology is conceived as a discipline and the way anthropologists are incorporated into medical practice settings outside the United States. Our search of the literature may also be impacted by what gets published and the language of publication. Moreover, the role of anthropology in medical education throughout the years has in some ways been delimited or constrained by the health systems of a country and competing traditional medical health systems such as we see in India and China. However, as the chapters in this volume reveal, there is significant involvement of anthropologists in medical education globally. The current integration of anthropological perspectives in medical education in the United States, for example, has been strengthened by discussions of health disparities, cultural competency and debates about universal health care. Furthermore, given the hegemony of the US biomedical allopathic medical model throughout the world, it is worth knowing with more depth the history of anthropological involvement in medical education in the United States (Baer et al. 1997).

Compilation and analysis of published articles by anthropologists over the past century has its limitations in properly reflecting the roles and contributions of anthropologists in medical schools. For this compilation we used electronic library web searches beginning with "AnthroSource," and "Anthropology Plus," then "Medline." Students in Wiedman's undergraduate medical anthropology courses and several graduate students wrote research papers elaborating on the careers of key anthropologists, which informed the content of this chapter. Bibliography software and qualitative research software were then used to search for key phrases and organize into categories and core themes.

The assembled publications under-represent the magnitude in the number and effectiveness of anthropologists as teachers and administrators in medical schools for several reasons. First, individuals may be totally dedicated to teaching and administration, and may not have time to publish. There may not be institutional incentives to publish, such as annual evaluations with an emphasis on teaching rather than on publishing. And even if they do publish, the topics are often in their specialized topics of study, most often not revealing their roles in medical education or even that they are anthropologists. Moreover, academic anthropologists may not be reflecting upon their roles in organizations, or find the time to report on their applied contributions. Also, while enculturating to their medical school roles, they often lose their identities as anthropologists, do not attend anthropology conferences, becoming affiliated with medical school professional organizations related to their job role. Finally, what the medical school culture accepts as contributions to the "clinical perspective," or "basic research" may limit their scope of publishing. In

"The Anthropology of Medicine," Romanucci-Ross, Moerman, and Tancredi (1983: 347) discern what is proper for medical school faculty to publish:

> The "field" of the art and science of medicine, then, is a culture, an island of cognition, affect, social structure and institutions, codified language; it has its boundaries which include members and exclude others. As an information system, the field of medicine is a relatively closed system of knowledge; it has many vested interests in remaining that way. Physicians who stray too far from the properly defined and encoded "clinical perspective," or from what is generally deemed to constitute proper "basic research," are likely to be shunned, or at least ignored, by peers and superiors.

Within these boundaries, explicit anthropological contributions to the generation of medical knowledge, be it clinical or basic research, or even educational research, often goes unpublished and unrecognized in the medical community. Numerous published articles recommend anthropologists involvement with medical schools, report on anthropologists evaluating aspects of the curriculum, or discuss the roles of anthropologists employed as medical school faculty, researchers, planners, or administrators. The challenge is to decipher from this literature the *actual* roles and impacts that anthropologists have had on the education of physicians.

Medicine and Early Anthropological Roles in Medical Education

It is not surprising that the early role of anthropologists in medical education were found in the field of physical anthropology in the teaching of anatomy and comparative human anatomy that Havelock Ellis was proposing in 1892. Early anthropological work was dominated by anthropometric methods measuring physical anatomical characteristics and comparative anatomy. The dominant theoretical paradigm was evolution of human biological characteristics to distinguish population differences. Evolutionary theory at the time attempted to explain these physical characteristics, as well as cultural differences, placing populations on a scale from savage to civilization. This evolutionary model was used by the Eugenics movement to justify racial segregation. Ellis was a key contributor to the eugenics movement, espousing the selection of desired heritable characteristics to improve future generations (Crozier 2008).

Counter to evolutionary theory, Franz Boas popularized the notion that "culture," learned and shared non-biological traits, as an explanation for the differences among individuals and societies. He formulated anthropology in the United States as a four field discipline: Cultural, Physical, Linguistics, and Archeology, at the turn of the twentieth century (Erickson and Murphy 2017). Boas was also a founder of the American Anthropological Association in 1902.

Founded in 1847, the American Medical Association (AMA), organized practitioners from a wide array of treatment modalities. Known as "regulars," or "allopaths" their theoretical model continued the ancient Greek philosophy of humoral medicine with a focus on the four humors; the body fluids of blood, phlegm, black biles, and yellow bile. Treatments involved restoring balance of the four humors such as wet-dry, hot-cold. Surgery and bloodletting with venipuncture were common interventions. Strong medicines produced the opposite of the symptoms emphasizing purging of the stomach and intestines. While "Allopathy" treated with opposites, "Homeopathy," treated with medicines producing similar symptoms. Originating in Germany, Homeopathy, used diluted medicines producing few side-effects. By the late 1800s both of these European health traditions were in competition with the US health traditions of Osteopathy and Chiropathy who focused treatments on the manipulation of the body. In France, with Pasteur's discovery of microorganisms as the cause of many diseases, and the introduction of sterile techniques, the "Germ Theory" became a major theoretical model for scientific medicine (Duffy 1993). Allopathy's transition from humoral medicine to an emphasis on science and biological causes of disease is the basis for the term "Biomedicine." Allopathy, and "Biomedicine" are used interchangeably throughout this chapter.

Scientific Medicine and the Consolidation of Biomedicine

Scientific medicine was introduced as a curriculum in the United States at Johns Hopkins University School of Medicine in 1893, requiring courses in science, anatomy, physiology, chemistry, while emphasizing clinical and laboratory research conducted with patients in an affiliated teaching hospital. This medical school curriculum became the basis of medical schools throughout the US. Training of physicians during this time was primarily in hospitals. The Johns Hopkins model shifted independent hospital-based training of physicians to university teaching hospitals where medical schools emphasized scientific research guiding medical students clinical procedures and interventions. Moreover, the AMA underwent a major reorganization in 1900 requiring physicians to be members of their local district medical society where monthly meetings presented medical reports and national organization news. To be recognized as members individual practitioners had to be non-sectarian physicians in good standing residing in the district, a graduate of a medical college recognized by the American Medical Association, and a legal practitioner in the state. By-laws and elected officers were required of the district or county level organizations, and these had to be affiliated with a state level organization who were affiliated with the National organization. This reorganization of AMA physicians led to nationally coordinated efforts to raise the quality of training and care provided by MDs, as well as the collection of dues to support the various AMA organizational levels and initiatives. Once organized, they then formulated ways to control the quality of the members by requiring physicians in 1903 to sign an ethics statement saying among other things, that they would not use "religion" or "faith" in their treatments, stating "It is inconsistent with the principles of medical science and it is incompatible with honorable standing in the profession for physicians to designate their practice as based on an exclusive dogma or a sectarian system of medicine." (AMA House of Delegates 1903) This ultimately removed religion and faith from the healing interventions of allopathic physicians who emphasized scientific biological medicine. Biomedicine claimed to be "secular" in other words, a system without spiritual or religious basis. By privileging "Biomedicine," "Secularism" and "Science," the AMA aligned with the US national political philosophy of separation of church and state (Asad 2003).

This historical process of biomedical professionalization, secularization and authoritative power, led to the exclusion of non-secular traditional healing systems where religion is integral. This emphasis on secular scientific explanations, excluding non-secular explanations for health and disease, is core to the biomedical resistance we see today to medical anthropology's emphasis on the importance of the patient's culture and healing systems in physician training in medical schools. For example, this political influence and power is manifested at the 1906 Oklahoma constitutional convention and during the first legislature in 1908 to exclude Native American medicine. Over 40 tribes from throughout the country were forcibly removed by the US military to Indian and Oklahoma Territories beginning in the 1830s. At the founding of the state of Oklahoma in 1907, Native Americans assertively expressed their concerns about laws that restricted their rights to Indigenous medicine and peyote. With the lobbying of secular allopathic physicians, legislators decided not to recognize Native medicine within the healthcare system, which they portrayed as religious beliefs. Ten years later, in 1918, Peyotists chartered the Native American Church with the state of Oklahoma, solidifying the distinction between scientific medicine and healing systems where religion is integral. This political and legal recognition of secular medicine to the exclusion of non-secular traditional medical systems by states, then influenced ethnic based forms of healing to be recognized as religions rather than health care systems (Wiedman 2012).

State laws and policies favoring secular biomedicine on who could practice medicine, then influenced the exclusion of many health cultures and traditions from the state recognized health system and payment for services. Biomedicine labeled these as "quacks." Not only traditional healers were marginalized, but also professionally organized medical systems such as Osteopathy, Chiropracty, Homeopathy, and Midwifery (see Chap.12 by Blonder). At this time, Chiropracty had the largest number of trained practitioners and the most training facilities around the country.

The Flexner Report

In 1906, the Flexner Commission, sponsored by the corporate based Carnegie Foundation, issued a report on how to improve the quality of American health care. The Flexner Report of 1910, based on the Hopkins model of medicine, was a defining moment in modern medical education. Based on a French/German model of medical education, it solidified a biomedical model and the pursuit of knowledge as the gold standard in US medical education, as compared to the well-being of patients (Bonner 2000). It set up a system of full-time academic medicine and medical teachers, which was criticized by some such as William Osler and Harvey Cushing as removing the study of medicine "from the realities and messy details of their patients' lives." (Duffy 2011) Privileging allopathy they recommended that only graduates of accredited AMA medical schools be licensed. Schools not receiving accreditation lost corporate and foundation contributions. By not receiving federal funding and student financial aid they lost students to AMA accredited schools. After the 1910 Flexner report, many non-allopathic training institutions closed. From 1910 on we have the hegemony of allopathy where all but allopathic physicians were considered legitimate by the state, insurance companies, and by the general population (Baer 2001). This exclusionary perspective of biomedicine makes it difficult for anthropology's expertise in comparative healing systems and health care to be valued in the medical school curriculum. It also constrained anthropologists attempting to insert patient and community perspectives into the medical school curriculum, or the building of new medical schools focused on community-based care.

While physicians at this time often practiced from their home office, or offices along main streets, they resisted the formation of publicly funded hospitals until the increase of incurable tuberculosis patients in the 1910s could not be adequately supported in their private facilities. Segregation of tuberculous patients in sanitariums began public funding of hospitals. Over the years, hospitals became the primary place for biomedical treatment with a sterile environment to control germs, centralized expensive technologies, and the treatment of many patients in a short periods of time. By the 1950s, following the Johns Hopkins Model of physician training, few medical schools were independent of hospitals, most were now connected to Universities with scientific research emphases. Medical school students took lecture based coursework, and then experienced hands-on patient care in a teaching hospital. This further removed the student physicians from real-life situations and communities of the patients, concentrating biomedical physicians in urban centers where hospitals and laboratory testing facilities provided the foundation for their type of care. Osteopaths and Chiropractors were more often the primary care providers in rural and poor areas. Allopathy or biomedicine, with a biological basis of care, became known as cosmopolitan medicine around the world. The historic consolidation of biomedicine in cosmopolitan university teaching hospitals, challenges the work of anthropologists to re-engage medical students in community-based care and the recognition of the larger social, political, economic, and cultural determinants of health (Starr 1982).

Early Contributions of Physical Anthropologists to Medicine

During this time period of the early twentieth century, anthropologists in medical education were primarily physical anthropologists teaching anatomy, and conducting research contributing to the understanding of diseases. For example, physical anthropologists demonstrated the correlation of sickle cell anemia with malaria and the development of agriculture in Sub-Sahara Africa and the Mediterranean (Livingstone 1958; Alland 1970). Anthropologists contributed to clinical diagnoses and interventions based on definitions of diseases and recognized standards of care. Kuru among the Fore of Eastern Highlands of New Guinea is an example of anthropology contributing to the discovery and definition of Prions in the 1970s. Kuru is an acute progressive degenerative disease of the central nervous system leading to death. Anthropological research contributed to "prions," a new category of neurological disease in the WHO International Classification of Diseases and Related Health Disorders (WHO 2018). Fieldwork among the Fore of New Guinea in 1961–1962 by cultural anthropologists Robert Glasse and Shirley Lindenbaum probed the historical memories of older Fore associating the disorder of Kuru with the custom of consuming brain matter during funeral rituals primarily by the women. Due to the long incubation period disease symptoms began to appear 20 years after this custom disappeared (Lindenbaum 1979, 2001). The most common form of prion disease is Creutzfeldt-Jakob disease in humans, and mad-cow disease. Gajdusek, D. C. and V. Zigas (1959) received the Nobel prize for their work in identifying prions, this new form of disease.

Shift from Physical Anthropology to Cultural Anthropology in the Practice of Medicine

A review of the literature shows a gradual shift from physical to cultural anthropology in the United States by the mid-twentieth century. We found, however, that anthropology was incorporated early in the curriculum of the Superior School of Rural Medicine (*Escuela Superior de Medicina Rural*) founded in Mexico City in 1938 (Castro Abitia and Manzano Zayas 1966). The school was established to train "physicians who will function as cultural agents in the rural environment, who will take an active part in the social transformation of Mexico." (Ibid p. 198) The changing roles of anthropology in Mexico medicine is highlighted in Chap. 9 by Maya and Vega.

Countering the biomedical focus on disease and the body, in 1948, WHO defined health as "....a state of complete physical, mental and social well-being and not merely the absence of disease or infirmity." WHO's broadening the definition of health began the process of reincorporation and legitimization of the excluded health professions, traditional medical systems, prevention and community medicine throughout the world. By the late 1950s, cultural anthropologists became more engaged in medical school curriculum. In 1953, William Caudill, one of the earliest sociocultural anthropologists to hold a position at a medical school (in the Department of Psychiatry and Mental Hygiene at Yale University) wrote an extensive review of the contributions of applied anthropology to understandings of disease since the 1800s (Caudill 1953). However, there was, as he noted in the journal *Science* a year earlier, little "intercommunication" between the fields of medicine and anthropology (Caudill 1952). Benjamin Paul (1956) outlined four aspirational contributions that continue to resonate with contemporary purposes for anthropology in training physicians. These are to communicate social science concepts in an understandable manner, instill respect for cultural differences, convey that culture is more than a collection of customs, and help the clinician realize how their cultural values and preconceptions impact their clinical practice.

Likewise, Hasan and Prasad (1961) argued the advantages of anthropology over other social sciences in medical education as it "bridges into the physical, biological, and social sciences and into the humanities, the workers in this field are in better position to have a comparable knowledge of medicine and public health and in turn can communicate their knowledge and experiences of socio-cultural and physiographic environments." (Hasan and Prasad 1961: 941) This is an important distinction for the advantages of anthropology in the field of medical education which continues to be debated today.

Several sociological studies in the late 1950s brought attention to the socialization of medical students into professional culture: Boys in White (Becker 1961), The Student Physician (Merton and Reader 1957), and Mastering Medicine (Coombs 1978). Two of the issues that these early studies of the medical education process noted was the homogenizing process of student recruitment, and the predominantly white male composition of medical school students. The homogenizing process of recruitment (Johnson 1991: 129) and the medical curriculum itself continues to be recurrent topics for anthropology publications. The profile of medical students continues to be very similar today, with the exception that more women now make up medical school classes.

Medical education is perhaps inevitably linked, among other things, to the systems of healthcare practice in which students are being trained to function. This is important to consider since anthropological roles in medical education are contingent on our understanding of the "culture of biomedicine" and the broader healthcare system. The 1960s saw several changes in the practice of medicine that opened the door for anthropologists increasing their role in medical education from physical anthropologists to cultural anthropologists. These included the growing recognition of the social and behavioral aspects of an individual's health leading more anthropologists, and behavioral scientists in general, to teach in medical schools. It was during the 1960s that the health care economy and infrastructure in the US transformed with the growth in voluntary health insurance, increased investment of private foundations, and the explosion of medical knowledge and technology (Weaver 1968: 1).

Even with this recognition of the importance of the behavioral sciences in medicine, a survey conducted in the early 1960s by Peter New and Thomas May (1965) identified only 24 anthropologists teaching in medical schools out of 353 social scientists teaching in 67 schools. More anthropologists were hired as researchers than as teachers. Thomas Weaver makes the distinction between the "anthropology of medicine" and "anthropology in medicine," the latter which he describes as "the applied or more directly related contributions made by anthropologists involved in research, teaching, administration, and consulting in medical and public health settings." The anthropology of medicine he defines as "basic or background anthropological contributions to the understanding of sociocultural factors in health and diseases which result from research by anthropologists who are usually outside of a formal medical setting." (Weaver 1968: 1) He articulated the purpose for anthropology in medical education as follows: "The goal of the medical anthropologist as a teacher in schools of medicine and public health is to demonstrate the cultural, social, and environmental factors which impinge on the health situation." (Weaver 1968: 5)

Building on experience over 10 years in medicine, nursing, nutrition and health science, Read (1970) similarly highlights the challenges of integrating medical anthropology into these settings. However, she also notes the value medical anthropology provides students with "a much needed release from cramming facts which have to be memorised. They can learn to take a "cool" look at a situation, to frame their own questions, to analyse and challenge their own and other people's ideas." (p. 165). She suggests a sequence for introducing anthropology in an "intelligible" way: (1) the hospital as a small society within a larger society, (2) "the roles of the personnel in hospitals and health service", (3) "health programs and health services as a form of social change" (p. 166), and (4) "the culture of a given community, and its culturally determined attitudes to health and disease" (p. 167). Read also notes the role medical anthropologists can play in finding common ground when students from different health disciplines come together. This continues to be an important role for anthropologists today (as highlighted in the chapters by Rubinstein and Lane, Chap. 14, as well as Martinez, Chap. 13).

These descriptions resonate even today, and are very similar to the goals that anthropologists who find themselves in medical teaching roles aspire to, as well as the roles that anthropologists are being asked to fulfill today and recent proposals for changing the preparation of future physicians. These include the American Association of Medical Colleges (AAMC) recommendations in 2012 on Behavioral and Social Foundations for Future Physicians and recent changes in medical entrance exams in the US in 2015, which we elaborate on further in this chapter.

Foundations of Theoretical Models in the 1970s

Several of the most quoted anthropology theoretical models to explain health and disease were formulated in the 1970 and 1980s. The "Disease—Illness" distinction and "Explanatory Models" are at the foundation of medical anthropology theory today and recurrently used by the authors throughout the chapters of this book. Horatio Fabrega, an anthropologist and psychiatrist who served as president of the Society for Medical Anthropology in 1972, defined the distinction between "disease" and "illness" terms where disease refers to "states that are biologically altered (i.e., chemical, physiological)" and illness refers to "the complex but socially defined state that forms the bases of decisions about medical treatment." (Fabrega 1973).

In 1973, anthropologist and psychiatrist, Arthur Kleinman began writing about medicine as a cultural system rooted in social and cultural contexts, stating that it is "important to recognize that medical systems are enmeshed within symbolic reality, and that they, in turn, give form to different kinds of symbolic realities within which illness and healing occur" and that these symbolic reality is transferred through enculturation. It is here that he first uses the term "explanatory models" which are used to "make sense of illness." He also pointed out the "hybrid quality of our contemporary care systems" and advocated for the comparative study of medical systems. Kleinman, who first trained as a physician and later obtained a master's in anthropology, was influenced by his ethnographic work on mental illness in Taiwan and China (Kleinman 1973b: 160–161, 1980). In 1974, he first presented on "explanatory models" in health care. He remains as one of the most influential anthropologists in medical education, and the explanatory model questions he outlined in the 1970s continues to be taught today in medical schools as part of how to elicit the patient's perspective (Kleinman 1983).

Kleinman (along with Benson) expanded the model in a 2006 article in the journal *PLOS Medicine* to embed the "illness narrative" in the social-structural context, incorporating the asking "what is at stake" for the patient or "the moral meaning of suffering," the relevance of ethnic identity, the role of stress in the patient's life, and cultural influences in the clinical encounter, including the culture of the provider. In this article, Kleinman was critical of the cultural competency approach that had become popular in medical education because it suggests that culture can be reduced to a technical skill and that a person can acquire enough knowledge about a group to be "competent" and that culture is made synonymous with ethnicity, race, or language, with beliefs and/or culture are held as static. He also noted that "culture" and "ethnicity" are not always central to a case. Moreover, discussions of cultural competency often exclude discussions of the culture of the provider.

Concomitantly, in a landmark 1977 *Science* article, psychiatrist and internist George Engel introduced the "biopsychosocial model" citing Fabrega's 1975 article (in the same journal) on the need for an ethnomedical science. Engel argued that "But the existing biomedical model does not suffice. To provide a basis for understanding the determinants of disease and arriving at rational treatments and patterns of health care, a medical model must also take into account the patient, the social context in which he lives, and the complementary system devised by society to deal with the disruptive effects of illness, that is, the physician role and the health care system." (1977: 132). His proposed model incorporates the role of biology, psychology, and socio-environmental factors in the experience of illness, as well as the role of the physician and health care system. Engel advocated for psychiatrists as well as other behavioral scientists to teach the model, with Family Medicine taking on a larger role in its teaching (Engel 1982).

The biopsychosocial model has been criticized as conceptually underdeveloped, not practically applicable, or testable (Farre and Rapley 2017) and excluding the centrality of the patient's experience (Butler et al. 2004). However, Engel's model has continued to be influential in medicine, particularly in primary care and family medicine. Though rarely cited in the anthropological literature, the biopsychosocial model gave support to anthropological perspectives on health and clinical ethnography in medical education (Kleinman 1982).

A large percentage of anthropology's contribution to health and healing is built upon Fabrega's illness—disease distinction and Kleinman's "Explanatory models." We can see their influence in Hazel Weidman's (1979) "Transcultural," and "Health Culture," models, James Dow's (1986) "Symbolic Healing" that applies to every patient-healer experience, Mark Nichter's (2010) discussion of "Idioms of Distress," portraying the verbal expressions of the patient, and Sue Estroff's "Chronicity", detailing the illness-self identity transformation. Their influence is also evident in Howard Stein's (1985: 56–77) psychoanalytical model of "Countertransference" which explores interpersonal transactions between the physician in training and the patient, illness stories and therapeutic emplotment. These were later developed by Mattingly (1998) using narration and cultural constructions to assess and adapt treatment care. Also by William Dressler's (2000) "Cultural Consonance theory" to recognize individual experience within the community's shared culture as explanations for depression and hypertension. Each of these are well developed anthropological theories that have clinical and individual treatment plan implications.

Community Medicine and Clinical Care

Community Medicine and Medical Education: 1960s–1980s

Greater demand for anthropological skills in medical education were facilitated by the community health movements of the 1960s and 1970s. Anthropologists became medical school experts in community health beliefs and practices, facilitators of medical school's engagement with the surrounding community, gaps between clinical medicine and community healthcare needs, placement of medical students in community-based training experiences, research and action programs in community-based health care systems, accessibility for economically and socially marginal, economic, and political power hierarchies (Pelto and Pelto 1978).

While the study of social organization has always been a focus of anthropology, the genre of community studies emerged with the notable works of Robert Redfield's "Tepoztlan: a Mexican Village" (1930), followed by a restudy of Tepoztlan by Oscar Lewis (1951). Solon Kimball and Conrad Arensberg research in the 1940s established a long line of community studies in the United States. In "Culture and Community," (1965) they compared southern US communities with other American communities presenting the perspective that the community is the level of analysis most suited for the study of human culture. Community modes of knowledge transmission, histories, language systems, ecology, and social organization provide residents with a template for thinking and a model of human interaction replicated in institutions such as schools and health care systems. Their focus on solving human problems in communities provided a knowledge base for anthropologists to bring theory and methods to clinics, hospitals and medical schools.

In response to the technical specialization of physicians and their reliance on urban hospitals, the US government began in the 1960s to fund neighborhood health centers, and community mental health facilities. The purpose of the Economic Opportunity Act of 1964 was to bring under one roof, accessible community health care with specialist and supportive services. Boards of Directors comprised of direct recipients of care, community organizations, and providers, in equal parts. Similarly, the Community Mental Health Centers Act of 1963 and legislation through the 1970s provided funds for mental health professionals, technical personnel, and construction of facilities in urban and rural locations (Bowers 1977: 174–177).

Until this time, persons with severe mental health issues were institutionalized in state mental hospitals. Due to this legislation the number of institutionalized people decreased dramatically, as community mental health facilities provided continuing care. This state supported community care model was problematic to biomedical health professionals who preferred private practice, authority, and control. It was during this time that psychotropic medications for depression and behavioral disorders became available enabling physicians to control prescriptions to those in the community. This shift of power to community-based care was responding to the calls for social justice by the civil rights movement and urban poor. It also provided employment for the many returning Vietnam veterans trained in medical support roles. To fill this gap, community medicine expanded with the training of Community Health Representatives (CHR), Physician Associates and Assistants (PA), and Advanced Nurse Practitioners (ARNP).

Anthropologists became the experts in community health beliefs and practices, and an increasing role in understanding the impact of "culture" on health. Transcultural psychiatry began to be formulated in the 1950s and 1960s focusing on cross-cultural variations in depressive symptomatology, suicide, psychotic disorders and personality with research from regions throughout the world (Kirmayer 2013). Cross-cultural anthropological research on culture-bound syndromes and ethnomedicine contributed to the knowledge and skills that anthropologists brought to medicine. Visual and applied anthropologist John Adair joined the Cornell-Navajo Field Health Research Project on the Navajo Reservation in Arizona, as chief anthropologist from 1953 to 1960. Along with many anthropologists providing anthropological insight, perspectives, and methodologies on ways to integrate traditional Navajo medicine with biomedicine. John Adair and Kurt Deuschle (1970) published the ground breaking book, *The People's Health*. A 1970s example of this teaching of anthropological perspectives to medical students is Ethel Nurge (1975) who offered a course "Blended Clinical Experience and Cultural Study of Certain Ethnic Groups." By focusing on the tribes of northwestern New Mexico, she organized information in a way for medical students to link biological, environmental, familial and social factors. More specifically, she linked diseases with beliefs and behaviors related to state of well-being, illness and therapy.

Within this mid-twentieth century context of health inequalities in access and affordability of biomedicine, we see a shift from cosmopolitan hospitals to neighborhood health centers. The limited number of physicians trained in allopathic medicine in the 1970s who were available, willing, and able to practice in rural areas or underserved communities outside the vicinity of cosmopolitan hospitals created the need to train a variety of health professionals in community medicine. This is the era when more Ph.D. anthropologists were graduating then the available number of anthropology department teaching positions, leading many into applied anthropology employment in health organizations, governments, non-profits, and corporations (Guerrón-Montero 2008). This was also a time of changing conceptions of doing "fieldwork." Laura Nader's (1972) "studying up" approach shifted cultural anthropology's research gaze to upper classes and elites. Anthropologists no longer needed to travel to faraway places to do their fieldwork; they turned to their own society and culture as research sites. Biomedicine came under ethnographic scrutiny and applied anthropology interventions.

With an increasing number of anthropologists engaged in health research, education and clinical applications, they organized professionally between 1967 and 1971 as a Section within the American Anthropological Association known as Society for Medical Anthropology (Weidman 1986). With this specialization and professional recognition, the employable roles at various levels of the health system grew in number. The early 1970s, with the initial efforts to bring together anthropologists with health interests, an extensive debate about naming, identity, and professional roles took place in the first editions of the medical anthropology newsletter, and at sessions at the annual conference of the American Anthropological Association. Hazel Weidman, as the first editor of Medical Anthropology News, which at the time was just several printed pages, hosted a lively dialog on the new roles for medical anthropologists. A 1974 Howard Stein letter in the Medical Anthropology news portrays the dialog at the 1973 AAA session as a time of professional role questioning, emerging identities, and conflicting positions on the futures of new professional roles and titles of "health," "medical," "clinical," anthropology were debated. Textbooks then became available faciltiating the teaching of medical anthropology (Foster and Anderson 1978; Logan and Hunt 1977; McElroy and Townsend (2015)).

As the number of students interested in this field grew, we see the initiation during the mid-1970s of academic departments with specialties in medical anthropology. Among the earliest of these was Columbia University in New York, the University of California at San Francisco, and the University of South Florida in Tampa. Graduates of these programs entered the employment sector with a professional identity and title of "medical anthropologist." Even with this rise in the number of medical anthropologists, a 1974 survey of medical school curriculum received 27 completed questionnaires revealing only one required anthropology course, 4 electives, and 13 lectures, mostly taught in first and second years (Rousch et al. 1976).

There are many other key figures that emerge in the history of anthropology in medical education during this era of the late 1970s and 1980s, including Stephen

Schensul, Paul Farmer, and Howard Stein. We cannot possibly go into depth about each contribution, but provide key references to rescue this history in the context of the continuing themes that anthropologists have contributed to medical education. Below we describe one example of the role of anthropologists in community medical education from this era, acknowledging that there are many other examples to learn from the chapters in this book.

Miami Health Ecology Project

Federal and foundation funding for studies to enhance behavioral sciences in medical education stimulated research and new approaches from the social sciences. However, the details and long-lasting impact of these approaches are often lost in our historical archives. A prime example is the Miami Health Ecology Project, led by anthropologist Hazel Weidman, a multi-year funded research project beginning in 1971 that identified the health beliefs and practices of the major ethnic groups in the neighborhoods surrounding the major public hospital in Miami: Jackson Memorial Hospital and the University of Miami (UM) Medical School. This was a concerted applied medical anthropological effort to have biomedicine recognize the importance of traditional medicine and healers in the provision of care; health systems that were disenfranchised with the 1903 AMA Codes of Ethics and lobbying of states to exclude non-biomedical healers.

The Miami Project, one of the first medical anthropology nationally funded longitudinal studies, had as its purpose not only increase the ethnic communities use of the hospital, but also train health professionals to be culturally responsive practitioners, and to change the institutional structures and organization of care. In the second multi-year funding cycle, Weidman and team applied the "Transcultural Health Care" model to initiate a cross-cultural training institute and to establish clinics located in the neighborhoods of discrete ethnic communities (Lefley 1975; Weidman 1979). Five central concepts guided this healthcare model: culture, health culture, co-culture, culture broker, and culture mediation (Weidman 1983a, b). She purposefully employed these concepts as strategies for perceptual and structural change in the organization and delivery of mental health care in the Miami multi-ethnic setting (Weidman 1975; Scott 1975).

Weidman formed the "Office of Transcultural Education and Research" in the UM Department of Psychiatry, bringing together anthropologists, psychologists, and social workers to implement the "health culture model" in the Medical School and Hospital. Social scientists, clinicians, and paraprofessionals of matching ethnicity to the populations served became a core of "culture brokers" with a service, teaching, and research role at the interface of the university, medical center, and community (Lefley and Bestman 1991). A strategy for structural change was to hire anthropologists as the culture brokers mediating between ethnic specific clinics and the hospital. Three anthropologists, Merci Cros Sandoval directed the Cuban Clinic, Claude Charles directed the Haitian clinic, and Dennis Wiedman directed the Anglo clinic (Wiedman 1984). By employing anthropologists in the medical school Weidman attempted to empower anthropologists within the biomedical system by institutionalizing the job category of "Clinical Anthropologist" (Weidman 1983a, b; Weidman 1985).

Hazel Weidman's "transcultural" and "culture broker" model is now used in diverse clinical, community, and global health applications. Visiting anthropologists observing and learning from this transcultural delivery of health care implemented this model in their own locations, for example, Stephen Schensul in Boston, and Paul Farmer's international health care provider "Partners in Health" (Mas 2019). Dennis Wiedman built upon this experience and cultural model of community based care, as lead academic planner at Florida International University in the planning of the new medical school: Herbert Wertheim College of Medicine. The Miami Project influenced the importance of "health culture" in other health professions as well (Lefley 1984; Lefley and Pederson 1986). Anthropologist Madeleine Leininger formed the "Transcultural Nursing Society," in 1974. Furthermore, the formation of the "Cross-Cultural Training Institute for Mental Health Professionals," extended training in culturally appropriate care to mental health professionals from 97 facilities throughout the nation (Lefley and Bestman 1991). Anthropologists continue to be instrumental in the planning and implementation of new medical schools with a community and population-based mission. (See for example Rushing and McMullin, Chap. 10; Wiedman Chap. 6; Wiedman 2016; Wiedman and Martinez 2017).

Clinical Anthropology: 1980s and Beyond

During the 1980s and 1990s, medical anthropology grew to be one of the largest sections of the American Anthropological Association and one of the areas of research garnering the greatest research grants and contracts. The diversity of research and applications elaborated and transformed as medical anthropologists added new knowledge to health and medicine. With the graduation of greater numbers of medical anthropologists from the specialized academic programs, there were wide ranging discussions in Medical Anthropology Newsletter, and journals about the roles and identities of anthropologists in the healthcare system. This was pivotal in the continuing employment of anthropologists, many of whom were not finding employment in the traditional professional role of college professor, but found opportunities in various positions that applied anthropological theory and methods.

The term "Clinical Anthropology" emerged in the early 1980s among anthropologists attempting to define their professional role within the hospital, clinic, and medical school settings. Early proponents of this role envisioned anthropologists as a direct care provider, clinic manager, evaluator, and educator, among others. A growing section of the American Anthropological Association, the SMA's newsletter became a point of convergence for many anthropologists involved with health issues, both within Departments of Anthropology and among those employed in medical settings in universities, hospitals, and public health organizations. Numerous articles starting in the mid-1970s envisioned the professionalization of the new role of "Clinical Anthropologist" and documented the rapid emergence of anthropologists with an interest in social and cultural aspects of medicine and the teaching of physicians (Kleinman 1977; Stein 1980). New professional roles for clinical applications of anthropology were discussed at the 1973 conference of the American Anthropological Association (Stein 1974). A July 1980, conference on clinical anthropology at the University of Illinois in Urbana culminated in the edited book *Clinical Anthropology: A New Approach to American Health Problems?* edited by Demitri Shimkin and Peggy Golde (1983). This enthusiastic formation of a new professional identity and role within the clinic, medical school, and health care system brought together anthropologists with diverse interests and training, as well as theoretical and methodological orientations.

By 1982, the various roles of clinical anthropologists were elaborated in the book *Clinically Applied Anthropology: Anthropologists in Health Science Settings,* by Noel Chrisman and Thomas Maretzki (1982). In this book, four chapters are devoted to medical school education and training: Robert Ness wrote about "Medical Anthropology in a Pre Clinical Curriculum," Howard Stein about "Ethnographic Mode of Teaching Clinical Behavioral Science,"Arthur Kleinman about "Clinically Applied Anthropology on a Psychiatric Consultation-Liaison Service," and Hazel Weidman wrote about "Research Strategies Structural Alterations, and Clinically Relevant Anthropology." Often referred to as "Clinically Applied Anthropology" today, anthropologists practice in the full range of health care settings, including hospitals, clinics, medical schools, health professional schools, and all kinds of healthcare delivery systems. As anthropologists become immersed within clinics or health systems, they apply anthropology data, theory, and methods that clarify specific clinical issues influencing changes in patient care and health care delivery systems (O'Rourke 1983; IResearchnet 2019; Chrisman and Johnson 1990).

Early debates concerned whether "clinical anthropologist" could refer to anthropologists as direct care providers who perform patient interventions. However, training for direct care provider roles did not develop in anthropology departments as stand-alone career tracks. Rather anthropology departments developed combined degrees with medicine, nursing, psychology, and occupational therapy. In this way, these combined degrees provide the legal liability and licensing credentials necessary for direct patient care. Major employment careers for clinically applied anthropologists are now established roles in nursing, occupational therapy, family medicine, and psychiatry, with MD/PHD programs graduating physician anthropologists.

Transcultural Nursing

For training of nurses, the work of anthropologists Pamela Brink and Madeleine Leininger introduced "transcultural nursing" as a distinct nursing specialty which focuses on global cultures and comparative cultural caring, health, and nursing phenomena. Madeleine Leininger is well known in nursing for her influential "Sunrise Model," that portrays the patient and nurse within the social, cultural, and economic conditions affecting clinical care (Leininger 1970, 1978). The primary aim of this specialty is to provide culturally congruent nursing care which recognizes and appreciates cultural differences in patient's values, beliefs, and customs affecting how they deal with illness, healing, disease, and deaths (https://tcns.org). Dr. Leininger founded the Transcultural Nursing Society in 1974–1975 with Pamela Brink (1976). Leininger (1989) in the first issue of the peer-review journal "Journal of Transcultural Nursing," describes these new roles in "Transcultural Nurse Specialists and Generalists: New Practitioners in Nursing." For over 35 years, the Council on Nursing and Anthropology (CONAA) has organized and supported nurse-anthropologists, nurses, health care professionals, anthropologists and health social scientists for scholarly and evidence-based practice initiatives.

Occupational Therapy

Occupational Therapy is a clinical profession closely aligned with anthropology. Dr. Geyla Frank et al. (2008) edited a special issue of the *NAPA (National Association for the Practice of Anthropology) Bulletin* focused on the collaborations and prospects of anthropology and occupational therapy, as well as how this clinical occupation incorporates critical medical anthropology (Frank et al. 2010). In collaboration with then NAPA President Dennis Wiedman, brought Occupational Therapy anthropologists into NAPA, a section of the American Anthropological Association, by initiating in 2007–2008 the NAPA-OT field school. The vision of the fieldschool serves to facilitate transdisciplinary learning among students in occupational therapy, global health, applied anthropology, and related fields. The NAPA-OT Field School in Guatemala nurtures leaders in applied medical anthropology and occupational therapy using a social justice framework. Students work intensively in clinical and community settings gaining skill in research, observation, communication, and transdisciplinary collaboration. Training emphasizes critical theories in applied medical anthropology, global health, approaches to social and occupational justice, and human rights. Occupational therapy students fulfill a portion of their Level II professional degree requirements. The goal is to promote social and occupational justice, enacting partnerships with NGOs (non-governmental organizations) in and around Antigua, Guatemala. Integrative field work within occupational therapy and anthropology, systematically refines a set of concepts, theories, bodies of knowledge, and tools for implementation as practitioners and researchers in real-world contexts (NAPA/OT Fieldschool 2019; http://napaotguatemala.org/).

Psychiatry

A large proportion of anthropologists employed in medical schools over the years are in departments of psychiatry. Psychological anthropology has long been at the theoretical foundation of anthropology, even before the culture and personality studies of Margaret Mead and Ruth Benedict. Alfred Kroeber practiced psychotherapy with his patients. Notable anthropologists employed in departments of anthropology during the founding years of the Society for Medical Anthropology were Arthur Kleinman and Hazel Weidman. "Transcultural Psychiatry" is a peer-reviewed academic journal initiated in 1963 publishes papers in the fields of cultural psychiatry, psychology and anthropology, as does the journal "Culture, Medicine and Psychiatry." Starting with a comparative approach focused on the diverse manifestations of mental disorders among different societies, this specialty broadened to incorporate social and cultural aspects of illness into the clinical framework with a focus on the illness experience. For example, a 2019 special issue of Transcultural Psychiatry focuses on "culture bound syndromes," and "idioms of distress," presenting a long line of anthropological research concerned with cross-cultural concepts, experiences of distress and clinical psychiatric applications. (Kaiser and Weaver 2019).

Family Medicine

Family medicine as a distinct speciality in MD training emerged during the 1970s era of training physicians to provide primary, family, and preventive community care. Anthropologist Howard Stein, a prolific scholar on the training of family medicine physicians, joined the Department of Family and Preventive Medicine at the University of Oklahoma Health Sciences Center in 1978. For more than 45 years he taught didactic seminars, conducted grand rounds presentations, and worked one-on-one with medical school residents and faculty. Working from a psychoanalytic and ethnographic approach his work helped physicians have access to the inner and interpersonal worlds of patients, faculty, and staff. In several books and many journal articles, he portrayed how he engaged with residents in grand rounds and rural clinics of western Oklahoma (Stein 1990b, Stein and Apprey 1985). His 1996 book *Prairie Voices: Process Anthropology in Family Medicine* is considered as a foundation for anthropology's role in Family medicine. A unique approach is his use of poetry. He would participate and observe a clinical doctor- patient experience, then in a few days present an original piece of poetry that captured the emotional, psychological and cultural aspects, resolving the awkwardness or surfacing meaningful healing moments. He pursued ways of learning something new that could improve the doctor-patient-family-staff relationship and in turn, all aspects of doctoring. In Chap. 15, Scott, Moralez and Andazola discuss integrating health equity across a family medicine residency program and present a historical view on the role of anthropologists in Family Medicine.

Medical Humanities

Traditionally, anthropologists in medical schools have worked within departments of psychiatry, pediatrics, family medicine, etc. As the numbers of anthropologists and other behavioral and humanities PhD faculty increased in the 2000s, medical and health humanities programs solidified as administrative structures within medical schools. Medical humanities including multi-disciplinary fields of humanities, arts, and social sciences advocate for the complexities of modern lives and illness experiences in the clinical encounter. Anthropologists are ideal collaborators in this multidisciplinary endeavor. Together emphasizing interdisciplinary goals, these faculty are now in positions to voice the humanistic values within physician training. The integration of humanistic epistemologies into medical education reiterates the tension between the individual patient and the sociocultural factors, the human experience, and technical biological competency, reductionism and scientism (see Rushing and McMillan, Chap. 10).

Medicine is fundamentally based on the Western humanist tradition that animates many medical humanities programs, and humanists within the discipline of anthropology. McDonald and Crowder in this volume (Chap. 11) present the tensions that anthropologists are faced with as new faculty in a Medical Humanities program where moral medical practices and teaching pedagogies build upon the western philosophy of the individual and self. Since the early 1900s, allopathic medicine has focused on the individual body, diseased part, and diseases. It is the individual patient's responsibility to follow the doctor's regimen in order to be healed. This aligns with the central humanist model of the autonomous self as a coherent and bounded individual with intentional thought, action, and belief. This gaze on the individual becomes problematic for anthropologists entering a medical humanities program as they question the hegemony of the humanist tradition that transforms differences in patients, communities, and cultures into familiar western epistemologies and ontologies. Anthropologists find themselves in a tense yet fundamental role in revealing the cultural specificity of the Western ideal of the self and related values of individualism. Drawing upon the large body of ethnographies on cultural variations of 'personhood,' and 'collective identities,' it becomes the role of anthropologists to integrate into medical education the biological, social, cultural, historical, political, economic, technological and environmental conditions that make possible the selves of patients, doctors, and also the broader constructions of the Western self.

MD/PhD in Anthropology Programs

Joint MD/ PhD programs have been training anthropologist physicians for several decades. Many of these program graduates are now in major roles in medical schools, medical professional organizations, and even CEOs of healthcare organizations. Physician/Anthropologists Dr. Paul Farmer and Jim Yong Kim are founders of one of the most well-known non-profit healthcare organizations, "Partners in Health," whose goal is to "draw on the resources of the world's leading medical and academic institutions and on the lived experience of the world's poorest and sickest communities" (Partners is Health 2019). Some of these graduates have gone on to highlight the contribution of anthropologists for clinical care. For example, "Case Studies in Social Medicine," initiated by the New England Journal of Medicine (Scott Stonington et al. 2018) , highlight the importance of social concepts and social context directly relevant in clinical medicine in language that physicians use. Discussions of real clinical cases translate theories and methods for understanding social processes in terms that can be readily used in medical education, clinical practice, and health system planning. Using case studies as a mode of communication, anthropologists introduce major points and perspectives that broaden the biomedical gaze on disease, physiology and specific body parts. Discussions of structural violence and structural racism resolve early critiques in the literature by critical medical anthropologists Singer and Baer that those working in the health care systems perpetuate inequities and often ignore the structural and political factors that cause the disparities (Singer and Baer 1995).

From these careers and examples, we can see how clinically applied anthropologists influence medical education at many levels by effectively conveying sociocultural explanations for the distribution of illnesses suffered by patient populations, access and response to care, and differential treatment outcomes as results of macro level social, economic, and political forces.

Continuous "Anthropological" Themes in Medical Education

Although there are many ways that anthropologists engage in medical education, in this section we focus on and summarize three main themes that are continually represented in the literature as major topics anthropologists bring to the medical school curriculum, resident training, and the clinical encounter: (1) the culture of biomedicine, (2) "cultural competence", and (3) community medicine/social determinants of health.

Culture of Biomedicine

A strength of social and cultural anthropologists engaged in medical schools is their emphasis on ethnography as a methodology to explore aspects of the clinical encounter within the context of biomedical culture (Stein 1982). With years of participating and observing medical school education, Stein (1990a) compiled one of the most comprehensive books on this topic: *American Medicine as Culture*. Stein develops chapters on values and meanings, metaphors and decision making, moralism and social control, group dynamics and practice, money and identities, socialization of becoming a physician, links between culture and the personality of the physician and patient. Interestingly, Janelle Taylor (2003: 559) suggests that medicine and medical practitioners do not see themselves within their own cultural paradigm, and that their view of other "cultures" places them in a privileged position with biomedicine as a "culture of no culture".

Atkinson and Pugsley (2005) provide a history of the ethnographic tradition in medicine, discussing a number of studies that have provided detailed and context-sensitive accounts of the everyday life of medical schools, medical practitioners, and medical students. In "The Demise of the Bumbler and the Crock: From Experience to Accountability in Medical Education and Ethnography," Janelle Taylor (2014) portrays the ethnographer of the 1950s as a clueless "bumbler" who, through experience, gains understanding and expertise and is transformed into a professional anthropologist. By the 2000s, the risks, rewards, and outcomes of ethnographic research rendered bumbling inadmissible in medical settings. Requiring the more rigorous training of anthropologists conducting ethnography in clinical settings and its use in medical school curriculum.

Ethnographic studies of health care systems around the world enabled the detailed analysis of the similarities and differences of patient—healers. Through cross-cultural comparisons, the cognitive, social, and material aspects of traditional healers and biomedical physicians can be better understood. It was through this comparative study of medical systems, that Arthur Kleinman (1973a, b) and many other anthropologists have contributed to an integrated approach to the study of the relationship of medicine and culture. Arthur Kleinman's *Patients and Healers in the Context of Culture* (1980) is now a foundation work in medical anthropology. From cross-cultural comparisons, James Dow (1986) proposed a universal process in the patient-healer relationships. Healers and the healed are embedded within specific symbols representing the healer's culture with the healer manipulating the transactional symbols to help the patient transact their own meanings and emotions leading to physical well-being.

Comparing the world healing systems, Pamela Erickson's (2008) book *Ethnomedicine* details aspects of the culture of biomedicine. A unique cultural characteristic of biomedicine is the primary healing occurs with the physician alone with the patient. Most ethnomedical systems are embedded in a social group setting where family and community members are present. From this cross-cultural perspective, Erickson contends that biomedicine, like any health tradition, is an "ethnomedicine" emerging from the cultural traditions of France, Britain, Germany and the US. Comparing ethnomedical systems, biomedicine focuses the training of medical students on seeing into the body, healing primarily through biological interventions using material culture items of surgery, prescription medicines, and injections. Many other ethnomedical systems address both disease and illness in a more holistic way, incorporating cognitive, symbolic, psychological, social, and economic factors affecting the physical conditions of the patient.

Based on their ethnographic study of the training of students at Harvard Medical School, Good and Good (1993) characterized the culture of biomedicine as based on the scientific search for value-free facts and the view of the person as a diseased body. Training focused on case histories of particular diseases. Biomedicine is about "entering the body" with technologies such as X-rays, CT scans, and lab tests. Good and Good provided an ethnographic example of the transition of medical students during the anatomy course where they dissected a human. This is the major time in the curriculum that students learn the "medical gaze" viewing the body, not as a person but as an object. Dissections violate the sanctity of the body. Students shift from seeing the person to seeing the organic body and its individual parts. The medical gaze reconstitutes the student, enabling them to function as biomedical practitioners, but limiting their cognitive perspective and explanations for the diseased body, discounting the larger social, cultural, political and economic factors for health and well-being. The "medical gaze," influences biomedical ways of seeing the body, a focus on specific diseased body parts, and a detached relationship with patients (Foucault 1973).

A recent example of anthropologists detailing even finer grained aspects of biomedical culture is analyses of medical school teaching of percussion touching. Harris (2016) contends that with the over reliance on technologies, physicians have become deskilled in sensory diagnosis with physical examinations. By ethnographically following how percussion is taught to and learned by medical school students, Harris suggests through this multi-sensory practice the student physician's boundaries and bodies blur. Learning percussion perpetuates diagnostic craft skills as a way of knowing the patient's and one's own living breathing body.

The "culture of biomedicine" is not only an important topic that anthropologists strive to insert into the medical school curriculum, it is important to teach in the graduate training of anthropologists who want to successfully work in medical schools.

From Cultural Competence to Cultural Humility and Integrative Medicine

Many of the themes we saw in early engagements of anthropology with medical education have persisted into recent times, but the language has transformed with the shifts and growing role of the social and behavioral sciences in medical education.

Anthropologists typically are called upon by medical schools to teach cultural competency and cultural sensitivity. Beginning in the late 1970s, U.S. health care educators sought to promote "cultural competency" to reduce racial and ethnic disparities in health outcomes. Cultural competency education was intended to sensitize health care practitioners to the needs of diverse individuals and communities whose beliefs, values, and customary practices often differed from those of the medical professionals serving them.

Culturally and Linguistically Appropriate Services (CLAS) Standards, originally released by the Office of Minority Health in 2001, now lists 15 requirements and recommendations for health care providers (Office of Minority Health 2018) based on the recognition of health disparities between the growing population of minorities in the US. In 2005, the AAMC set forth a definition of cultural competency as "a set of congruent behaviors, knowledge, attitudes, and policies that come together in a system, organization, or among professionals that enables effective work in cross-cultural situations." It "combines the tenets of patient and family-centered care with an understanding of the social and cultural influences that affect the quality of medical services and treatment" (AAMC 2005). The AAMC later released the Tool for Assessing Cultural Competency Training (TAACT) in 2006, which was revised in 2008 (Lie et al. 2008).

In 2011, an AAMC report outlined core behavioral and social science competencies for future physicians. Interestingly, the role of anthropology as a discipline is quite narrowly conceived to the role of culture and community in health. According to the AAMC 2011 Report, the contribution of Anthropology to medical education is to: "Accurately describe the influence and potential implications of culture and community context on health behaviors, beliefs and outcomes, as well as how physicians should appropriately integrate this knowledge into patient care." Meanwhile, anthropologists are doing ethnographic research that can inform what the document calls "Health Care Goal Attainment," including the categories identified as mind-body interactions, health promotion and wellness, treatment adherence, chronic illness management, and healthcare team efficiency.

As of 2018, the Liaison Committee on Medical Education, the accrediting body for allopathic medical schools in the United States and Canada, published the following 2018 standard on "Cultural Competence and Health Care Disparities," stated: "The faculty of a medical school ensure that the medical curriculum provides opportunities for medical students to learn to recognize and appropriately address gender and cultural biases in themselves, in others, and in the health care delivery process." (AAMC, March 2018) The recommended instructional content includes "the manner in which people of diverse cultures and belief systems perceive health and illness and respond to various symptoms, diseases, and treatment," "basic principles of culturally competent health care," "recognition and development of solutions for health care disparities," "meeting the health care needs of medically underserved populations," and "the development of core professional attributes (e.g., altruism, accountability) needed to provide effective care in a multidimensional and diverse society" (AAMC, March 2018).

Janelle Taylor (2003: 555) offers a critical perspective on medical education and the institutional culture of medicine, arguing that they both tend to systematically foster "essentialist" cultural concepts in educating medical students who then apply these notions to patients. Taylor maintains that while cultural competence spawned positive transformative changes in medical education for immigrant communities, such as expanding professional training, providing translation services, and holding seminars, it has also run the risk of only understanding culture from a simplistic and harmful perspective. Taylor claims that, "cultural 'humility' ought to replace cultural 'competence' as the goal of multicultural education in medicine." Her reasoning is that cultures are multifaceted and constantly changing things, therefore placing the medical practitioner in a situation of lifelong learning which requires a disposition of humility, not competence. In 2011, Good et al. published a volume "Shattering Culture: American Medicine Responds to Cultural Diversity," based on ethnographic studies of health-care settings with a focus on the recent preoccupation with cultural competence. Around this time period, the Journal of Culture, Medicine and Psychiatry published two special editions (Holmes et al. 2011; Willen and Carpenter-Song 2013) that highlight experiences of anthropologists teaching medical students, as well as ethnographic research on medical education largely around the topic of cultural competence. As already noted, educational efforts at cultural competency have been increasingly critiqued for inadvertently stereotyping diverse patients into homogenous communities, and ignoring the broader social and structural determinants of health. The notion of being able to teach cultural competence in medicine has been critiqued by many, including Kleinman and Benson (2006) who point out the concept of cultural competency suggests culture can be reduced to a technical skill, portrays culture as static, and makes culture synonymous with ethnicity, race, or language, i.e. "Chinese believe x. . .Mexicans believe y." Furthermore, they note that it excludes a discussion of the culture of the provider.

The field of cultural competency has moved from a list of "traits" toward an attitude of "open-mindedness" (Jenks 2011), or "self-reflective practice" (Bullon 2013), largely based on the original critique by anthropology of biomedicine. However, anthropologists continue to be challenged as to how to effectively teach complexity of the culture concept and help medical students and physicians alike achieve "cultural competency" in a medical education environment where the focus is on "memorization of facts." There remains two major frameworks for cultural competence in biomedicine: (1) the categorical approach in which providers learn about an array of values, beliefs, and behaviors attributed to certain cultural groups, and (2) the cross-cultural approach "which seek to modify a doctor's interactions with *all* patients rather than just with those who appear culturally "different" from the health care provider" (Shaw and Armin 2011). However, as the field moves more towards "open-mindedness," "cultural humility," and "self-reflection," the political and socio-historical contexts that produce inequalities between different "cultural" groups continue to be lost (Jenks 2011; Shaw and Armin 2011).

Beyond the issues of "cultural competency," countering the biomedical gaze on disease and one organ system, anthropological engagements with integrative medicine emphasize treating the whole person in a holistic, patient-focused approach to health care and wellness including mental, emotional, functional, cultural, spiritual, social, and community aspects. Integrative medicine aims for well-coordinated culturally appropriate care between different kinds of health providers and institutions. Medical anthropologist Hans Baer (2004) details how the integration of traditional and biomedicine would be beneficial to communities. The World Health Organization (WHO) by the early 2000s recognized that to rely upon biomedical physicians to provide care throughout the world would be impossible given the very limited number of trained physicians graduated each year. This is especially so in rural and under-developed parts of the world where physicians do not prefer to live and work. In 2007, the WHO strategic plan put forth strategic goals, policies and ways to implement integrative medicine where traditional community health people, knowledge, and resources are recognized as important health care providers along with biomedical physicians and health professionals. This strategy was refined further with the WHO "Traditional Medicine Strategy 2014–2023" supporting member states in developing proactive policies and implementing action plans that strengthens the role of traditional medicine in keeping populations healthy.

Since the 1980s, we see complementary and alternative medical systems (CAM) have gained significantly in public use and recognition. The US government's National Institute of Health (NIH) began recognizing the multitude of healing traditions in 1991 with the establishment of the Office of Alternative Medicine, then renamed in 1998 as the National Center for Complementary and Alternative Medicine, as the Federal Government's lead agency for scientific research on complementary and alternative health approaches. Countering 100 years of biomedical hegemony, NIH changed the name to the National Center for Complementary and Integrative Health (NCCIH) in 2014. This name and mission change acknowledges the importance of the political, economic, and social determinants of health. It encourages health professionals and the training in medical schools to include well-being of patients beyond what occurs in the physician offices to include the work of self-empowered individuals within their communities, prevention and public policies (Witt et al. 2017).

From Culture and Communities to Social Determinants of Health and Structural Violence

Numerous publications have recently emerged that further open the door for anthropologists to play a greater role in medical education. Over the last 20 years there has been a newfound interest in allopathic medical education towards incorporating social and behavioral competencies in medical curricula in order to address the social determinants of health and population health (see Maeshiro 2008), as well as teamwork and communication. This coincides with a renewed emphasis on social responsibility and social accountability (Boelen and Woolard 2009) including an emphasis on serving and addressing the needs of local communities. Cuff and Vanselow (2004) noted that:

> Skills in the behavioral and social sciences are essential for the prevention of many chronic diseases and for effective management of patients with these diseases. . . . In addition, good communication skills and the cross-disciplinary education discussed in this report will improve their ability to relate to their colleagues in medicine, as well as other professionals.

Since the onset of the cultural competency movement, health practitioners have tended to focus primarily on cultural barriers to health care framed in terms of race and ethnicity, to the neglect of negative political and economic forces that compounded discrimination. In 2011, the AAMC published a set of behavioral and social science in medicine, competencies, including to "Accurately describe how social determinants of health influence health outcomes and how physicians can incorporate this knowledge in the care of patients." Anthropological work in public health from the 1970s influenced the emergence of social determinants of health as an explanatory model (Foster 1978). While this topic was "assigned" to Sociology and Psychology as the fields best equipped to teach this material, anthropologists find themselves immersed in this topic and grappling how to convey this complex material in a way that is digestible by medical students, many of which have limited exposure to the social and behavioral sciences. The social determinants of health may be simply stated as the economic and social conditions that influence the health of people and communities (Commission on Social Determinants of Health 2008). The role of the social determinants of health gained saliency in medicine and public health through the work of Michael Marmot, a social epidemiologist who would later become the head of the British Medical Association. His study of health among British civil servants, published in the medical journal *The Lancet*, showed a steep inverse association between social class, assessed by grade of employment, and mortality from various diseases (Marmot et al. 1991). Marmot would later outline the determinants of health, including stressors, early life experiences, social exclusion (including poverty), working conditions, unemployment, social support, access to health promoting food and transportation, among other things, for the World Health Organization (Wilkinson and Marmot 2003).

In the 1990s, physician and anthropologist Paul Farmer warned that concentrating exclusively on "culture" mis-recognizes the pathological effects of social inequality, politics, and human rights. He eloquently brought the political science and human rights concept of "structural violence" (Farmer 1999) to clinical attention by documenting the ways in which policies, market forces, and institutional arrangements disproportionately shorten the lives of the poor. His work reinvigorated the field of global health and enlivened a generation of idealistic health profession students and clinicians to mobilize practically and politically for the transfer of medical resources to resource-poor nations and underserved domestic populations. Importantly, the concept of structural violence has been instrumental in defining access to health care as a human right (Singer and Baer 1985; Farmer 2003; Farmer et al. 2006; Bourgois et al. 2017). Engaging anthropology at the national policy level, Sandra Lane, one of the authors of Chap. 14, chaired the National Academies of Engineering, Sciences and Medicine committee that wrote: *A Framework for Educating Health Professionals to Address the Social Determinants of Health*.

This broader health professional discussion of social determinants of health shifted anthropological medical school teaching and research efforts on how to document the ways in which economics, policies, market forces, and institutional systems disproportionately affect clinical care and medical education. Merrill Singer and colleagues developed the concept of "syndemics" in the early 1990s as a set of closely interrelated endemic and epidemic conditions, all of which are strongly influenced and sustained by a broader set of political-economic and social factors. The synergy among epidemics make each worse. (Singer 1994, 2009). Now a widely used concept in epidemiology and public health, "syndemics" challenges the clinical diagnoses and treatments of diseases as distinct entities.

Medical school entrance exams (MCAT) now require students to have a basic knowledge of social and behavioral sciences and humanities. Two new content areas: (1) Psychological, Social, and Biological Foundations of Behavior; and (2) Critical Analysis and Reasoning Skill, are an opportunity for anthropologists to prepare pre-medical students for the practice of medicine in the twenty-first century. The sections test students' knowledge of the social and behavioral determinants of health, as well as their critical reasoning skills needed for medical school (AAMC 2012). This greater emphasis in social and behavioral sciences, is increasing enrollments in anthropology courses by pre-med majors.

Because of these efforts, many clinicians have become aware of the negative health effects of political and economic forces outside the clinic, but may feel helpless in the face of these social structural forces and consider them to be beyond the purview of clinical practice. Others continue to interpret nonadherence to treatment protocols and inability to pursue healthy lifestyle modifications to be the willful moral choices of their patients rather than effects of social structural inequalities (Stonington and Coffa 2019). As a result, clinicians sometimes become frustrated by their patients or subject to burnout. The continued challenge of anthropologists in medicine is to synthesize these complex issues and provide tools to think about them and address them to a clinical audience.

Clinical anthropologists, Phillipe Bourgois, Seth Holmes, Kim Sue, and James Quesada (2017) developed a "Structural Vulnerability Scale," an assessment tool to help clinicians articulate and address the effects of detrimental social structures on patient care. In this way anthropologists are responding to the call for ways to implement "structural competency" in clinical medicine. This clinical assessment tool operationalizes the concept of structural vulnerability, highlighting the pathways through which specific local hierarchies and broader sets of power relations may exacerbate an individual patient's health problems. The goal is to facilitate an applied pragmatic approach to intervening on these forces, identifying obstacles to healthy lifestyles, treatment adherence outside the clinic, while facilitating access to care inside the clinic. The Structural Vulnerability Scale begins with the awareness that all individuals live within diverse but identifiable power relationships. Social hierarchies limit access to resources, shaping decision making and behavior in ways that are sometimes beyond the individual's capacity to control or change. The structural vulnerability assessment tool helps identify where extra support should be mobilized with physician referrals to clinic staff, community agencies and resources (Bourgois, et al. 2017: 3, 23, 24).

Conclusions

From this history we learn that anthropologists in the United States have a long history of engagement with medical education. With this broad perspective from the 1890s to the present, recurrent patterns of engagement emerge in areas of medical education in which anthropologists have and can make an impact. We can also learn lessons on how to continue and improve upon our roles.

Employable roles of anthropologists in US medical schools have transitioned from physical anthropologists teaching comparative anatomy in the 1890s, to the great diversity of employable roles today. With the shift to social and cultural anthropology in the 1970s, we see a blossoming of anthropologists engaged in almost every aspect of medical schools and clinical care. Psychiatry and Family Medicine were the first departments in medical schools where social and cultural anthropologists found a home. In more recent years, with the rising acceptance of psychology, sociology, anthropology, philosophy, ethics, and behavioral medicine, completely new departments are being established to complement traditional medical school departments. Over the past 15 years we see variations on department names such as "Society and Medicine," "Health Humanities," and "Medical Humanities" where medical professionals with the Ph.D. are integrated into the medical school administrative structure.

From this history we see the multitude of ways that anthropologists contributed to medical education. Primary among these is a focus on the clinic and the community. Clinical contributions range from the patient-doctor encounter, relationships, communications, cultural sensitivity, symbolic healing, explanatory models, and the culture of biomedicine. Anthropologists bring a 100 years of research and theoretical perspectives on community, social structures, and the family that can inform the practice of medicine. When training new physicians, the anthropologist brings to the medical school curriculum a broadening of the biomedical perspective to include the patient's social, cultural, and economic conditions within the community, the national and international connections. Expanding the biomedical focus on the body and disease, anthropologists call for attention to the patient's health culture, political, and economic factors, many of which cause structural violence, factors for health inequalities and poor health outcomes. Research methods and theoretical perspectives that focus on the clinic, the community, and the culture of medicine are some of the skills that anthropologists bring to employable roles in medical education and the training of physicians in medical schools.

Scientific reductionism transforms complexity into simplicity. Allopathic physicians and biomedicine in general prefer short, concise answers, formulas or models. Anthropologists tend to communicate theoretical paradigms, concepts, and explanatory theories in long written and spoken narratives expressing the humanistic, social and cultural contexts of patients and communities. For medical students and physicians to understand anthropology's theories and perspectives, clinically applied medical anthropologists reduced concepts to more easily and more quickly understandable phrases and models. During this history of anthropology in medical education, we see anthropology's primary theoretical constructs of "culture," "social structures," "social and cultural contexts," and "explanatory models," transformed into succinct check lists of attributes that clinicians could easily use during the clinical encounter and for medical students to memorize. Through this history we see "cultural sensitivity," and "cultural competency," in many cases are reduced to culture trait lists for each of the ethnic groups in a service area. Considering the infinite diversity of cultural and individual health experiences, "cultural humility," in more recent years is the realization that the physician needs to continually be learning the life experiences of their patients. Similarly, the emphasis of anthropologists on the larger social, political and economic contexts of a patient, family, and community are reduced to "social determinants of health" studied using easily obtainable census, social, economic, and population data summarized from internet computerized data sets rather than ethnographic studies. Oftentimes, culture and ethnicity are not even represented. Likewise, "Structural Violence," is transformed into the physician and medical school curriculum as "Health Disparities." The recent development of the Structural Vulnerability Scale is an example of how anthropologists can build upon the utilitarian reductionism of medicine to integrate topics beyond biomedicine by developing a list of questions to be asked of patients. These questions then provide behavioral information for physicians to use to better understand the life circumstances of a patient and ideally, enabling them to better devise a treatment plan with referrals to support staff, social service providers, housing and economic resources.

"Cultural competency," "Social Determinants of Health," "Health Disparities" "Transcultural Health Care," are examples of major contributions of anthropology reduced to very simplified forms for implementation in clinical care. They are now required topics in the medical school curriculum and the MCAT testing of pre-med majors. These phrases derived from anthropological basic research and deep historical theoretical perspectives are reductionistic transformations adopted by other academic and clinical disciplines of medicine, psychology, psychiatry, social work, nursing, among others. Applied medical anthropologists enthusiastically collaborated with other disciplines as they addressed critical health issues in federal and foundation funded research and interdisciplinary team training. Often it was not anthropologists, but other disciplines that obtained the funding to develop training workshops, programs, online learning modules translating anthropological contributions into the specific language and models for the educating of their students and practitioners. These contributions of anthropological theories, methods, and procedures are frequently unrecognized by contemporary health practitioners. The resistance that many in biomedicine may have towards anthropological perspectives on culturally appropriate care can be traced to the professionalization of allopathic medicine in the early 1900s. Most important was the alignment of the AMA as providing secular medicine, declaring all other health traditions as quacks, and those faith-based as a religion rather than a medical system. Political lobbying resulted in non-secular, traditional medicines excluded from state recognition and funding. Anthropology has a continuing challenge to facilitate the training of Integrative Medicine, and the importance of the non-secular, faith, and religion in patient's lives. Recently, Roberts (2016) criticized medical anthropologists for often taking the secular approach to research and education. She challenges the profession toward a non-secular medical anthropology, reincorporating god, gods, faith and beliefs into medical education.

Erasure of the history of anthropological contributions is a form of cultural appropriation by academic and professional groups. This erasure should be viewed within the hegemonic and highly structured allopathic medical systems where physicians are the dominant voice with economic and policy authority. Cultural group erasure is a recurrent feature of stratified societies and organizations where those in power control the narrative, discourse, and what they consider as truth (Foucault 1973). Anthropologists, now placed in medical school departments of Health Humanities, Philosophy, and Ethics with other Ph.Ds, distinct from departments with MDs, is an example of this social stratification of medicine where lower status results in less power and authority to influence the training of future physicians. We hope this chapter highlights the valuable contributions that anthropologists have and can make to medical education, and that it provides a foundation for how anthropologists can be better integrated as medical school faculty and take academic leadership roles where they can make a difference.

Acknowledgements We would like to acknowledge the contributions of many Medical Anthropology students at Florida International University who engaged with the medical education literature in their course projects helping enrich this history. Special thanks to Dr. Catherine Mas for going above and beyond her role as peer-reviewer for the chapter and engaging in a continued dialogue with us on the history of anthropology in medicine.

References

Adair, John, and Kurt Deuschle. 1970. *The people's health: Medicine and anthropology in a Navajo community*. New York: Appleton-Century-Crofts.

Alland, Alexander. 1970. *Adaptation in cultural evolution: An approach to medical anthropology*. New York: Columbia University Press.

American Medical Association. 1903. *Proceedings of the American Medical Association House of Delegates*, May 16, 1903.

Arensberg, Conrad, and Solon Kimball. 1965. *Culture and community*. New York: Harcourt, Brace & World.

Asad, Talal. 2003. *Formations of the secular: Christianity, Islam, modernity (cultural memory) in the present*. Stanford: Stanford University Press.

Association of American Medical Colleges (AAMC). 2005. *Cultural competence education for medical students*. Washington, DC: American Association of Medical Colleges.

———. 2011. *Behavioral and social science foundations for future physicians*. Washington, DC: Association of American Medical Colleges.

———. 2012. *MCAT 2015: A better test for tomorrow's doctors*. Washington, DC: Association of American Medical Colleges.
Atkinson, P. and L. Pugsley. 2005. Making sense of ethnography and medical education. *Medical Education* 39(2): 228-234.
Baer, Hans A. 2001. *Biomedicine and alternative healing systems in America: Issues of class, race, ethnicity, and gender*. Madison, WI: The University of Wisconsin Press.
———. 2004. *Toward an integrative medicine: Merging alternative therapies with biomedicine*. Walnut Creek, CA: AltaMira Press.
Baer, Hans, Merrill Singer, and Ida Susser. 1997. *Medical anthropology and the world system: A critical perspective*. Westport, CT: Bergin & Garvey.
Bartlett, F.C. 1923. Obituary of William Halse Rivers Rivers 1864–1922. *American Journal of Psychology* 34 (2): 275–277.
Becker, Howard. 1961. *Boys in white: Student culture in medical school*. New Brunswick, NJ: Transaction Books.
Bernard, Alan. 2000. *History and theory in anthropology*. Cambridge: Cambridge University Press.
Boelen, Charles, and Bob Woollard. 2009. Social accountability and accreditation: A new frontier for educational institutions. *Medical Education* 43 (9): 887–894.
Bonner, Thomas Neville. 2000. *Becoming a physician: Medical education in Britain, France, Germany, and the United States, 1750–1945*. Baltimore: Johns Hopkins University Press.
Bourgois, Phillipe, Seth Holmes, Kim Sue, and James Quesada. 2017. Structural vulnerability: Operationalizing the concept to address health disparities in clinical care. *Academic Medicine* 92 (3): 299–307.
Bowers, John Z. 1977. *An introduction to American medicine, 1975*. Rockville, MD: U.S. Dept. of Health, Education, and Welfare, Public Health Service National Institutes of Health, Washington.
Brink, Pamela. 1976. *Transcultural nursing: A book of readings*. Englewood Cliffs, NJ: Prentice Hall.
Bullon, Antonio. 2013. Learning by teaching an unsuccessful "cultural sensitivity" course. *Culture, Medicine, and Psychiatry* 37 (2): 280–287.
Butler, Christopher C., Martyn Evans, David Greaves, and Sharon Simpson. 2004. Medically unexplained symptoms: The biopsychosocial model found wanting. *Journal of the Royal Society of Medicine* 97 (5): 219–222. https://doi.org/10.1177/014107680409700503.
Castro Abitia, Hector, and Gonzalo Manzano Zayas. 1966. The teaching of anthropology in a department of preventive medicine. *The Milbank Memorial Fund Quarterly* 44 (2): 198–210.
Caudill, William. 1952. Anthropology in medicine. *Science* 30 (1952): 3.
———. 1953. Applied anthropology in medicine. In *Anthropology today*, ed. A.L. Kroeber, 771–806. Chicago: University of Chicago Press.
Chrisman, Noel J., and Thomas M. Johnson. 1990. Clinically applied anthropology. In *Medical anthropology: Contemporary theory and method*, ed. Thomas M. Johnson and Carolyn Sargent. New York: Praeger.
Chrisman, Noel J., and T.W. Maretzki. 1982. Anthropology in health science settings. In *Clinically applied anthropology: Anthropologists in health science settings*, ed. Noel J. Chrisman and T.W. Maretzki, 1–34. Boston: Kluwer.
Commission on Social Determinants of Health (CSDH). 2008. *Closing the gap in a generation: Health equity through action on the social determinants of health*. In *Final report of the Commission on Social Determinants of Health*. Geneva: World Health Organization.
Coombs, Robert H. 1978. *Mastering medicine: Professional socialization in medical school*. New York: Free Press.
Crozier, Ivan. 2008. Havelock Ellis, Eugenicist. *Studies in History and Philosophy of Science Part C: Studies in History and Philosophy of Biological and Biomedical Sciences* 39 (2): 187–194.
Cuff, Patricia A., and Neil A. Vanselow. 2004. *Improving medical education: Enhancing the behavioral and social science content of medical school curricula*. Washington, DC: The National Academies Press.

Dow, James. 1986. Universal aspects of symbolic healing. *American Anthropologist* 88: 56–69.
Dressler, William W., and James R. Bindon. 2000. The health consequences of cultural consonance: Cultural dimensions of lifestyle, social support, and arterial blood Pressure in an African American Community. *American Anthropologist* 102 (2): 244–260.
Duffy, John. 1993. *From humors to medical science: A history of American medicine*. 2nd ed. Urbana: University of Illinois Press.
Duffy, Thomas P. 2011. The Flexner report—100 years later. *The Yale Journal of Biology and Medicine* 84 (3): 269–276. https://www.ncbi.nlm.nih.gov/pmc/articles/PMC3178858/.
Ellis, Havelock. 1892. The place of anthropology in medical education. *The Lancet* 140 (3598): 365–366.
Engel, George L. 1977. The need for a new medical model: A challenge for biomedicine. *Science* 196 (4286): 129–136.
———. 1982. The biopsychosocial model and medical education: Who are to be the teachers? *New England Journal of Medicine* 306: 802–805.
Erickson, Pamela. 2008. *Ethnomedicine*. Long Grove, IL: Waveland Press.
Erickson, Paul A., and Liam Donat Murphy. 2017. *A history of anthropological theory*. 5th ed. Toronto: University of Toronto Press.
Fabrega, Horacio. 1973. Toward a model of illness behavior. *Medical Care* 11 (6): 470–484.
———. 1975. The need for an ethnomedical science. *Science* 189 (4207): 969–975.
Farmer, Paul. 2003. *Pathologies of power: Health, human rights, and the new war on the poor*. Berkeley: University of California Press.
———. 1999. *Infections and inequalities: The modern plagues*. Berkeley: University of California Press.
Farmer, Paul E., Bruce Nizeye, Sara Stulac, and Salmaan Keshavjee. 2006. Structural violence and clinical medicine. *PLoS medicine* 3 (10): e449–e449.
Farre, Albert, and Tim Rapley. 2017. The new old (and old new) medical model: Four decades navigating the biomedical and psychosocial understandings of health and illness. *Healthcare* 5 (4): 88. Multidisciplinary Digital Publishing Institute. https://www.ncbi.nlm.nih.gov/pmc/articles/PMC5746722/
Foster, George. 1978. Medical anthropology: Some contrasts with medical sociology. In *Health and the human condition: Perspectives on medical anthropology*, ed. Michael H. Logan and Edward E. Hunt, 2–10. North Scituate, MA: Duxbury Press.
Foster, George M., and Barbara Anderson. 1978. *Medical anthropology*. New York: Wiley.
Foucault, M. 1973. *The birth of the clinic: An archaeology of medical perception*. New York: Pantheon Books.
Frank, Geyla, P. Block, and R. Zemke. 2008. Anthropology, occupational therapy and disability studies: Collaborations and PROSPECTS [Introduction to special theme issue]. *Practicing Anthropology* 30 (3): 2–5.
Frank, Geyla, C. Baum, and M. Law. 2010. Chronic conditions, health, and well-being in global contexts: Occupational therapy in conversation with critical medical anthropology. In *Chronic conditions, fluid states: Chronicity and the anthropology of illness*, ed. L. Manderson and C. Smith-Morris, 230–246. New Brunswick, NJ: Rutgers University Press.
Gajdusek, D.C., and V. Zigas. 1959. Kuru: Clinical, pathological and epidemiological study of an acute progressive degenerative disease of the central nervous system among natives of the Eastern Highlands of New Guinea. *The American Journal of Medicine* 26 (3): 442–469.
Good, Byron, and Mary-Jo Devecchio Good. 1993. Learning medicine: The constructing of medical knowledge at Harvard Medical School. In *Knowledge, power and practice*, ed. S. Lindenbaum and M. Lock, 81–107. Berkeley: University of California.
Good, Mary-Jo DelVecchio, Sarah S. Willen, Seth Donal Hannah, Ken Vickery, and Lawrence Taeseng Park, eds. 2011. *Shattering culture: American medicine responds to cultural diversity*. New York: Russell Sage Foundation.
Guerrón-Montero, Carla María. 2008. *Careers in applied anthropology in the 21st century: Perspectives from academics and practitioners*. Malden, MA: Blackwell.

Haddon, A.C., and F.C. Bartlett. 1922. Obituary of William Halse Rivers Rivers, M.D., F.R.S., President of the Royal Anthropological Institute, Born 1864, Died June 4, 1922. *MAN* 22: 97–104.

Harris, Anna. 2016. Listening-touch, affect and the crafting of medical bodies through percussion. *Body & Society* 22 (1): 31–61.

Hasan, K.A., and B.G. Prasad. 1961. Place of anthropology in medical education. *Journal of Medical Education* 36: 940–942.

Holmes, Seth M., Angela C. Jenks, and Scott Stonington. 2011. Clinical subjectivation: Anthropologies of contemporary biomedical training. *Culture, Medicine, and Psychiatry* 35 (2): 105–112.

IResearchnet. 2019. *Clinical anthropology*. http://anthropology.iresearchnet.com/clinical-anthropology/. Accessed 20 Aug 2019.

Jenks, Angela. 2011. From "Lists of Traits" to "Open-Mindedness": Emerging issues in cultural competence education. *Culture, Medicine, and Psychiatry* 35 (2): 209–235. https://doi.org/10.1007/s11013-011-9212-4.

Johnson, Thomas M. 1991. Anthropologists in medical education: Ethnographic prescriptions. In *Training manual in applied medical anthropology*, ed. Carol E. Hill. Washington, DC: American Anthropological Association.

Kaiser, Bonnie N., and Lesley Jo Weaver. 2019. Culture-bound syndromes, idioms of distress, and cultural concepts of distress: New directions for an old concept in psychological anthropology. *Transcultural Psychiatry* 56 (4): 589–598.

Kirmayer, Lawrence J. 2013. 50 years of transcultural psychiatry. *Transcultural Psychiatry* 50 (1): 3–5.

Kleinman, Arthur M. 1973a. Some issues for a comparative study of medical healing. *International Journal of Social Psychiatry* 19 (3–4): 159–165.

———. 1973b. Toward a comparative study of medical systems: An integrated approach to the study of the relationship of medicine and culture. *Science, Medicine and Man* 1 (1): 55–65.

———. 1974. Explanatory models in health care relationships. In *Health of the family. National Council for International Health*, 159–172. Washington, DC: National Council for International Health.

———. 1977. Lessons from a clinical approach to medical anthropological research. *Medical Anthropology Newsletter* 8 (4): 11–15.

———. 1980. *Patients and healers in the context of culture: An exploration of the borderland between anthropology, medicine, and psychiatry*. Berkeley: University of California Press.

———. 1982. Clinically applied anthropology on a psychiatric consultation-liaison service. In *Clinically applied anthropology: Anthropologists in health science settings*, ed. Noel J. Chrisman and Thomas W. Maretzki, 83–116. Boston: Kluwer.

Kleinman, Arthur M. 1983. The cultural meanings and social uses of illness: A role for medical anthropology and clinically oriented social science in the development of primary care theory and research. *The Journal of Family Practice* 16 (3): 539–545.

Kleinman, Arthur, and Peter Benson. 2006. Anthropology in the clinic: The problem of cultural competency and how to fix it. *PLoS Med.*. Available from http://www.plosmedicine.org/article/info%3Adoi%2F10.1371%2Fjournal.pmed.0030294.

Lefley, Harriet P. 1975. Approaches to community mental health: The miami model. *Psychiatric Annals* 5 (8): 26–32. https://doi.org/10.3928/0048-5713-19750801-06.

———. 1984. Cross-cultural training for mental health professionals: Effects on the delivery of services. *Hospital Community Psychiatry* 35 (12): 1227–1229. https://doi.org/10.1176/ps.35.12.1227.

Lefley, Harriet P., and Evalina W. Bestman. 1991. Public-academic linkages for culturally sensitive community mental health. *Community Mental Health Journal* 27 (6): 473–488.

Lefley, Harriet P., and P.B. Pedersen. eds. 1986. Cross-cultural training for mental health professionals. Springfield, IL: Charles C Thomas.

Leininger, Madeleine M. 1970. *Nursing and anthropology; Two worlds to blend.* New York: Wiley.
———. 1978. *Transcultural nursing: Concepts, theories, and practices.* New York: Wiley.
———. 1989. Transcultural Nurse Specialists and Generalists: New Practitioners in Nursing. *Transcultural Nursing* 1 (1): 4–16.
Lewis, Oscar. 1951. *Life in a Mexican village: Tepoztlan restudied.* Urbana: University of Illinois Press.
Liaison Committee for Medical Education (LCME). 2018. *Functions and structure of a medical school: Standards for accreditation of medical education programs leading to the MD degree.* March. http://lcme.org/publications/#Standards
Lie, D., J. Boker, S. Crandall, C. DeGannes, et al. 2008. A revised curriculum tool for assessing cultural competency training (TACCT) in health professions education. *MedEdPORTAL* 4: 3185. https://doi.org/10.15766/mep_2374-8265.3185.
Lindenbaum, S. 1979. *Kuru sorcery: Disease and danger in the New Guinea highlands.* Palo Alto, CA: Mayfield.
———. 2001. Kuru, prions, and human affairs: Thinking about epidemics. *Annual review of anthropology* 30: 363–385.
Livingstone, Frank B. 1958. Anthropological implications of sickle cell gene distribution in West Africa. *American Anthropologist* 60: 533–562.
Logan, Michael H., and Edward E. Hunt. 1977. *Health and the human condition: Perspectives on medical anthropology.* North Scituate, MA: Duxbury Press.
Maeshiro, Rika. 2008. Responding to the challenge: Population health education for physicians. *Academic Medicine* 83 (4): 319–320.
Marmot, Michael G., Stephen Stansfeld, Chandra Patel, Fiona North, Jenny Head, Ian White, Eric Brunner, Amanda Feeney, and G. Davey Smith. 1991. Health inequalities among British civil servants: The Whitehall II study. *The Lancet* 337 (8754): 1387–1393.
Mas, Catherine. 2019. *The culture brokers: Medicine and anthropology in global Miami, 1960–1995.* Ph.D., Department of History, Program in the History of Science and Medicine, Yale University.
Mattingly, Cheryl. 1998. *Healing dramas and clinical plots: The narrative structure of experience.* New York: Cambridge University Press.
McElroy, Ann, and Patricia K. Townsend. 2015. *Medical anthropology in ecological perspective.* Boulder, CO: Westview Press.
Merton, Robert King, and George G. Reader. 1957. *The student-physician: Introductory studies in the sociology of medical education.* Cambridge, MA: Harvard University Press.
Nader, Laura. 1972. Up the anthropologist—perspectives gained from studying up. In *Reinventing anthropology*, ed. Dell H. Hymes, 284–311. New York: Pantheon Books.
NAPA/OT Fieldschool. 2019. National Association for the Practice of Anthropology and Occupational Therapy fieldschool. http://napaotguatemala.org/. Accessed 3 Sept 2019.
New, Peter Kong, and J. Thomas May. 1965. *Report on teaching of social sciences in medical and public health schools.* Presented at the business meeting of the medical sociology section of the American Sociological Association. Chicago. August 30, 1965.
Nichter, Mark. 2010. *Idioms of distress revisited. Culture, medicine and psychiatry* 34 (2): 401–416.
Nurge, Ethel. 1975. Anthropological perspective for medical students. *Human Organization* 34 (4): 345–352.
Office of Minority Health. 2018. National standards for culturally and linguistically appropriate services in health and health Care (The National CLAS Standards). https://minorityhealth.hhs.gov/omh/browse.aspx?lvl.2&lvlid.53.
O'Rourke, Thomas W. 1983. How can the health professions use anthropology? The health education perspective. In *Clinical anthropology: A new approach to American health problems?* ed. Peggy Golde and Demitri B. Shimkin, 293–303. Lanham, MD: University Press of America.

Partners in Health. 2019. https://www.pih.org/. Accessed 26 Aug 2019.
Paul, Benjamin D. 1956. Anthropology and public health. In *some uses of anthropology: Theoretical and applied*, ed. Joseph B. Casagrande and Thomas Gladwin. Brooklyn: Theo Gaus' Sons.
Pelto, Pertti J., and Gretel H. Pelto. 1978. Medicine, anthropology, community: An overview. In *Health and the human condition: Perspectives on medical anthropology*, ed. Michael H. Logan and E. Hunt Edward, 401–406. North Scituate, MA: Duxbury Press.
Read, Margaret. 1970. Some problems in teaching medical anthropology. *Social Science & Medicine* 4: 163–167.
Redfield, Robert. 1930. *Tepoztlan—A Mexican village*. Chicago: University of Chicago Press.
Rivers, William Halse. 1916. Medicine, magic and religion. *Lancet XCIV* 59–65: 117–123.
Rivers, W.H.R. 1968(1914). Kinship and social organization. London: Athlone Press.
Roberts, Elizabeth. 2016. Gods, germs, and petri Dishes: Toward a nonsecular medical anthropology. *Medical Anthropology* 35 (3): 209–219.
Romanucci-Ross, Lola, Daniel E. Moerman, and Laurence R. Tancredi, eds. 1983. *The anthropology of medicine: From culture to method*. South Hadley, MA: Bergin & Garvey.
Rousch, Robert E., Debbie Kothmann, and Janet M. Schreiber. 1976. Medical anthropology in the curriculum. A revisit to the subject. *Journal of Medical Education* 51: 119–124.
Scott, Clarissa. 1975. Competing health care systems in an inner city area. *Human Organization 34* (1): 108–110.
Shaw, Susan J., and Julie Armin. 2011. The ethical self-fashioning of physicians and health care systems in culturally appropriate health care. *Culture, Medicine, and Psychiatry* 35 (2): 236–261.
Shimkin, Demitri Boris, and Peggy Golde. 1983. *Clinical anthropology: A new approach to American health problems?* Lanham, MD: University Press of America.
Singer, Merrill. 1994. AIDS and the health crisis of the US urban poor: The perspective of critical medical anthropology. *Social Science and Medicine* 39 (7): 931–948.
———. 2009. Introduction to syndemics: A critical systems approach to public and community health. San Francisco: John Wiley & Sons.
Singer, Merrill, and Hans A. Baer. 1995. *Critical medical anthropology*. Amityville, NY: Baywood Press.
Starr, Paul. 1982. *The social transformation of American medicine: The rise of a sovereign profession and the making of a vast industry*. New York: Basic books.
Stein, Howard F. 1974. Letter. *Medical Anthropology Newsletter* 5 (3): 15–16.
———. 1980. Clinical anthropology and medical anthropology. *Medical Anthropology Newsletter* 12 (1): 18–19.
———. 1982. Ethnographic mode of teaching clinical behavioral science. In *Clinically applied anthropology: Anthropologists in health science settings*, ed. Noel Chrisman and T.W. Maretzki, 1–34. Kluwer: Boston.
———. 1990a. *American medicine as culture*. Boulder: Westview Press.
———. 1990b. *The psychodynamics of medical practice*. Oakland, CA: University of California Press.
———. 1996. *Prairie voices: Process anthropology in family medicine*. Westport, CN: Bergin & Garvey.
Stein, Howard, and Maurice Apprey. 1985. *Context and dynamics of clinical knowledge*. Charlottesville: University Press of Virginia.
Stonington, Scott, and Diana Coffa. 2019. Structural iatrogenesis: A 43-year-old man with "opioid misuse." Case studies in social medicine. *New England Journal of Medicine* 380: 701–704. https://doi.org/10.1056/NEJMp1811473.
Stonington, Scott D., Seth M. Holmes, Helena Hansen, Jeremy A. Greene, Keith A. Wailoo, Debra Malina, Stephen Morrissey, Paul E. Farmer, and Michael G. Marmot. 2018. Case studies in social medicine-attending to structural forces in clinical practice. *New England Journal of Medicine* 379 (20): 1958–1961.

Taylor, Janelle S. 2003. Confronting "culture" in medicine's "culture of no culture". *Academic Medicine* 78 (6): 555–559.

———. 2014. The demise of the bumbler and the crock: From experience to accountability in medical education and ethnography. *American Anthropologist* 116 (3): 523–534.

Taylor, Rex, and Annelie Rieger. 1984. Rudolf Virchow on the typhus epidemic in Upper Silesia: An introduction and translation. *Sociology of Health and Illness* 6 (2): 201–217.

Virchow, Rudolph. 1848–1849. *Die Meizinishe reform. Eign Wochenschrift*, 10 July 1848–29 June 1849. Berlin: Druck & Verlag von G. Reimer.

Weaver, Thomas. 1968. Medical anthropology: Trends in research and medical education. In *Essays on medical anthropology*, 1–12. Athens: University of Georgia Press, Athens.

Wiedman, Dennis. 1984. Directing geriatric health care: Some practical issues. *Practicing Anthropology* 6 (3):7–8.

———. 2012. Upholding indigenous freedoms of religion and medicine: Peyotists at the 1906–1908 Oklahoma constitutional convention and first legislature. *American Indian Quarterly* 36 (2): 215–246.

———. 2016. Strategic Planning. In *Anatomy of a dream: The making of the FIU Herbert Wertheim College of Medicine, 2006–2016*, ed. Thomas Breslin and Barbara Roller, 30–41. Gainesville: University of Florida Press.

Weidman, Hazel H. 1975. Concepts as strategies for change. *Psychiatric Annals* 5: 17–19.

———. 1979. Transcultural view—Prerequisite to interethnic (intercultural) communication in medicine. *Social Science & Medicine* 13 (2B): 85–87.

———. 1983a. The mediating person—Bridges between cultures. *American Anthropologist* 85 (2): 445–447.

———. 1983b. Research, service and training aspects of clinical anthropology: An instructional overview. In *Clinical anthropology: A new approach to American health problems?* ed. Peggy Golde and Demitri B. Shimkin, 119–153. Lanham, MD: University Press of America.

———. 1985. Clinical anthropology and public-health anthropology—A commentary. *Human Organization* 44 (1): 80–81.

———. 1986. On the origins of the SMA. *Medical Anthropology Quarterly* 17 (5): 115–124.

Wiedman, Dennis, and Iveris L. Martinez. 2017. Organizational culture theme theory and analysis of strategic planning for a new medical school. *Human Organization* 76 (3): 264–274.

Wilkinson, Richard G., and Michael Marmot, eds. 2003. *Social determinants of health: The solid facts*. Geneva: World Health Organization.

Willen, Sarah, and Elizabeth Carpenter-Song. 2013. Cultural competence in action: "Lifting the hood" on four case studies in medical education. *Culture, Medicine, and Psychiatry* 37 (2): 241–252.

Witt, Claudia, Delia Chiaramonte, Suan Berman, Margaret A. Chesney, George A. Kaplan, Kurt C. Stange, Steven H. Woolf, and Brian M. Berman. 2017. Defining health in a comprehensive context: A new definition of integrative health. *American Journal of Preventive Medicine* 53 (1): 134–137.

World Health Organization (WHO). 2014. *WHO traditional medicine strategy 2014–2023*. https://www.who.int/medicines/publications/traditional/trm_strategy14_23/en/

———. 2018. *ICD 11—International classification of diseases and related health problems*. Geneva: World Health Organization. https://www.who.int/classifications/icd/en/.

Dennis W. Wiedman, PhD, is Professor of Anthropology, Department of Global and Sociocultural Studies. Florida International University. Miami, Florida. He received his Ph.D. in Anthropology from the University of Oklahoma in 1979 where he trained in medical anthropology at the University of Oklahoma College of Medicine. Employment in the Department of Psychiatry at the University of Miami School of Medicine in the Office of Transcultural Education and Research grounded him in clinical anthropology as Director of a Department of Psychiatry community mental health unit. He is the Founding Director of the FIU Global Indigenous Forum with the mission to bring the Indigenous voice to FIU, South Florida, and the world. His research interests include Native American health, type II diabetes, organizational culture, applying anthropology, and directing culture change. He specializes in social and cultural factors for the global pandemic of Type II diabetes and metabolic syndrome. He teaches courses in medical anthropology, anthropological theory, and ethnohistorical research methods. During more than a decade in the FIU Provost Office he was the Assistant to the Provost, University Accreditation Officer and first Director of Program Review. As lead strategic planner for the university's first major strategic plan he had a key role in planning and envisioning the new FIU Medical school incorporating medical anthropology principles and a community focus. He served on the Executive Board of the American Anthropological Association (AAA) in the practicing/professional seat, and was President of the National Association for the Practice of Anthropology (NAPA). Throughout these academic, applied, and practicing leadership experiences, he consistently published on organizational culture theory and analysis in leading journals and book chapters.

Iveris L. Martinez, PhD is Professor, Archstone Foundation Endowed Chair in Gerontology, and Director of the Center for Successful Aging at California State University, Long Beach. She was a founding faculty member of the Herbert Wertheim College of Medicine (HWCOM) at Florida International University where she served as chief of the Division of Medicine and Society and chaired the admissions committee for the college for 5 years. Between 2007 and 2018, she taught the first year introductory course and other course content on health disparities, cultural competency, and social determinants of health at HWCOM, as well as led an annual interprofessional clinical workshop across the health sciences. An applied anthropologist, she has received funding from the National Institutes of Health, the Macarthur Foundation, and others for her community-based research on social and cultural factors influencing health, with an emphasis in aging, Latinos, and minority populations. Her current research interests include improving services for caregivers of persons with Alzheimer's, reducing social isolation in aging, as well as interprofessional efforts to create age-friendly communities. She previously served as the Chair of the Board of the Alliance for Aging, Inc., the local area agency on aging for Miami-Dade and Monroe Counties, and President of the Association for Anthropology, Gerontology, and the Life Course. She holds a joint Ph.D. in Anthropology and Population and Family Health Sciences (Public Health) from Johns Hopkins University.

Chapter 3
Beyond Moralism in Medical Education: The Making of Physician-Anthropologists for the Study of Good Care in France

Samuel Lézé

> *How many things were articles of faith to us yesterday, which are fables to us today?*
>
> *Michel de Montaigne*

A Brief Introduction to French Medical Folklore

First day at the Faculty of Medicine, term 1, October 2004: I was aware that the first-year lecture was to take place in a 1000-seat amphitheater. I already had experience with audiences accustomed to listening to lectures in the humanities. But I had not imagined the room would have such an impressive volume: a floor the size of a concert hall or at the Opera. Before going into the room, you had to go see the porter to get a microphone—an essential item. He coldly handed it to me with a disturbing sentence: "if necessary, call me using the telephone on the desk at this number . . .—What could I need?—You will see. . .".

Entering the amphitheater, which was quickly filling with students, I went to the podium to put down my notes. On my left was a disarticulated skeleton with a paper plane on its side. On my right, a video projector for the slide presentations. Behind me, a green chalkboard with some vestiges of inscriptions. On the ceiling, were many stuck paper planes as well as blobs of wet paper and chewing gum. There was no chair on the podium. So I went to get one from the main floor. To put my notes into order and to acquire a concentrated air, I needed to sit down and to plunge myself into the first sentences of the course. As the buzz of the huge hall began to diminish, 5 min before the beginning of the class, a group of ten "Santards" entered silently. Santards are young officers from the School of Health of the Armies, a French tradition dating from the late nineteenth century. The first ranks were kept vacant for them. I did not know that I was going to have students in the military garb.

S. Lézé (✉)
Department of Human Sciences, ENS de Lyon, France
e-mail: samuel.leze@ens-lyon.fr

I. L. Martinez, D. W. Wiedman (eds.), *Anthropology in Medical Education*,
https://doi.org/10.1007/978-3-030-62277-0_3

It was then that a clamor began to be heard: "Where is the teacher?" Where is the teacher? "Where is the teacher?" From the upper levels of the amphitheater, a chorus of voices shouted *Carré!* (In slang, literally: "square"—referring to students repeating the first year after having failed it) and a *bizuth* (meaning a first-year student) responded *bizuth*! As I tapped on my microphone to give the signal that class was beginning, I started the class by reading my text without adjusting my voice to the hubbub. Immediately, an incredible silence fell: I could almost hear students breathing in the first row. I observed that the whole class was copying my lecture to the letter. The reactions of the students indicated to me that I should not go too fast, and even, that I had to dictate as a lesson! Because I was dictating, it was possible to interrupt me. The audience reacted to some of my comments and tried to dialogue certain words. For example, when I mentioned an important aspect that might be useful for the eliminatory exam, there was a swirling movement in the heart of the group accompanied by a hissing sound "ssssss!" When I spoke of a more technical aspect that could be forbidding, they used humor as a "safety valve" when I pronounced the formula "therapeutic process" (in French: "processus"), a student immediately shouted a mirror repetition: *suce!* (Sucks). When I talked about nursing work (expressed through the stereotype of "the female nurse"), the mostly masculine audience stopped the course with a "mmmmum!", and other interjections. That is not all.

After 15 min, a *Carré* gave a signal and the course stopped for 2 min to sing: "Flame Captain, you're not from our galaxy", a song popularized by "Space Opera", a Japanese cartoon of the 1980s but who originated from an 1940s American comic. It kind of served as a "break" within the 2-h course. Some of the pandemonium that happens in medicine courses has been filmed and is even broadcasted on YouTube. The course resumed without any more ado, and 15 min later came another even more theatrical interruption. Two "carrés" gave a shout and lifted a (consenting) "bizuth" onto the podium to lower his trousers, the whole production accompanied by a bawdy song. He ended up tied up and taped to a chair and the "carrés" laboriously heaved him and his chair onto my desk. At the end of the song, everything was quickly put back into place after general applause (including mine) and I could continue my class, still going slowly enough to leave time for the "note taking", everything was scrupulously well noted and retained, including my extemporaneous comments. At the end of the class, I was applauded. I had the unpleasant impression of not having managed to give my full lecture, of having given something close to dictation, concentrated as I had been on the "balance of power" rather than the content, and constrained by a standard format inadequate to the critical content that I professed to be offering. Lost in my reflections on the situation, I did not see that four students were waiting for me.

I was indeed awaited by four very worried *bizuths*. They wanted to know if it was possible to have the written version of my course, especially if I could print it "to learn it by heart". Although I had explicitly said that there was nothing to "learn by heart", they wanted to learn the "summary" of all the topics that could appear in the qualifying exam. I was physically escorted to the photocopy room because the last time they had asked, the text had been stolen by *Carrés*. This is only a rumor of course. The circulation of false information circulates constantly and adds to the already burdensome atmosphere of teaching humanities at the medical school. One of the "bizuths" told me in the underground corridors, before reaching the copy room, that he was "taking the exam" and was anticipating the next class with great interest. He told me that the previous week, a lecturer had lasted only 15 min and had left threatening to make up all the classes he could not teach on the very day of the qualifying exam.

Why have I not talked about the course content yet? Because the situation first appeared to me as *ethnographic*. In my field notes of that period, which were devoted to the clinical work at a day hospital for psychotic adolescents, I wrote that same evening and I kept it more than 10 years later: the teaching situation gave rise to an observation of a *space*, a *temporality*, a *hierarchy* and a foreign *lexicon*. A participation that reveals many unspoken rules because of the very disruption it causes. Without gaining familiarity with these codes, how to teach correctly in this situation? How not to remain a strange anthropologist holding foreign speech in the middle of this medical "folklore"? And then, how can one not judge that it is impossible or inadmissible to teach under these state-of-war conditions between *carrés* and *bizuths*? There is the dilemma of "discipline": How to have a course be heard through all this mayhem? How to make audible the voice of anthropology, lost in this mass education, this "hostile" public, especially in a section of "human sciences" mixed in with historians, philosophers and caregivers. What does all this mean for my lecture on *symbolic efficiency* and the notion of a *therapeutic system* (Csordas and Kleinman 1990) that I had prepared so well, perhaps to no avail, with the naive scruples of the beginner?

In rereading my notes today, it is possible to say that at that time, a medical professor was someone who was older than me and who, unlike me, did not sit down and read his notes. He was someone who stayed standing and lectured without notes, scrolling down a power-point and commenting on visuals, using a certain eloquence in front of a room that he kept his eyes on. He talked to the audience as needed by quickly adding "keywords" to the board. His eloquence implied a solid balance, which included using irony towards the "carrés" that he cruelly crushed: a "carré" must listen twice as much as a "bizuth" because he or she has failed once already. He also knew how to frustrate them by circumventing the opportunities for heckling, that is to say by avoiding saying certain words. Paradoxically, he was a professor who, though without ever saying so explicitly, never stopped communicating with his body that the most important thing to understand is that medicine cannot be learned during the university lectures, cluttered as they are with formulas and abstractions. Real medicine will only be learned in the future at the hospital. The Faculty of Medicine separates those who will become practitioners from those who will languish for another year in this hell or, worse yet, will have to leave, covered in shame, to attend the Faculty of Sciences or the nursing school.

Humanities as Moral Education

The specificity of this pedagogical scene can be better understood if it is contextualized not only within the general organization of medical education in France, but also within the organizational culture of each specific medical school (Wiedman and Martinez 2017) beyond the "folklore" that can be judged as an obstacle to overcome. In the common understanding, the "folklore" of the *Carabin* (an ironic term synonymous with medical students) is reduced to a set of "rites of passage": the now forbidden "hazing", obscene or macabre jokes, bawdy songs, memorable "parties", on the sidelines of the "official" training course, from the first year to the internship (a national ranking competition distinguishing generalists from specialists). Thus, how to analyze the place of the humanities in France since their introduction into the faculties of medicine in the 1990s? In France, the carabin's moral career has at least two *turning points* that are decisive and structuring in his or her access to the doctor profession, medical training, and clinical practice.

First, since 1971, access to true medical training involves passing through a competitive examination rather than a simple testing process. There is a quota of the number of places allocated to the 34 faculties of medicine, a "*numerus clausus*". Between 1972 and 1992, the number of places at the national level dropped from 8500 to 3500. But for the 2012–2013 academic year, the number was 7492 places for 55,696 students registered and for 2017–2018, 8205 for 59,753. If the amphitheater seems to be frenetic, that is because of the 800 students enrolled in the first year at the time, only 80 will be able to attain the second year of the courses and really begin their medical training—or about 15% and 25% of registrations. The first year is a year of selection and successive reforms have focused on transforming it into "training" to avoid the waste of an entire academic year for so many students (Déplaude 2015). Hence the majority of students cannot imagine preparing for the competitive exams without resorting to a private preparatory school supervising the cramming of students, including in the humanities. This private preparation is often criticized by academics. The annual amount is around 4000 euros. This is the place where the "courses" are transcribed and distributed in the form of "cards" that put all the information of the course into "tables". The training is done by transfers of "repetitions" and exercises from the annals (or "colles", literally "glue" for "a trick question").

Second, for over 200 years, since 1802, the last competitive examination at the end of the sixth year before Residency, "Internat" (now called "Epreuves Classantes Nationales, ECN"), has been perceived as the great "rite of passage". It can either evoke the national placement competition that ranks students and allows for their classification into generalists (around 4000 places) or specialists (around 4000 places), or it can evoke a long-term internship in various departments of a *hospital*, within the public health system which is public in France (Lézé 2014). Medicine is not learned at the University. After becoming a "clinician", the profession and the art of healing are really learned at the bedside of the sick. The head of the clinic, a more or less charismatic character, is always idealized by interns. It is within this practical context that the budding doctor takes on the final competitive struggle to access the specialized training set up between 1982 and 1984. It is also within this context that we find with even greater amplification the *carabin* folklore which can be studied ethnographically to understand how a French doctor is made produced (Godeau 2007).

It was only in 1992, thanks to a former dean of the Faculty of Medicine at Necker Hospital in Paris, a pediatrician, that the first year of the courses included training in "General Culture" to counterbalance the place of biology in medicine. After strong protest, the name was changed to "the Human and Social Sciences" through the Ministerial Order of May 2, 1995 (which concerned the humanities and social sciences module of the first year of undergraduate medical studies, PCEM1). The latter was not just a surface reform, it now became the subject area with the strongest grade weight! (Visier 2011: 143–44). Thus it became possible to fail the entire competitive exam by failing this subject. The reform of 2009 increased the numbers even more because the first year became a core year of coursework common for all the health professions (medicine, pharmacy, odontology, maieutics, physiotherapy). It became necessary to build new amphitheaters to accommodate the doubling or tripling of the student numbers, with some medical schools even distributing recorded courses. With the Ministerial Order of October 28, 2009, The HSS become the "Unité d'Enseignement" (teaching unit) number 7 (UE7) "Health, Society, Humanity" (SSH) whose main objective is to give a "culture of health" in order to provide the health professions with a common culture and deontology (Visier 2011: 144–45). Depending on the medical school, doctors, philosophers, anthropologists or sociologists organizing the courses on this subject vary greatly, despite the creation of a reference handbook and the National College of Teachers of SHS in Medicine in 2008 (Mouillie et al. 2011). The reform of 2019 announced, however, that as of September 2020, there would be an end to the *numerus clausus* so as to "stop wasting human potential" according to a striking formula in the Health System Organization and Transformation bill of March 26, 2019.

Two other factors are decisive in explaining that the humanities have increased the anxiety level of the students in this competitive struggle. First, this is the only test that does not rely on "memorization" but on "reflection". The assessment of other subjects is done with Multiple Choice Question (MCQ) Exams, which can be corrected by an automated computer system and not on a test paper written by hand. This aspect not only leads to constant doubt about the objectivity and fairness of the evaluation, but also to uncertainty about what should be learned by heart. The first explicit objective of this test, however, is to evaluate, at the end of high school, basic skills in "the capacities of analysis and reflection of the student". Moreover, it is often one form or another of a "dissertation", the classic exercise required in the high school French and philosophy classes. The subject may be: "Can happiness be prescribed?", "Is aging a disease?", or "Can we say anything to a sick person?" This essay has an introduction (with a "problematization", or thesis statement), a dialectic development exploring and debunking the first idea, which is always bad, in two or three main paragraphs in the body of the essay ("thesis", "antithesis" with or without "synthesis") and in the best cases a conclusion that is not a summary, but an opening out of the subject. But the "memorization" of the courses can give the catastrophic result of transforming the "reflection" into a mere presentation of "keywords" which, in the best cases, is based on "definitions". But cases where students merely parrot the things heard during the lecture on "care for the patient", "the caregiver *must* preserve the autonomy of the patient", and "vulnerability *must* lead to solicitude" all shows the inculcation of a spiritualistic morality of the self against positive knowledge (which like the "dissertation" was derived from the nineteenth century world view, Goldstein 2005) to the detriment of an ethical reflection on the limits of the biosciences.

It is, therefore, a true moral education of the "future" doctor that takes place through the introduction of the humanities in medicine. The paradoxical goal of the humanities is to encourage students to reflect on a medical practice that they do not yet have nor will perhaps ever have, from the perspective of the various disciplines of humanities, ranging from the history of medicine to the anthropology of health systems, to the major ethical questions confronting medicine. In other words, to instill *doubt* (but in fact, moral certainties) at the very moment when the identification with the role of doctor is the strongest (Lézé and Masure 2007). Anthropology is thus lost in the midst of various disciplines, which are themselves lost in the middle of the courses devoted to anatomy, cell biology, or biochemistry. But the message is all the more paradoxical because medicine cannot be identified with the totality of its knowledge either, and so it is also lost in the midst of science and in the midst of a central political value of contemporary societies, "Health". Perhaps the greatest paradox, as some students sometimes remark, is that the subject which is the farthest away from the biosciences is the one that presents the questions posed by the practical and real practice of medicine. Basically, the guiding principle is always the famous "doctor-patient relationship" and the sociocultural factors that condition or challenge it: scientific progress, ethical limits, legal codification, or political events (including public health).

Beyond a Chorus of Complaints in Medical Education

From these two descriptions, it is easy to grasp to what extent medical folklore and organizational culture of a local medical school can cause dissatisfaction or irritation (Tarot 1999). There is a situational incongruity. But, deep down, where to locate this incongruity? In the ordered disorder of the heckling or in the disorder that can cause an almost inaudible anthropological discourse? What is the meaning of "inaudible" here? Literally too quiet to be heard? It all depends on the perspective rendering a moral evaluation. Is it found in the stern look of the professor whose moral expectation is to have docile "good students" who might identify with him and thus spare him from the heckling. In his perplexity at seeing his teaching reduced to cramming, dogmatism or a patchwork of opinions with regard to real knowledge (Visier 2011: 145)? For can an anthropology course be based on "facts" to be learned if there is never any questioning of the values, norms and emotions that arise during caregiving? What is the best strategy (Rice and McCurdy 2002)? Or, does this evaluation lie in the equally demanding look of the student whose moral expectation, within the framework of the preparation of one of the most competitive university programs in France, is to have a "good teacher", one who masters a "medical discourse" that can be adopted so as to immediately identify the symbolic boundary that truly separates them from students from other faculties? An exchange on an internet medical tutoring forum of the Faculty of Lille in September 2010 shows this situation well:

> Hi, **Welcome to the magical world of SHS, where the more you think you have succeeded, the lower your ranking**. Now about your method, ask yourself if you have chosen the right keywords, the right ideas. I'm not sure that everything synthesized on a card is a good thing because if you are missing keywords or important ideas you will (pass necessarily for 'exam) **but hey there are so many things that come into account in the grade** (syntax, grammar, conjugation, etc. ...) and any **without real (scale)? on this matter, it's very difficult to (train) study, so the best is still to learn one's course by heart +++ and to pray.** Finally, I say that, I was not more successful in the exam than you with this method, but I know people for whom it worked very well. **This is the course that selects the most and the one about which we know the fewest things** but hey it's like that, the only thing to do is to limit the damage and to get points elsewhere and take advantage of the 2nd quad with the MCQ to raise your grade and really work hard at the biophysics. It is there also that the selection will be played mainly with our dear Pr. Huglo. **In short, SHS is a dogma in University**. If there is a method that works, that is a good question. Maybe some people have good grades who will certainly enlighten you better than me. (emphasis added)

It should not be forgotten that anthropologists can be even more critical and their moral expectation is also *loyalty* to their discipline. The fear of "dilution", when attaching oneself to academic reproduction with courses of authentic anthropology cannot be dispensed with the mythology of the exotic terrain and some picturesque anecdotes, with or without the help of Malinowski and Radcliffe-Brown. Likewise, doctor colleagues may feel threatened to preserve the *esprit de corps* of students belonging to their faculty. Thus, a professor of medicine could say to the professor of anthropology, who is their colleagues in a medical faculty: "You have destabilized *my* students. But perhaps that was your goal?" (Goubert 1987: 59).

These various forms of complaining, regarding the inhumanity of the first year of medicine, are part of a rhetorical repertoire that is constantly re-enacted. Recently, the film *Première année* (The Freshman) (2018) by Thomas Lilti, has just released this rhetorical repertoire more widely. A striking scene delivers, for example, a well-known joke: "How can you tell a prep student from a med one? Make them learn the phone book. The first will ask *why*, the second by *when*." While anchored nevertheless in the same substance, a *moral consensus* on the necessity for the humanization of medicine, all the way from medical studies to clinical practice at the hospital. The complaining doctors and the lamenting of the humanities faculty complement each other very well. They are sometimes indistinguishable. In France at least, the "science of man" was in the nineteenth century a theoretical goal for medicine and philosophy as an ideal *synthesis* of the complete man: a body and a spirit, a physiology, and a psychology. The two disciplines tried to obtain the monopoly of synthesis by appropriating physiology or psychology and by accusing each other of "reductionism" (Azouvi 1995).

It is the same updated creed that is found in doctors' fears of *dehumanization* linked with the technological, economic and legal rationalization of caregiving (Mattéi et al. 1997: 3–26). This fear is always expressed in the name of a "person" who has two components: the body and the mind (Mattéi et al. 1997: 12). This anti-dualism is in perfect harmony with the spontaneous holism of the humanities (Hemmings 2005), which seems to compete only to impose "good" as a higher morality. Paradoxically, therefore, the medical ideal of introducing humanities, in order to "humanize physicians", is a medical idea that seems perfectly immune to the analysis of the humanities in the race for moralism, as well as the majority of positive values that are currently in health policies before being in this moral education: the autonomy of the person. Anthropology, however, continues to concretely show the limits or paradoxes of this moral value of "autonomy", especially in psychiatry (Pols et al. 2017), where chronicity is a very important, sometimes hopeless, clinical reality (Bister 2018).

It has become a "cliché" of contemporary medical education to criticize the bad training given in the past. Indeed, the patient-physician relationship in the clinical encounter is a basic *moral relation* between two roles with a set of Rights and Obligations or a set of moral Norms and Values. Parsons (1951) developed the concept of "Sick Role Mechanism" in defending the ideal patient-physician relationship, a "paternalism" in the name of what is "good" for patients from the point of view of the physician. But the term was almost synonymous with professionalism. The patient was under the control of the doctor to achieve healing. Sixty years later, the term has undergone a reversal of value (Burnham 2014). For the sake of patients, this moral relationship has gradually become the model to be criticized and avoided. As a result, during this period, there was a profound change in the grounding of medical authority. Paternalism is no longer the best moral attitude to convey good care. This is another moral consensus between the physician and the social scientist. This critical history is well-known and provides the questionable foundations of bioethics (McCullough 2011). However, two issues are not so clear. This narrative is a *moral history* about what "good care" is. At the same time, this moral history is becoming a version of *moral education* in medical training supported by social scientists, specifically by medical anthropologists, Medical humanities, including bioethics. As in many research protocols, the humanities still have a small place, that of "moral guarantee" (Van den Hoonaard 2011). Medicine requires a service that the humanities gives it too easily, in a perfect "pre-established harmony", including in criticism.

The French translation of this criticism of paternalism is interesting to highlight because since the development of the famous myth of the "Paris School of the medicine" in the nineteenth century (Hannaway and Laberge 1998) until now, medical training in France has had the ambition to protect and illustrate the centrality of the clinical encounter, known as the "Clinic" (or the art of "seeing, hearing, feeling" a sick person), a local variant of medical paternalism and humanism. This claim is supported by the following argument: good experience of patient pathologies gives the best first-hand knowledge in order to ground its medical judgment. The basis of this claim is simply that "experience" is a valuable source of knowledge. The defense of this *art* of "seeing, hearing, feeling" against biology, is a commonplace of medical discourse and a specificity that seems to be particularly French. However, there is a variant of this defense of the clinical practice in the United States linked to the threat of losing a moral vision of good mental health care due to economic rationalization (Ware et al. 2000).

However, this claim is trivial because everywhere in the world it is claimed that the clinical years of training are the most crucial in the subsequent practice and attitude of the physician towards patients. These years are an important moment of socialization where chief physicians are informal clinical models. It is the model of the "patient-centered medicine", valued in a local form by the idea of a "clinic of the singularity" (a subjective listening to patients and not only an objective observation). However, it is in this period of transition between a medical student and doctor that both *reflexivity* in complex situations and *reflexes* of reduction of clinical uncertainty occurs (Schön 1983). In this "hidden curriculum" (Lempp and Seale 2004), the student can learn both the best and the worst practices and local mistakes (Chadalavada and Bewley 2011), yet it is also the place where clinical authority develops. But this clinical authority is today challenged by Evidence-Based Medicine (EBM) and Ethics (that experience of the patient is valuable) during medical education. This tension is particularly strong for interns in psychiatry. Why Psychiatry rather than Nephrology? As a case study, psychiatry is certainly the medical specialty where the *gap between theory and practice* is experienced as difficult to assume in particular in order to judge what the good care is (Mattingly 1998). A care that is also the subject of much polemic about semiology, since psychoanalysis has become less and less the reference model (Paris 2005; Lézé 2010, 2013). Moreover, French psychiatry has long been acculturated through the human sciences and the suspicions regarding biology by Phenomenology, Lacanian psychoanalysis and the psychiatric reception of Michel Foucault's critical thought.

The Making of Physician-Anthropologists in Psychiatry

Whose side are anthropologists on regarding this moral issue: preserving the heritage of an endangered local moral practice (the "clinic"), or converting the science student to a new medical humanism between Evidence-Based Medicine (EBM) and Ethics? Neither. Quite the contrary. I believe that the contribution of the anthropologist is rather to be beyond moralism, not to give moral lessons, but to offer doctors tools to analyze the moral questions arising in clinical practice. Training physicians in social and cultural anthropology could more broadly produce physician-anthropologists and develop a medical anthropology of proper caregiving worthy of interest for anthropology *and* medicine.

Where to locate this training? In the two strategic moments of medical training that I have described before: First, still and always in the first year of medicine, despite the dogmatic framework and the teaching conditions. This is difficult work, but if the teaching is focused by medical anthropology on clinical case studies rather than philosophical discussions on abstract ethical dilemmas, then the teachers who teach the subject convey important notions even if they take the form of basic definitions. In all this, something remains in the student's mind. This "something" is actualized precisely at the time of the discovery of the clinical work during the last 4 years of internship and so, 5 years after this coursework in humanities. While meeting with my first medical students in the Amphitheater, I also met with interns, most in psychiatry and internal medicine, who needed no moral lessons to take reflective distance from their experience of the dogmatism of biomedicine (Schön 1983). On the contrary, they might have seemed a little too demanding of the social sciences and "criticism". Many *Medical Humanities* Master's programs (organized by philosophers or by social scientists) recruit even greater numbers in this public every day by paying attention to a form of *hybridity* since they are programs open to humanities students, who will never become doctors. Now, as explained before, one of the most represented medical specialties of medicine in these courses is psychiatry and this experience is very instructive for the development of a teaching strategy of medical anthropology in medicine.

Instead of repeating the usual complaints about this medical education, I want to describe how despite these organizational constraints, young students in medicine learn to take an anthropological distance from biomedicine, which will be particularly important during their clinical internship. In truth, this distance is already germinating for every medical student in the discovery of "somatoform disorders". Some students may consider this subject as a waste of time rather than an "interesting case" (i.e. a "Crock", Becker 1993) or a case for consultation-liaison psychiatry. The others are thus interested in Human Sciences (history, psychology or ethnography) because of this curious semiology.

In that situation, as a teacher and researcher in medical anthropology, I would like to explain two processes. First, how do psychiatrists, among other examples of physicians, become anthropologists and how are they integrated into my team as anthropologists. How is anthropological knowledge produced within this current of thought not oriented directly for clinical insight, but for a medical anthropology focusing on *moral criteria*, go beyond what is "bad" or "good", and understand *clinical judgment* in psychiatry and a local clinical authority (Mattingly 1998). The Physician-Anthropologist helps to study *moral economies of good care* and as a result the development of *better clinical insight*. This is a strategy that is worthy of interest both for a medical anthropology *and* psychiatry by making the two disciplines more attentive to the borders between the Clinic and Criticism (Chrisman and Maretzki 1982; Morgan 1990). The study of good care is therefore not only a concern for moral anthropology (Fassin and Lézé 2014), but also for psychiatry which wants to better understand the concrete, sometimes involuntary clinical consequences of "good" care that derives its value from a notion of an abstract "Good".

Two illustrative examples show the significance of the anthropologization of medicine, specifically psychiatry, after the medicalization of anthropology (Morgan

1990). These examples concern two child psychiatrists who are members of my "Dire la Santé Mentale" (DSM) team. Of course, this acronym is an ironic reference to the "American Bible of Psychiatry" (Diagnostic and Statistical Manual of Mental Disorders) with a new French content focusing on what is at stake in conflicts between clinicians in order to "Speaking mental Health" (Literally "Dire la Santé Mentale"). These two child psychiatrists are members because they are primarily anthropologists and not only child psychiatrists. It is up to them to defend the contribution of anthropological training in medicine, and their backgrounds help to better understand the scope of anthropology in psychiatry:

Our first colleague, Yannis Gansel, passed the medical examination in 1995 about 2 or 3 years ago after the introduction of the humanities in medicine. Within that context, he had to attend 10 h of lectures and read two books (Foucault's *The Birth of the Clinic*, and Canguilhem's *The Normal and Pathological*). He approached it like the other subjects, by "memorizing" without his classes providing him with any "reflexivity". His point of view is that training in the humanities at the beginning of the curriculum is of little interest. It should come later when students have experienced clinical work. It is also during his internship (i.e. Residency) that he experienced the biologization of training in psychiatry, where psychiatry teachers trained in psychoanalysis were retiring and those from the neurosciences were taking their places. From 1999 onward, before his clinical internship, he wanted to understand this war between different schools of thought where the "old guard" wanted him to "choose a camp". In 2004, he did a master's degree in the history of science and that's how he really became acquainted with the social sciences through readings, including my ethnography of French Psychoanalysts (Lézé 2010) and Tania Luhrman's ethnography of medical education for psychiatrists in the US (Luhrman 2000). His medical thesis was on the reception of the Diagnostic and Statistical Manual of Mental Disorders in France. Having become a hospital practitioner in child psychiatry, his practice puzzled him and he undertook a doctorate in medical anthropology with Richard Rechtman at the Ecole des Hautes Etudes en Sciences Sociales (EHESS) on the subject of "complex cases" in child psychiatry and the management of "difficult adolescents". To approach this issue, the epistemological history approach, combined with ethnography, shows the formation of a "concern for adolescents" as well as the clinical development of the concept of "containment" (Gansel and Lézé 2015; Gansel 2019). He joined the DSM team as a research associate in 2017.

Our second colleague, Mathias Winter, after following a classical humanities program, including coursework in philosophy and a master's in cognitive science at the Ecole Normale Supérieure de Lyon, turned to medicine because he felt that there was a "bridge" between this institution and the local medical school without going through the competitive examination of medicine. Indeed, entering my academic institution (ENS) involves an even more difficult competitive examination, which makes it possible to obtain the status of student-civil servants during 4 years. However, within the French epistemological tradition, medicine can be seen, according to Canguilhem's motto, as a "foreign matter" good to think anthropologically and offering practical and concrete problems. During his internship, Winter turned to psychiatry, in continuity with his training in French historical epistemology (Canguilhem, Foucault), and his master's degree in cognitive science. It was at the time of his medical thesis on autism that the question of a thesis in the humanities and a return to the ENS arose. The choice of medical anthropology (and its link to epistemology), provides a research perspective on clinical work in child psychiatry and an interesting approach for studying controversial conceptions of the "good" treatment of autism. Mathias's work is currently being carried out at the margin or in addition to participation in "classical" (biomedical) clinical research. He joined the DSM team as a PhD student in 2016.

Doctors becoming anthropologists is an old idea, at the very origin of medical anthropology. However, if we consider the exemplary careers of Arthur Kleinman in the US, Roland Littlewood in the UK, or Didier Fassin and Richard Rechtman in France, they remain exceptions in the medical world. Of these remarkable exceptions, it may be possible to make a rule for medical studies. What anthropology can bring to medicine is not a "moral guarantee" or morality to "humanize" an increasingly specialized and technical discipline, nor to valorize against medicine, the point of view of patients, which would be today more humane and skilled. Whether medical or not, medical anthropology can focus on clinical judgments to analyze the *moral components*, coming from the clinical situation or health policies. Anthropological knowledge may or may not be useful in clinical practice but, is medicine nothing but an anthropology? Is it an unfortunate anthropology, caught in a tension between physiology and psychology, between the singular and the general, between theory and practice?

Conclusion

Teaching Medical Humanities at the medical school is a social role much like the social roles we study as anthropologists. Thus, when the anthropologist takes on this role, he or she fulfills the function of *cultural intermediary* of a moral economy of the humanities composed of obligatory norms (e.g. "Critical thought"), of desirable values (e.g. "the Person"), and expected effects (e.g. "Empathy for suffering"). This role is the perfect protection to cling to as a missionary, among the savages who are obviously faithless and lawless. Nevertheless, did one become an anthropologist to teach the values of the humanities as a form of Moralism? Although I have clearly answered *no* to this question, it immediately raises two problems in the teaching of Social and Cultural anthropology in medical school.

First, is substituting irony for criticism a way of cynically escaping any form of morality by accessing a position "outside the game"? Montaigne would answer ironically that "on the highest throne in the world, we still sit only on our own bottom". Indeed, analyzing morality does not imply being able to evade it in the name of neutrality or impartiality. On one hand, neutrality is an epistemic norm founded in a moral value that can easily become merely an empty rhetorical norm, just like irony. On the other hand, the ethnography of morality in clinical settings is also a moral attitude starting from the "doubts" of the ethnographer (or the doctor) rather than "certainties". An epistemic norm (the obligation of "the description of obligations", desirability, emotions) *morally and logically* rejects a moral norm (the moralism of the obligation to adhere to the norms of humanism). Therefore, the ironist does not cultivate doubt for doubt's sake, he also doubts his doubt, because we have to decide *how and what to teach* (or to cure) in situations of uncertainty and the risk of being wrong. That's why when you are lost in the middle of the forest, it is rational to have a *temporary* certainty: let's go straight, we will eventually leave the forest!

Secondly, is favoring the "becoming anthropologist" of the doctors (whether psychiatrists or not) a work of moral conversion? Doctors do not become anthropologists when they learn a new moral discourse, whether it is critical or not, because he already has a solid "pragmatic idealism" (Becker et al. 1992) that can easily be enriched by the vocabulary and references of the humanities. According to my experience, doctors logically become an anthropologist when they want to analyze the unexpected anthropological problems they encounter at the very heart of clinical work and semiology. Like the anthropologist, they may have to endorse a *provisional morality* (to decide without being duped) in the face of the doubt they encounter situations of uncertainty. The main maxim of this provisional morality would be: "when the accumulation of clinical experience is not enough to reduce the gap between theory and practice, between knowledge and a case, the experience becomes ethnographic and the objectivation of what serves as a *guide to practice* (i.e. a moral economy) then becomes necessary".

The heart of the medical *art* is to decide in a situation of uncertainty. There are many ways to reduce the various forms of clinical uncertainty: by learning by heart biology or lessons of morality. But today's faith is a future fable. If it is easy to behave in good manners (or clinical guidelines) as a means of easing our consciences, it is much more difficult to act appropriately and make sure. Morality, thus implies an endless anthropological analysis that temporarily amplifies doubt, whereas decisions are to conclude based on certainty, just as temporary. In the end, medical anthropology radically transforms *the epistemic regime of this certainty*. This is not a moral certainty acquired by mere imitation, but a rational certainty that is the fruit of an objectivation and the subject of an active decision.

Acknowledgements This study was supported by "The Battle for the Science of Man" Research Program (BATTMAN) funded by the LabEx COMOD, Lyon University (2017–2020). I am very grateful to Iveris L. Martinez, Dennis Wiedman, Layla Roesler, Delphine Antoine-Mahut, and the two anonymous reviewers for their relevant and stimulating comments on the manuscript, English language editing, and proofreading. Thanks to Yannis Gansel and Mathias Winter for sharing with me their medical education experiences.

References

Azouvi, François. 1995. *Maine de Biran: La Science de l'Homme* [Maine de Biran: The Science of Man]. Paris: Vrin.

Becker, Howard S. 1993. How I learned what a crock was. *Journal of Contemporary Ethnography* 22 (1): 28–35.

Becker, Howard S., Blanche Geer, Everett C. Hughes, and Anselm L. Strauss. 1992. *Boys in white: Student culture in medical school*. New Brunswick: Transaction.

Bister, Milena D. 2018. The concept of chronicity in action: Everyday classification practices and the shaping of mental health care. *Sociology of Health and Illness* 40: 38–52.

Burnham, John. 2014. Why sociologists abandoned the sick role concept. *History of the Human Sciences* 27 (1): 70–87.

Chadalavada, Sucharitha, and Susan Bewley. 2011. Absorbing bad practice. *British Medical Journal* 342: d2503.

Chrisman, Noel J., and Thomas W. Maretzki, eds. 1982. *Clinically applied anthropology: Anthropologists in health science settings*. Boston: Reidel.

Csordas, Thomas, and Arthur Kleinman. 1990. The therapeutic process. In *Medical anthropology: Contemporary theory and method*, ed. T. Johnson and C. Sargent, 11–25. New York: Praeger.

Déplaude, Marc-Olivier. 2015. *La hantise du nombre: Une histoire des numerus clausus de médecine* [The obsession with numbers: A history of *numerus clausus* in medicine]. Paris: Les Belles Lettres.

Fassin, Didier, and Samuel Lézé, eds. 2014. *Moral anthropology. A critical reader*. London: Routledge.

Gansel, Yannis. 2019. *Vulnérables ou dangereux? Une anthropologie du souci des adolescents difficiles* [Vulnerable and dangerous? An anthropology of the care of difficult adolescents]. Lyon: ENS Editions.

Gansel, Yannis, and Samuel Lézé. 2015. Physical constraint as psychological holding: Mental-health treatment for difficult and violent adolescents in France. *Social Science & Medicine* 143: 329–335.

Godeau, Emmanuelle. 2007. *L'esprit de corps: sexe et mort dans la formation des internes en médecine* [Group spirit: sex and death in the formation of medical interns]. Paris: Les Editions de la Maison des Sciences de l'Homme.

Goldstein, Jan. 2005. *The post-revolutionary self. Politics and psyche in France, 1750–1850*. Cambridge: Harvard University Press.

Goubert, Jean-Pierre. 1987. "Introduction d'une approche de sciences sociales dans une faculté de médecine parisienne" [Introduction to a social science approach in a Parisian medical school]. In *Étiologie et perception de la maladie dans les sociétés modernes et traditionnelles* [Etiology and perception of illness in modern and traditional societies], ed. Anne Retel-Laurentin, 59–61. Paris: L'Harmattan.

Hannaway, Caroline, and Ann F. Laberge, eds. 1998. *Constructing Paris medicine*. Amsterdam: Rodopi Press.

Hemmings, Colin P. 2005. Rethinking medical anthropology: How anthropology is failing medicine. *Anthropology & Medicine* 12 (2): 91–103.

Lempp, Heidi, and Clive Seale. 2004. The hidden curriculum in undergraduate medical education: Qualitative study of medical students' perceptions of teaching. *British Medical Journal* 329 (7469): 770–773.

Lézé, Samuel. 2010. *L'autorité des psychanalystes* [The authority of psychoanalysts]. Paris: Puf.

———. 2013. Qu'est-ce que la psychiatrie aujourd'hui? [What is psychiatry today?]. *L'information psychiatrique* 89 (2): 115–119.

———. 2014. France. In *Cultural sociology of mental illness*, ed. Andrew Scull, 316–317. London: Sage.

Lézé, Samuel, and François Masure. 2007. Taquiner la raison. [Tormenting reason]. *L'Homme* 184 (4): 191–201.

Luhrmann, Tanya M. 2000. *Of two minds: The growing disorder in American psychiatry*. New York City: Alfred A. Knopf.
Mattei, Jean-François, Etienne, Jean-Claude, and Chabot, Jean-Michel. 1997. *De la médecine à la santé. Pour une Réforme des Etudes Médicales et la Création d'Universités de la Santé* [From medicine to health: for a reform of medical studies and the creation of health universities]. Paris: Flammarion.
Mattingly, Cheryl. 1998. In search of the good: Narrative reasoning in clinical practice. *Medical Anthropology Quarterly* 12 (3): 273–297.
McCullough, Laurence B. 2011. Was bioethics founded on historical and conceptual mistakes about medical paternalism? *Bioethics* 25 (2): 66–74.
Morgan, Lynn M. 1990. The medicalization of anthropology: A critical perspective on the critical-clinical debate. *Social Science & Medicine* 30 (9): 945–950.
Mouillie, Jean-Marc, Lefève Céline, and Visier Laurent, eds. 2011. *Médecine et sciences humaines. Manuel pour les études médicales* [Medicine and human sciences: manual for medical studies]. Paris: Les belles lettres.
Paris, Joel. 2005. *The fall of an icon: Psychoanalysis and academic psychiatry*. Toronto: University of Toronto Press.
Parsons, Talcott. 1951. *The social system*. New York: Free Press.
Pols, Jeannette, Brigitte Althoff, and Els Bransen. 2017. The limits of autonomy: Ideals in care for people with learning disabilities. *Medical Anthropology* 36 (8): 772–785.
Rice Patricia, C., and W. McCurdy David, eds. 2002. *Strategies in teaching anthropology*. Upper Saddle River: Prentice Hall.
Schön, Donald. 1983. *The reflective practitioner: How professionals think in action*. New York: Basic Books.
Tarot, Camille, ed. 1999. Les sciences humaines en médecine: la médecine dans les sciences humaines? [Human sciences in medicine: medicine in human sciences?] *Mana* 6.
Van den Hoonaard, Will C. 2011. *Seduction of ethics: Transforming the social sciences*. Toronto: University of Toronto Press.
Visier, Laurent. 2011. Vingt ans d'enseignement des sciences humaines et sociales dans les études médicales en France. [Twenty years of teaching human and social sciences in medical schools in France]. *Bioethica Forum* 4: 143–148.
Ware, Norma C., William S. Lachicotte, Suzanne R. Kirschner, Dharma E. Cortes, and Byron J. Good. 2000. Clinician experiences of managed mental health care: A rereading of the threat. *Medical Anthropology Quarterly* 14 (1): 3–27.
Wiedman, Dennis, and Iveris L. Martinez. 2017. Organizational culture theme theory and analysis of strategic planning for a new medical school. *Human Organization* 76 (3): 264–274.

Samuel Lézé, PhD taught the first-year introductory course in Humanities at Lyon Medical School between 2004 and 2006 as Assistant Lecturer. He received his Ph.D. in Social Anthropology from the School for Advanced Studies in Social Sciences (EHESS, Paris) in 2008. After completing a 2-year postdoctoral fellowship on a research program about moral anthropology with Didier Fassin at Institute for Interdisciplinary Research on Social Issues (IRIS), French National Centre for Scientific Research (CNRS, Paris), he was appointed Associate Professor at the École Normale Supérieure de Lyon in 2010. Between 2012 and 2016, he was a scientific expert at the Public Health National Committee in charge of the evaluation process (CSS9—National Institute for Health and Medical Research, INSERM). His research is particularly oriented towards clinical judgment formation in mental health care (from private practice to public institutions such as hospitals, prisons, trials, and education) since the nineteenth century. In 2015, he developed the DSM (Dire la Santé Mentale) team at Institute of History of Representations and Ideas in Modernities (IHRIM) to integrate psychiatrists and psychologists in Medical Anthropology and Humanities.

Chapter 4
Managing Uncertainty: Collaborative Clinical Case Conferences for Physicians and Anthropologists in Japan

Junko Iida and Hiroshi Nishigori

The State of Anthropology in Medical Education in Japan

In 2017, anthropology and sociology were first incorporated into the model core curriculum of Japanese medical education as "social sciences relevant to medicine". These subjects have been taught before at some medical schools in Japan, mostly as elective subjects, but now they have become compulsory components of medical education. Two factors helped lead to this change. The first factor is the change in disease structure in Japan: as a super-aging society, increasing numbers of people are suffering from chronic rather than acute diseases. As a result, physicians are involved less in curing diseases at hospitals and more in providing care in local communities, where they often face sociocultural problems.

The second factor is the current international interest in incorporating behavioral and social sciences in medical education. Japanese medical education has been strongly affected by medical education in the United States. The Educational Commission for Foreign Medical Graduates (ECFMG), the nonprofit organization that provides certification of the qualifications of international medical graduates before they enter U.S. graduate medical education, announced in 2010 that starting in 2023 physicians applying for ECFMG Certification will be required to graduate from a medical school that has been appropriately accredited through a formal process that uses criteria comparable to globally accepted criteria, such as those developed by the World Federation for Medical Education (WFME) (ECFMG 2018;

J. Iida (✉)
Comprehensive Education Center Faculty of Health and Welfare, Kawasaki University of Medical Welfare, Kurashiki, Japan
e-mail: iida@mw.kawasaki-m.ac.jp

H. Nishigori
Center for Medical Education, Graduate School of Medicine, Kyoto University, Kyoto, Japan
e-mail: hiroshi.nishigori@gmail.com

I. L. Martinez, D. W. Wiedman (eds.), *Anthropology in Medical Education*,
https://doi.org/10.1007/978-3-030-62277-0_4

WFME 2019). Following that announcement, the Japan Accreditation Council for Medical Education (JACME) was established in 2015 and it issued *Basic Medical Education: Japanese Specifications, WFME Global Standards for Quality Improvement*. All 82 Japanese medical schools nationwide are currently under evaluation to receive the "international accreditation of medical education" based on the "global standards" that incorporate the social sciences, including medical anthropology.

However, as very few Japanese people, including physicians, are familiar with anthropology, it is not easy to incorporate social sciences into medical education in an effective way. While the social sciences are seen to play an important role in medical education, barriers to their implementation remain in many countries (Benbassat et al. 2003; Isaac and Rief 2009; Litva and Peters 2008). Previous studies have pointed out that one of the main factors in the unsuccessful introduction of social sciences is the fact that medical students often fail to perceive the relevance of the social sciences for clinical practice. On the other hand, it is also suggested that social science education during the clinical clerkship period could promote an understanding that social sciences are clinically relevant (Benbassat et al. 2003). However, physicians who teach medical students during clinical clerkships or bedside-based clinical training in undergraduate medical education may have received little or no instruction in social sciences. Likewise, social scientists tend to lack experience in clinical medicine. To overcome these barriers, collaboration between social scientists and physicians is necessary (Litva and Peters 2008; Satterfield et al. 2010).

Being aware of the need for collaboration, the authors of this chapter, an anthropologist (Iida) and a general practitioner/medical educator (Nishigori), conducted various collaborative activities with other physicians and anthropologists. Among these activities, this chapter focuses on the Collaborative Clinical Case Conferences (CCCC) for physicians and anthropologists that was developed in process. In a CCCC, a medical student or a physician presents a case from clinical practice in which it was difficult to use biomedical knowledge to understand or deal with the issues it presented. Participants, including anthropologists, discuss the case, and one or more anthropologists comment on the case. While it is an examination of a case involving a patient's life and social relations rather than a "clinical case," after repeated discussion with the anthropologists and physicians who participated in CCCC, we have elected to use the term "clinical case conference," which is familiar to physicians, in order to express CCCCs' clinical relevance.

This chapter describes how anthropologists and physicians collaborated together to develop CCCC, the structure of these conferences, and how these conferences have been replicated by physicians, medical students, and anthropologists. Through this description, this chapter not only suggests a model of clinically relevant anthropology education for (future) physicians, but also explores the variability of anthropology (Ito 2016), examining what form of anthropology has been created in the practice of collaboration with physicians.[1]

---

[1]This chapter is a revised version of a Japanese paper (Iida and Nishigori 2019).

Confronting Uncertainty

Many physicians have a sense of uncertainty in their clinical practice. In Japanese, the word *moyamoya*, which also means "misty, foggy, and murky," is often used to express this sense of uncertainty. It includes an uncomfortable feeling in the absence of clear answers, due to a lack of conviction in the determination or decision one has made, or due to the inconsistency between one's logical judgment and emotion. The clinical process inevitably involves uncertainty for the physician because there is a gap between the probability-based judgments that biomedicine relies upon and the circumstances of an individual case (Montgomery 1991). Illness experience allows for various interpretations, judgments, and choices. Physicians in Japan increasingly have *moyamoya* today because of the aging society, the increase in chronic diseases, and the resulting shift to home care.

In clinical situations that require clear and quick assessment, however, an uncertain feeling is rarely verbalized because physicians are often negatively evaluated for having such feelings. Despite the fact that many physicians have uncertain feelings, they either keep it to themselves, stop thinking about it because there are no clear answers or solutions, or pretend not to notice it. While uncertainty is difficult to deal with in the context of biomedicine, it is accessible through anthropology, which explores uncertain and complex human behavior in everyday life. Our experiences with CCCCs demonstrates that anthropology can provide the viewpoints and frameworks that allow practitioners to verbalize their uncertain feelings and consider the issues in the social and cultural contexts in which they occur. CCCCs aim to help participants confront the feelings of uncertainty that they usually ignore, and discuss these feelings with other participants, including anthropologists, to realize the possibility and importance of viewing the phenomena from perspectives different from those in the health profession.

While our efforts share similarities with quite a few previous works, they are different from those works. Kathryn Montgomery, for instance, pointed out that the inevitability of uncertainty in medicine resulted in the use of cases that have a narrative structure, as the foundation of consideration, description, and education (Montgomery 1991). Although narrative-based approach, which is interpretive, is often applied in the analysis of the cases in CCCC, other anthropological concepts and perspectives are also introduced. While narrative (based) medicine (Greenhalgh and Hurwitz 1998; Charon 2006) and patient-centered medicine (Stewart et al. 2013) incorporated human and social sciences in general, especially in family medicine, CCCC is a collaborative activity between anthropology and all clinical departments. General practitioner, Cecil Helman's textbook on medical anthropology (2007) includes a variety of cases in clinical situations; however, the cases are introduced as examples of theoretical concepts. In contrast, CCCC starts with a case and anthropological concepts follow the case. On the one hand, the structure of CCCC is very similar to the "Case studies in social medicine" in the *New England Journal of Medicine*, although we noticed this fact after developing CCCC. On the other hand, this chapter also describes and examines exactly how CCCC was held and what kind of interactions and reactions occurred. While there have been practical reports on social science education for medical students through case conferences (e.g., Priel and Rabinowitz 1988), the aspect of how they (re)shape anthropology has not been examined sufficiently. Therefore, this chapter explores CCCC's impacts not only for physicians, but also for anthropologists.

Beginning Collaboration Between Physicians and Anthropologists

Over a decade ago, the authors of this chapter never expected to be involved in each other's discipline to the extent that they are today. After meeting at the University of Oxford in 2006, the accumulation of dialogue and exchange between them resulted in a variety of collaborative activities in research and education. That process, which is described below, can be regarded for Iida as a shift from the "anthropology *of* medicine" to "anthropology *with* medicine/medical education" (Ingold 2018).

Nishigori first became interested in anthropology, which he knew nothing about before visiting the UK, while mingling with doctoral students in anthropology at Oxford. After returning to Japan, the continued dialogue between the authors inspired research on physical examinations and the doctor-patient relationship (Iida 2013; Iida and Nishigori 2016). This represented Iida's first experience in conducting fieldwork in the realm of general and family medicine at medical institutions (including a university hospital, a community hospital, and a clinic) in Japan, thanks to Nishigori's introduction. Although Iida experienced a series of culture shocks during this research, it was a valuable experience that transformed her previous image of the world of medicine and physicians. While general and family physicians were extremely busy from early morning until late at night with enormous amounts of work, they were struggling with problems including issues in patients' daily lives and social relations that biomedicine could not solve. When we told them about anthropology and our research topic, a number of physicians expressed their interest. Some physicians said they had wanted to study anthropology in college, while others said that they did not understand the importance of the humanities and social sciences when they were students. Some physicians who knew that anthropology is regarded as one of the "ologies" of primary health care (Greenhalgh 2007) and that anthropological concepts were included in family medicine in North America (McWhinney and Freeman 2009; Stewart et al. 2013) were studying anthropology on their own. There was even a study group reading Arthur Kleinman's books.

Through the process described above, we became convinced of the affinity between primary care and anthropology, as well as the possibility of our collaboration in medical education. Initially, following Nishigori's interest, we collaboratively held workshops on qualitative research for physicians to identify physicians' interests in qualitative research. Second, to educate medical students and physicians, not only in the methodology, but also in the perspectives and ideas of anthropology, we developed CCCC workshops at a medical school and at the annual conference of the Japan Primary Care Association (JPCA), which garnered a much better reaction than expected. Ethnography and CCCCs then became key for incorporating anthropology education into medical school, although we did not initially expect these results.

Accordingly, Iida did not intend to work in medical education at first, but gradually found herself involved in medical education through the process of responding to collaborators' questions and requests and through discussions with collaborators and research participants in the field. Through their presence, these "strangers," physicians and anthropologists, demanded a "response" and "correspondence" from each other (Ingold 2018: 26–27).

The Structure of a Collaborative Clinical Case Conference

CCCCs were devised through dialogue between the authors. They have been undertaken by many physicians and anthropologists and have been repeatedly evaluated and improved. We have conducted CCCC as part of a study titled "The development of a collaborative clinical case conference by health professionals and social scientists as a method of incorporating behavioral and social sciences into medical education" after passing the ethical review at Kyoto University. Japanese medical schools use a 6-year European model of undergraduate education. Their programs include 4 years of preclinical studies and 2 years of clinical clerkship rotations in various clinical departments. From 2015 to 2018, we conducted seven CCCCs for medical students who were in the second half of the process of clinical clerkship at three medical schools. During the same period, we held seven CCCCs for physicians as part of the annual JPCA meeting and its related events and three CCCCs at other institutions, including a family medicine clinic and a university hospital. About 170 students and 310 physicians in total have participated in CCCCs, while 28 physicians and 19 anthropologists have participated in them as staff members (facilitators and lecturers). While we have held CCCC mainly for medical students and physicians thus far, sometimes other health professionals such as pharmacists and nurses also participate. A CCCC takes place in a classroom when held at a medical school, in a seminar room at a JPCA conference, and a meeting room at a clinic or a hospital. The structure of a CCCC is as follows.

Selection of a Case

Before each CCCC, a medical student or physician chooses one or several cases that are difficult to address through biomedical knowledge and sends them to anthropologists. If several cases are proposed, anthropologists choose a case to discuss, consulting with physician staff. In the process of repeated discussions among anthropologists who have participated in CCCCs, it has been recommended to generally choose cases following the criteria below.

First, a case that can be linked to anthropological discussion should be chosen. For example, cases that could be productively analyzed using anthropological (and sociological) concepts and ideas such as narratives, contexts, social roles, and gift exchange can be shortlisted. While physicians often propose cases that can be discussed in interprofessional conferences which are usually held only among health professionals such as nurses, pharmacists, physiotherapists and social workers, we attempt to choose those cases that could benefit from anthropological perspectives in their analysis.

Second, a case in which the anthropological discussion based on the case would be easy for beginners to understand should be chosen. Even though a case can be linked to anthropological concepts, the case should not be chosen if the discussion will be too difficult for those who have little knowledge of the humanities and social sciences.

Third, a case that might offer useful ideas and perspectives for future medical practice should be chosen. If possible, it is better to avoid highly unusual cases and to choose a common case similar to those that many physicians might experience.

Fourth, a case that is of interest to participants, including both (future) physicians and anthropologists, should be chosen. It is ideal to choose a case in which students and physicians will see their own problems reflected, and as a result, the case will provoke active discussion.

Although the following criteria are not indispensable, the fifth criterion is that cases should ideally involve background knowledge that the presenter is likely to have. As described later, anthropologists ask the presenter to add information about the social and cultural aspects of the case. Therefore, it is better to choose a case whose context the presenter would be familiar with.

Finally, we did not choose cases that fit the "stereotype" of anthropology. Anthropology is often connected with cases of patients from abroad and psychiatric cases, and it may work well in analyzing these kinds of topics. However, now that familiarity with anthropology is very low among physicians in Japan, we avoided these stereotypical cases as we were afraid of leading to misunderstanding on the part of beginners that the scope of anthropology is limited to these specific areas. In fact, we found that anthropology can be applicable for analyzing many other kinds of cases in medical practices.

Therefore, the case selection process is a very important phase in searching for the common ground between anthropology and clinical problems. Thus, anthropologists examine which cases they can use to encourage particular kinds of engagement by physicians. They consider which materials will make for good anthropological "dishes," giving physicians a taste of what it means to be "anthropological" and letting them experience how they might "cook" these dishes themselves in their own practices.

Enrichment of the Sociocultural Aspect of the Case

Next, a student or physician prepares the presentation of the case and sends the provisional slides to anthropologists via email. Although the slides they make for CCCC include a more detailed description of the social background of the patient compared to clinical conferences held only among doctors where diagnosis and treatment were discussed, the initial presentation tends to have insufficient information about the sociocultural aspects of the cases to sufficiently deepen the discussion. Therefore, anthropologists ask the presenter via email to add more context about the patient's social relations and life history to their presentation slides before the CCCC, (re)collecting data from the patient, family, other professionals, and clinical records if necessary. The presenter revises the slides and sends them to anthropologists again. Interestingly, students and physicians can generally comply with anthropologists' requests to some extent. All student presenters have been able to contribute additional information, even though students have little clinical experience and they cannot go back to the clinical field of the cases to collect data during their clinical clerkship rotations. Although medical students and physicians have information about sociocultural aspects, they tend to overlook its importance and do not initially include it in their slides.

If a presenter can add slides containing additional information to the original version of the presentation before CCCC, it is possible to conduct small group discussions in a two-step process at the CCCC. In that case, the first step follows the original version of presentation, in which participants are asked to think what else they should know when considering the problem, and after the presentation of additional information, participants deepen the discussion in the second step. This process enables medical students and physicians to experience the shift or expansion of their viewpoints towards the social and cultural aspects of a case. However, if a presenter cannot add much information, or if the time for the CCCC is short, we simply ask the presenter to revise the original slides to add information.

A medical student or physician also presents a question at the end of the case presentation. It addresses the aspect about which the presenter feels uncertain or *moyamoya*, which is also the point examined in small group discussions in a CCCC. Staff members (both anthropologists and physicians) should help the presenter in this process, because it can be difficult, especially for beginners, to form such a question. The question should be as simple as possible, because an overly complicated question is difficult to discuss at a conference, and while it needs to be based on the case presented, it also needs to present an opportunity for anthropological analysis. For example, "Why did this patient do (or not do) this?" "What should we (physicians) do in this case?" are some of the typical questions at CCCCs.

In the correspondence between anthropologists and (future) physicians before a CCCC, a clinical case is revised according to anthropological perspectives to essentially become a sociocultural case. Physicians are limited in their ability to collect data on the social and cultural aspects of a case. However, quite a few physicians said that anthropologists' requests made them reexamine clinical records or collect additional information from patients, family members, and other professionals, resulting in the shift of their viewpoints to realize what they did not notice beforehand. Junichiro Miyachi, a family physician who has collaborated with us to hold CCCCs, points out that "the phase of data collection based on anthropologists' requests is an opportunity for physicians to learn the basics of social scientific exploration of phenomena, experiencing the ethnography process in a highly compressed timeframe under the guidance of anthropologists."

On the Day of a CCCC

At each CCCC, after a short introductory lecture on anthropology and a case presentation, participants, including anthropologists, discuss the questions raised in the presentation in small groups. In a group discussion, anthropologists play the role of facilitators. Next, a representative from each group shares what they discussed with other groups. If additional information is presented, further small group discussions follow. Finally, comments on the case are given by anthropologists, and a further question-and-answer session is provided. We have conducted trials of between 1.5 and 4 h for each case. A conference length of 1.5 h is too short for experienced physicians, while medical students can hardly continue discussion beyond that. Based on our experiences of trial and error, we think that the appropriate length of a CCCC is about 1.5 h for students and 3 h for physicians.

In a CCCC for primary care physicians in particular, anthropologists are often surprised by the active discussions. Physicians' lack of information to answer the question makes them consider various possibilities. For example, in a CCCC for physicians, a family physician presented a case of a 75-year-old man who had suffered from chronic obstructive pulmonary disease (COPD) for 10 years who began living in a nursing home due to the progression of respiratory insufficiency. This patient snarled at staff when he had difficulty breathing during excretion, even saying that he wanted to die, while he insisted on excreting by himself. At the end of the case presentation, the family physician asked, "Why was this patient obsessed with excreting by himself despite his condition?" In the discussion, there were various comments and questions including the following:

- Did the members of his team of caregivers share their interpretations of his excretion with each other?
- The weakening of his physical function might have transformed his feeling of "death as recognition" into "death as body." That experience might have made him equate having his bodily needs attended to with death, linking his fear of death with his attacks against staff.
- He might have past experiences related to his obsession about excretion, including his childhood experiences as well as his friend's or relative's experience of providing caregiving.

- To receive assistance from others with his bowel functions could be regarded as an experience of "loss." If that is true, it is necessary to know his past experience of loss and his interpretation of it.

Through discussions like this, participants gradually realize that the possibility of the patient's narratives and behaviors have meanings in the context of his/her life story and social relations, including those with physicians.

Anthropologists' comments presented at the end of the CCCC are not the answers to the question or solutions to the problem, but the introduction of ideas that might be useful in the consideration of the problem or questions that shift physicians' viewpoints. As they do not actually observe the case but simply examine the case presented from a physician's point of view, anthropologists have limited information on which to base their comments. In providing perspectives and ideas that physicians would not recognize on their own, however, anthropologists try to help medical students or physicians learn or notice something new. Physician staff members asked anthropologists to use the simplest language possible, making it easy for beginners to understand, while showing references to demonstrate that the comments are based on academic evidence. As a result of following this suggestion, anthropologists noticed quite a few participants saying they learned that there is an academic discipline that provides suggestions for considering various matters that might have concerned them, although they had never discussed these issues thoroughly. Some participants even purchased the books referenced by the anthropologists while listening to their lectures.

If two anthropologists can provide comments, they can expose participants to a variety of viewpoints. In our experience, three commentators is too many according to the feedback from participants and staff. Medical students and physicians tend to think that there is only one correct answer, while many problems have several correct answers in the medical field. The variety of comments in group discussions as well as anthropologists' lectures enable (future) physicians to recognize the possibility of various perspectives. In the CCCC described above, for instance, first, our anthropologist colleague Yosuke Shimazono introduced the idea of the experience of illness as the transformation of life as well as the idea of excrement as something that threatens the boundary of the body, proposing a hypothesis that the patient was obsessed with excretion because dependence on others for controlling excretion symbolizes heteronomy. Next, another anthropologist, Akinori Hamada, pointed out that how people attend to the patient affects what kind of existence he "becomes"—e.g., the patient thinks that through physiotherapy he can maintain autonomous self, while nursing care intervention transforms the self into "that which is supported"—concluding that it is the way of living rather than death that is more important for the patient.

On the other hand, the presentation of different perspectives might confuse participants and exacerbate uncertain feelings. It is thus important to find the common ground between contradicting comments as the take home message. In the case above, for example, both Shimazono and Hamada focus on the transformation of self, although from different perspectives, it suggests the importance of exploring not in a universal medical framework, but in the context of the patient's social relations and life story. The process of finding the common ground between anthropologists' contradicting comments would also provide anthropologists an opportunity to consider what is the essence of anthropology that should be conveyed to (future) physicians.

Cases and Comments

Tables 4.1 and 4.2 show the 28 cases examined in CCCCs thus far and anthropologists' comments on them. While various cases have been examined, some common characteristics can be found.

First, many cases examined by both students and physicians concerned the difficulties in understanding a patient's or family's narratives and behaviors that deviated from biomedical judgment or common sense (S4, S5, S10, D3, D4, D5, D6, D7, D10, D11, D12, D13). Many anthropologists' comments on them suggested the possibility that apparently irrational narratives and behaviors have meanings in the context of patients' lives and social relations.

Second, the cases chosen by students included four cases regarding the difficulties of taking care of patients who were unlikely to be cured (S6, S9, S12, S13). In their comments on them, anthropologists pointed out that there should be different approaches to care depending on each patient's social context, and they sometimes introduced anthropological ideas about care.

Third, students' cases also included the ones concerned with their feeling of disorientation when faced with the possibility of various options and values (S1, S2, S14). Anthropologists' comments on them again referred to contextual factors, as well as to the necessity of viewing the knowledge of physicians and patients relatively, as students tend to see patients as having insufficient knowledge for decision making. The second and third categories can be seen as reflecting the puzzlement of students who have just encountered issues in clinical settings that they cannot fully address using their medical knowledge from textbooks.

No practicing physicians focused on this kind of puzzlement, though some of them presented questions about the extent of medical interventions and of physicians' roles (D2, D9). Both of these cases were presented by family physicians, reflecting on their close relationship with the patient's family and life to consider the appropriateness of medicalization as well as the extent to which a physician should get involved. In the CCCCs that examined these cases, some anthropologists introduced the idea of gift exchange as a way to explore the physician-patient relationship, while others pointed out the significance of providing care according to the phenomenological situation of the patient.

Anthropologists' comments transform participants' perceptions of the cases or introduce ideas from outside of the medical field that might lead to new understandings or hypotheses by (future) physicians. Anthropologists' questions that examine issues that physicians have taken for granted have particular impacts. For instance,

Table 4.1 Cases examined and anthropologists' comments (for students)

	Dates	University	Case summary (questions)	Anthropologists' comments
S1	Jan. 8, 2015	A	The reason why the reactions to illnesses such as cancer and AIDS differ depending on country and person	Different perceptions of illness and death among diverse social, cultural, political, and economic contexts
S2			End-of-life decision making when a physician, patient, and the patient's family have different opinions	The importance of collaborative decision making, rather than divided decision making (i.e. informed consent), based on the difference of quality, not quantity, of knowledge between physician and patient
S3			Decision making about a dementia patient who has no family	Social relationships with people other than family
S4	Oct. 30, 2015	A	A pregnant woman with uterine cancer who wants to give birth to her child	The idea of narratives and their social and cultural contexts
S5			An autistic child who often enters an expressway to see cars	Dominant story, alternative story
S6			Conversation with a cancer patient in the ward	Physician-patient relationship, transformation of conversation frame
S7	July 1, 2016	B	Conversion of a patient's word "tottering" into a biomedical term	Word meaning, connotation, illness narratives
S8			The gap between video-reviewed objective evaluation and self-evaluation	Observation exercise, physical examination and physician-patient relationship
S9	Oct. 27, 2016	A	The appropriateness of IC for a patient with metastatic tumors of multiple organs and her satisfaction with her care	The idea of narratives and their social and cultural contexts
S10			An autistic person who often calls for an ambulance	(no time for comments on this case)
S11	Oct. 17, 2017	A	To what extent is a medical student a professional?	Legitimate peripheral participation
S12			The appropriateness of the care for a terminal lung cancer patient who wanted to go home but died in a hospital without sufficient pain control	Logic of choice and logic of care
S13	July 28, 2018	C	How to take care of a stroke patient after an operation for the prevention of cerebral aneurysm who makes negative comments	Disease and illness, explanatory models, illness as the shrinking of lifeworlds, and the care for this condition

(continued)

Table 4.1 (continued)

	Dates	University	Case summary (questions)	Anthropologists' comments
S14	Oct. 16, 2018	A	Decision making based not on rational and scientific judgment but on the emotions and feelings of patients and family	Knowledge in clinical practice differing from scientific knowledge
S15			How illness affected the patient, family, and her partner's life	Illness experience as a story with no conclusions yet drawn

while the physician who presented the D3 case on a patient who expressed a positive reaction to a stoma focused only on the patient's reaction, anthropologist Yosuke Shimazono asked, "Why did the doctor feel this reaction was awkward?" Yusuke Hama, who commented on the D7 case of the woman who rejected medical interventions but complained of mental and physical symptoms after her husband developed dementia, asked, "What is the woman trying to protect?" Although they seem like simple questions, they impacted physicians to the extent that one of the participants said he was "struck by lightning."

Comments and discussions in CCCCs are not limited to the discipline of medical anthropology but are often based on cultural anthropology. They are not necessarily based on up-to-date anthropological discussions, but on basic or classic ones. To situate phenomena in social and cultural contexts, for example, is a basic practice for anthropologists. For many physicians who have never been trained to do so, however, anthropological viewpoints and concepts are fresh, and some of them said that they felt "relieved" to learn about them. In repeatedly staging CCCCs, anthropologists realized the significance of situating phenomena in sociocultural contexts for physicians.

Reaching a National Audience: CCCCs at the Japanese Primary Care Association (JPCA) Annual Meeting

We have improved the content and structure of CCCCs based on the comments from the feedback sheets that participants submitted after almost every CCCC. This feedback can be regarded as part of the correspondence between anthropologists and (future) physicians involved in "shaping the anthropology we do." The following is a summary of the feedback from the participants in the CCCCs related to JPCA (Pre-congress workshops of the annual meetings, workshops in Continuing Professional Development Autumn Seminar and the Annual Forum of the Osaka Branch) held for seven times involving approximately 230 participants. (Feedback for other events will be described later.)

First, we asked what participants expected from CCCC. The most frequent answer was that they thought they could learn something useful for their clinical practice. For example, a physician who works at a hospital wrote, "As I often experience cases that are difficult to deal with from a strictly biomedical point of

Table 4.2 Cases examined and anthropologists' comments (for physicians)

	Dates	Event	Case summary (questions)	Anthropologists' comments
D1	Jun. 12, 2015	JPCA pre-congress workshop (WS)	End-of-life care for a Buddhist monk: Was it affected by his expected role?	Conflict between social role and individual life, different perceptions of death over time, anthropological studies on death in Japan, the process of dying
D2			The appropriateness of medical intervention for a family in which everyone has a disability or disease	Similarity of the case description to ethnography, recovery of patients' agency
D3	Nov. 8, 2015	JPCA Continuing Professional Development Autumn Seminar	A patient who expressed a positive reaction to a stoma	Life history, gap between discourse and behavior, asymmetric relationship between physician and patient, boundary of the body and pollution
D4			A family devoted to religious activity while neglecting an elderly family member	Cultural competence, new religion, secularism, power of sisterhood, gap between family ideology and reality
D5	Feb. 10, 2016	Family medicine conference	A house with too many accumulated things	Relationship between the family and local community, relation between family history and the house
D6			A woman who complains of mental and physical symptoms after her husband developed dementia, while rejecting medical interventions	Relationship among family members, systematic perspectives
D7	June 10, 2016	JPCA pre-congress WS	Deadlocked physician-patient relationship (the aftermath of the case above)	Family history and social relationship (from the role of mother to the role of wife), what the patient protects
D8	Nov. 6, 2016	JPCA Autumn Seminar	An outpatient with SLE who came to a university hospital to ask for a second opinion	The logic of patients and logic of physicians (department), narratives searching for a story of illness
D9	May 12, 2017	JPCA pre-congress WS	Care by a physician for a patient with progressing disease	Gift exchange and physician-patient relationship, illness as an experience of "I no longer can" physically and socially and the care to create a new "I can"

(continued)

Table 4.2 (continued)

	Dates	Event	Case summary (questions)	Anthropologists' comments
D10	July 22, 2017	The 65th Seminars & Workshops on Medical Education	Conflict between a COPD patient's respiratory discomfort and the respect for his will to excrete by himself	The transformation of the self through excretion care, the impacts on a patient's life accorded by treatment choices
D11	Nov. 12, 2017	JPCA Autumn Seminar	A pharmacist who insisted that a steroid worsened her mother's condition and wanted to use a supplement with no biomedical effect	Coexistence of knowledge about plural options of treatment for an individual, "subjunctivizing" elements in illness narratives
D12	Jan. 27, 2018	JPCA 4th annual forum of Osaka branch	A patient who refrains from taking drugs linking various symptoms with side effects as well as from dialysis to avoid becoming a family's burden	Relational autonomy, local biologies, patient's perception of the personal (=social) body being threatened by the use of blood transfusion, dialysis, and drugs
D13	Feb. 24, 2018	Seminar for junior residents	A patient with diabetic nephropathy who stopped taking the previous doctor's drugs according to his own decision and gave many gifts to a junior resident	Difference of adherence from intelligence, gift exchange

view, I wanted some clues to help me think outside the box or improve the situation somewhat." Other participants, especially those engaged in community medicine, also expressed similar expectations for tips to solve the problems that they encounter in daily clinical practices.

The second question was about what they were satisfied with in the CCCC. Many positively commented on their first encounter with anthropology, appreciating the new perspectives they learned. At the same time, some of them reflected on their practice, wondering if their treatments are really appropriate for patients. Many participants commented positively on the discussion about non-biomedical issues or about their *moyamoya*, which they do not usually have the opportunity to discuss deeply. Comments such as "The CCCC provided me with many frameworks for verbalizing my practices that I usually take for granted" suggest that they felt anthropological frameworks are useful. Some mentioned that the communication with people from different disciplines was fruitful, while others wrote that they liked the structure of CCCC.

As a point that needs improvement, many participants, especially those who took part in a 90-min CCCC, wrote that the time allotted for the CCCC was too short. We also received some suggestions that it would be better to further assess and exclude the possibility of organic diseases before discussing the social aspects of the cases. We therefore decided to ask participants for biomedical questions after the case presentation so that they could concentrate on social aspects later. In addition, some suggested that anthropologists should speak more in group discussions. This seems to reflect the difficulty some (especially younger) anthropologists had in stopping (older) physicians from talking, although the basic role of the facilitators was to adjust the course of discussion when it became too focused on the biomedical aspect of the case. Quite a few participants requested handouts, particularly references. However, those who were not used to anthropologists' descriptive presentation style complained of "too many letters per slide." Some participants also commented that they did not understand anthropology itself, which was a limitation of these case-based sessions. While initially the introductory lecture on anthropology was given at the end of CCCCs, we decided to do it at the beginning, following the participants' feedback as well as the experience that the discussion tended to focus on biomedical aspects. Furthermore, although most participants understood that the purpose of CCCC was not to eliminate their uncertain feelings, there was a comment that "those who search for the 'answer' might be frustrated."

When asked what they learned at the CCCC, many participants wrote about the concepts and key words they first encountered, such as "physician's logic and patient's logic (in their lifeworld)," "plot of a story," "plural hypothesis," and "gift exchange." Many participants referred to the affinity between family medicine and anthropology, which is natural because anthropological ideas such as "disease and illness" as well as "explanatory models" are incorporated in the "patient-centered clinical method" of family medicine. On one hand, there is a positive aspect in family physicians recognizing this affinity; on the other hand, it is possible that this affinity makes them use frameworks that they already know, including "care and cure," and lose their interest in learning anthropology. There were also comments that fundamentally question the scope of medicine and the role of a physician. From these comments, we could learn that there is a tacit rule in the medical field that physicians should not concern themselves with non-biomedical matters, and that some physicians are not satisfied with that rule. We could also learn about physicians' suffering in the medical world that evaluates nonintervention negatively.

Only a few participants expressed suspicions of the anthropological approach, writing that they felt it subjective and without scientific evidence. Many requested similar conferences on various cases in diverse fields of medicine. While there is room for improvement, it is thus possible to conclude that CCCCs for primary care physicians generally meet participants' expectations.

Staff's Reflections

After almost every CCCC, we had a staff reflection meeting and we recorded our discussions. The following presents relevant reflections of the staff who participated in the JPCA-related workshops.

Physician Staff's Reflections

Physicians who presented cases learn various things not only in the process of preparation but also from the discussions and anthropologists' comments at CCCCs. A family physician, for example, said that she was "saved" by the CCCC because she found a way to "keep an eye on" a patient and her family rather than trying to "solve" what she thought was a "problem," understanding that there was a context for their behavior that was difficult to understand. Another family physician pointed out that while a conventional case conference usually exclusively focuses on the patient, CCCC deals with the culture surrounding the patient as a whole, including the role of physicians.

On the other hand, Nishigori, an author of this chapter and an internist, noticed an aspect of CCCC that is similar to a case conference of internal medicine where diagnosis and treatment are discussed. While anthropologists and other participants ask a presenter various questions in CCCC, the presenter cannot reply to all of the questions, thus realizing that he/she should seek information on other aspects of the case to examine the problem. Similar realizations happen between a presenter and his/her instructors in a diagnostic inference case conference. It would be possible to see that CCCC is an opportunity for training for physicians in acquiring anthropological perspectives in a structure similar to that of diagnostic inference training. A family physician pointed out that physicians need not only knowledge but also training to incorporate anthropological approaches in family medicine, and CCCC can be an opportunity to provide that training.

Nishigori also suggested that CCCC could be applied in other specialties, including rheumatology, endocrinology, gynecology, and pediatrics. He pointed out that patients with health problems in these specialties also surely have socio-cultural problems to be discussed with anthropologists.

Anthropologists' Reflections

We have organized CCCCs while trying to recruit one or two new staff members if the schedule allows. Every anthropologist who first participated in a JPCA-related CCCC has expressed their surprise at participants' enthusiasm and active discussions. Comments on the affinity and possibility of collaboration between anthropology and primary care are also often heard.

We also discuss anthropologists' comments and lectures. As described earlier, one case usually includes several points to discuss, making various comments on diverse aspects possible. Anthropologists' different comments are thus interesting for other anthropologists as well. The same is true for the "introductory lecture on anthropology." Answering the question, "What is anthropology?" for those who know nothing about anthropology in only about 10 min, in a manner that will properly direct the discussion without providing an "answer" to the discussion question and in front of other anthropologists, is not easy. Different anthropologists have given diverse introductory lectures thus far, such as a lecture focusing on methodology, theory, and the differences from other disciplines. Listening to another anthropologist's lecture and examining the lecture with other staff members, including physicians, is also an opportunity for anthropologists to learn from each other.

Further Expanding the Impacts

When anthropology was incorporated into the model core curriculum of Japanese medical education in 2017, we believed that CCCCs described above could be a model for providing anthropological education for medical students relevant to clinical practice. Our experience, however, was limited to the field of primary care and to medical schools whose teaching staff had a strong interest in anthropology. It is therefore our task to examine if this method is effective for anthropology education for all students at all medical schools in Japan and for physicians in other departments. The following describes one of our trials in this regard.

Trials at C Medical School

After the revision of the model core curriculum, Iida was asked by C Medical School, where she had taught medical anthropology as a "liberal arts" elective for first-year students from 2009 to 2017, to teach it as a required subject. Based on her experiences thus far, she proposed a class related to clinical clerkships. Similar to many other medical schools in Japan, at C Medical School, students start learning clinical medicine by clinical clerkships in the last term of the fourth year to round every department until the first term of the sixth year. As a result, it was determined that she would teach an 8-h class on medical anthropology (basic course) for first-year students and a 9-h class on medical anthropology (advanced course) for fifth-year students.

Consulting with Nishigori, Iida next sought a collaborator at the medical school. Nishigori and Iida knew from past experience that there might be faculty members who were interested in the social sciences in the community medicine department, which was related to primary care. She thus asked the medical school to introduce some faculty members in the community medicine department, and she met two physicians from the department of general practice. The two faculty members expressed interest in her proposal to conduct CCCC in the class for fifth-year students and agreed to cooperate with her.

The two medical school faculty members also proposed to hold a CCCC for junior residents before the class and agreed to select a case presenter as well as physician facilitators. In Japan, after passing the National Examination for Medical Practitioners, graduates from medical schools must participate in a residency for

5 years. We decided to hold a CCCC as a seminar for junior residents in the first 2 years of their residency at C Medical School Hospital. Participants at this CCCC, however, reacted differently from those at the CCCCs we had before. Discussions in some groups were not active. While some participants were listening to the anthropologists' lectures with attention, others were not. One of the factors that might have led to the negative reactions was that this seminar was obligatory for all junior residents, while participation was voluntary in the CCCCs we had before. Another factor was that it seemed to be difficult for participants to understand how anthropology is useful, as it does not directly contribute to problem solving; it seemed the junior residents with little clinical experience were interested in clinical techniques that they could implement immediately. However, the most critical factor was that we did not sufficiently provide for physician facilitators' understanding. It was not enough that only half an hour was spent on explaining the tasks required to first-time facilitators just before the CCCC. In the meeting after the CCCC, quite a few facilitators criticized that "no answer" to the question was shown in the CCCC. We recognized that we should have let facilitators know beforehand as part of their faculty development that the purpose of a CCCC was not to solve the problem (that causes uncertain feelings). We feel it is necessary to set clearer goals for CCCC when training facilitators in the future.

Based on this experience, Iida and one of her collaborators at C Medical School, asked some of the junior residents and former graduate students, who participated in the CCCC, to become facilitators for fifth-year students. Beforehand, Iida and her collaborators carefully explained to the facilitators what the CCCC entailed. The CCCC was held on the last day of the class. A case was selected from the cases involving the uncertainty (*moyamoya*) felt during clinical clerkship and which were reported by all the students on the first day of the class. On the day of the CCCC, 98 students were divided into 20 groups and each facilitator participated in two groups. As a result of the careful preparation, discussions were relatively smooth and active. However, the second discussion based on the presentation with additional information was not active in some groups, as the case presenter, a medical student, could only add little information. The question for the group discussion, "If you are the doctor in charge of this patient, what would you do?" was overly vague.

For first-year students, who had no clinical experience, Iida decided to give lectures after presenting (fictitious) cases and having students discuss them, to help participants experience the class as clinically relevant. She used manuscripts of a textbook on anthropology and sociology for physicians and medical students that was in the process of being co authored by physicians and anthropologists and being edited by Iida and Nishigori (2021). The manuscript/textbook is a product of an Inter-University Research Project "A collaborative project on medical anthropology education for health professionals" at the National Museum of Ethnology. Every chapter of the textbook follows the same structure as a CCCC (i.e., case presentation, questions, additional information, questions, and anthropological commentary). The cases include those examined in the past CCCCs, those experienced and reported by physicians, and those written by anthropologists and edited by specialists in the related field of medicine. In the class, when distributing worksheets about the first case presentation and question, Iida asked students to discuss the question as well as what other information they should consider. Next, after handing out worksheets providing additional information and questions and asking them to further discuss, she gave them a lecture introducing anthropological perspectives that could be applied in examining the case. Students' reactions were better than she expected. Many students actively participated in the discussion. On the feedback sheets, 19 out of 136 students commented that they liked the class because it was based on case studies. Fifteen students wrote that the class was good because they could learn about the viewpoints of disciplines other than medicine. Ten students wrote negative comments, including "not interesting." Students were evaluated through a multiple-choice test and essay writing. Some students claimed the evaluation criteria of essay writing were unclear and subjective, although the evaluation criteria were based on a rubric and was explained. More exploration and improvement of evaluation methods are necessary.

The Variability of Anthropology

A collaborative clinical case conference held jointly by physicians and anthropologists is, as described above, an opportunity for anthropologists and (future) physicians to consider and discuss social and cultural problems that (future) physicians feel uncertain in clinical situations and learn from each other. It was created through a collaboration between physicians and anthropologists and has been improved through its repeated staging for primary care physicians and medical students. In CCCCs, anthropology has provided frameworks for situating phenomena in socio-cultural contexts and for verbalizing social and cultural phenomena. CCCCs have been highly appreciated, especially by primary care physicians. The important point is that case-based approaches begin not from anthropological concepts but from clinical situations, bridging the gap between medical discipline and anthropology.

Of course there are some limitations of CCCC. Only a few hours of CCCC may not be enough for (future) physicians to acquire anthropological perspectives. Information gathered and presented by physicians might not be enough either for the analysis of social and cultural aspects, which may thus only be a suggestion of possibilities. As mentioned above, more examination of evaluation methods for medical students, as well as more collaborations between anthropologists and physicians in various clinical fields, are also necessary.

CCCCs are not only opportunities for anthropologists to make comments and analyze cases or educate medical students and physicians, but also an opportunity for anthropologists to learn. Anthropologists who participate in CCCCs, inevitably consider how anthropology can contribute to medicine and health professions while they consider what it is like to be "anthropological" in the process of dialogue with (future) physicians.

The most important value of CCCCs might be, however, the fact that physicians and anthropologists share a time and space to discuss the same problems. They learn from each other's attitudes and *how* they speak in addition to, or even more than, *what* they say. When we started holding CCCCs, the first thing that physicians pointed out about anthropologists was that anthropologists' comments often have "preliminaries" and "excuses." These devices are necessary for anthropologists to relativize what they are going to say: for example, saying, "Although there are several other perspectives..." in acknowledgement of other anthropologists' different opinions. In contrast, an anthropologist described the way physicians go straight to the point as "they put it into high gear from the beginning." While some of the students and physicians who first heard anthropologists' way of speaking expressed their irritation, many reacted warmly. Those who had many experiences of collaboration with anthropologists pointed out their understanding that this discursive style was related to the anthropological approach. On the other hand, anthropologists learned that they (sometimes) need to neglect small points and speak directly when they talk to physicians. CCCCs were also an opportunity for staff as well as for participants to realize their own habits that they are usually unaware of through dialogue with people in a different field. This realization emerges not from a textbook but from the lived experience of sharing time and space with one another.

Anthropology can be regarded as "a practice of education" (Ingold 2018: 62–63). As Jackson describes, a field transforms an anthropologist; of his field, Sierra Leone, he writes "[Sierra Leone] transformed me, shaping the person I now am and the anthropology I do" (Jackson 2012: 28). CCCCs play a role in shaping the anthropology "done" by the anthropologists who participate in them.

While it is already suggested in other fields (Ito 2016), it is possible that the field of anthropologists' activity will also transform or be expanded. In this aging society, where health professionals face an increasing number of sociocultural problems surrounding the people for whom they provide care to, someday we might be able to see many anthropologists working in the field of health and medicine. As Ingold observed (Ingold 2018: 65), anthropology's engagement with medicine/medical education is a never-ending process of growth and discovery for both anthropologists and physicians.

Conclusion

This chapter demonstrated that CCCC is effective as an opportunity for (future) physicians to know that anthropological knowledge and perspectives are useful in clinical situations. They provide an opportunity, not only for teaching anthropology to (future) physicians but also for anthropologists to learn from the practice to create a new form of anthropology. It is suggested that CCCCs could provide both health professionals and anthropologists with a model for collaborating with each other in clinical as well as educational contexts.

Acknowledgements We thank all the people who participated in the collaborative clinical case conferences. This work was supported by a Grant-in-Aid for Scientific Research (18H00782).

References

Benbassat, Jochanan, Reuben Baumal, Jeffrey Borkan, and Rosalie Ber. 2003. Overcoming barriers to teaching the behavioral and social sciences to medical students. *Academic Medicine* 78 (4): 372–380.

Charon, Rita. 2006. *Narrative medicine: Honoring the stories of illness*. New York: Oxford University Press.

Educational Commission for Foreign Medical Graduates (ECFMG). 2018. *Medical school accreditation requirement for ECFMG certification*. https://www.ecfmg.org/about/initiatives-accreditation-requirement.html. Accessed 28 Jan 2019.

Greenhalgh, Trisha. 2007. *Primary health care: Theory and practice*. London: Blackwell.

Greenhalgh, Trisha, and Brian Hurwitz. 1998. *Narrative based medicine: Dialogue and discourse in clinical practice*. London: BMJ Books.

Helman, Cecil G. 2007. *Culture, health and illness*. London: CRC Press.

Iida, Junko. 2013. Physical examination as the "laying on of hands": The doctor-patient relationship in general and family medicine. *Japanese Journal of. Cultural Anthropology* 77 (4): 523–543. (in Japanese).

Iida, Junko, and Hiroshi Nishigori. 2016. Physical examination and the physician-patient relationship: A literature review. *MedEdPublish* 5 (3): 14. https://doi.org/10.15694/mep.2016.000100.

———. 2019. Exploring social and cultural problems in clinical situations together: Collaborative clinical case conference by health professionals and anthropologists. *Contact Zone* 11: 392–425. (in Japanese).

———, eds. 2021. *Anthropology and sociology for physicians and medical students: Learning through clinical cases*. Kyoto: Nakanishiya. (in Japanese).

Ingold, Tim. 2018. *Anthropology and/as education*. London: Routledge.

Isaac, Mohan, and Winfried Rief. 2009. Role of behavioural and social sciences in medical education. *Current Opinion in Psychiatry* 22 (2): 184–187.

Ito, Yasunobu. 2016. "Ethnography" in Japanese corporate activities: A meta-anthropological observation on the relationship between anthropology and the outside. In *Enterprise as an instrument of civilization: An anthropological approach to business administration*, ed. Hirochika Nakamaki, Koichiro Hioki, Izumi Mitsui, and Yoshiyuki Takeuchi, 55–72. Tokyo: Springer.

Jackson, Michael. 2012. *Lifeworlds: Essays in existential anthropology*. Chicago: University of Chicago Press.

Litva, Andrea, and Sarah Peters. 2008. Exploring barriers to teaching behavioural and social sciences in medical education. *Medical Education* 42 (3): 309–314.

McWhinney, Ian R., and Thomas Freeman. 2009. *Textbook of family medicine*. 3rd ed. New York: Oxford University Press.

Montgomery, Kathryn. 1991. *Doctor's stories: The narrative structure of medical knowledge*. Princeton: Princeton University Press.

Priel, Beatrice, and Betty Rabinowitz. 1988. Teaching social sciences in the clinical years through psychosocial conferences. *Journal of Medical Education* 63 (7): 555–558.

Satterfield, Jason M., Shelley R. Adler, Carrie H. Chen, Karen E. Hauer, George W. Saba, and Rene Salazar. 2010. Creating an ideal social and behavioural sciences curriculum for medical students. *Medical Education* 44 (12): 1194–1202.

Stewart, Moira, Judith B. Brown, Wayne Weston, Ian R. McWhinney, Carol L. McWilliam, and Thomas R. Freeman. 2013. *Patient-centered medicine: Transforming the clinical method*. 3rd ed. Boca Raton: CRC Press.

World Federation for Medical Education (WFME). 2019. *ECFMG 2023 announcement*. https://wfme.org/accreditation/ecfmg-2023/. Accessed 28 Jan 2019.

Junko Iida, PhD is Professor of Anthropology at the Faculty of Health and Welfare, Kawasaki University of Medical Welfare, Japan. She also teaches at Kawasaki Medical School. She was a visiting research fellow at the Institute of Social and Cultural Anthropology, University of Oxford, in 2006–2007. Her research interests has been in Thai traditional medicine, local healing practices in northern Thailand, physical examination and doctor-patient relationship, palliative care in Japan, as well as anthropology education for (future) health professionals. She is a member of the Behavioral and Social Sciences Committee of the Japan Society for Medical Education, as well as the Collaborative Committee on Anthropology Education for Health Professionals of the Japanese Society of Cultural Anthropology. Recent publications include the following: "The sensory experience of Thai massage: commercialization, globalization, and tactility", in Kalekin-Fishman, D., Low, K.E.Y. (eds.) Everyday Life in Asia—Social Perspectives on the Senses, pp. 139–156. Ashgate (2010); "Holism as a whole-body treatment: the transnational production of Thai massage." European Journal of Transnational Studies 5(1), 81–111 (2013); "Tying the hand: life sustaining technique in northern Thailand." Asiatische Studien 71(1), 305–326 (2017).

Hiroshi Nishigori, MD is the Professor at the Center for Medical Education, Nagoya University and a Visiting Project Leader Professor, Medical Education Center, Graduate School of Medicine, Kyoto University, Japan. He is a general internist who graduated from Nagoya University School of Medicine in 1998. He is a Fellow of the Japanese Society of Internal Medicine, certified in 2004, and a Diplomate in Primary Care of the Japan Primary Care Association, certified in 2011. He obtained a Master's degree in medical education from the University of Dundee in 2008, a PhD degree in general medicine from Nagoya University Graduate School of Medicine in 2008, and a PhD degree in health professions education from Maastricht University in 2020. He was a visiting research fellow at the University of Oxford in 2005–2006. His specialty is medical education as a social science, and his research interests include medical professionalism (especially altruism and work ethics), hypothesis-driven physical examination (HDPE), and behavioral and social sciences (especially cultural anthropology) in medical education. He is working as an editor of the Journal of Medical Education (Japan), is a member of the Behavioral and Social Science Committee under the Japan Society for Medical Education, a core member of the APME-Net (Asian Pacific Medical Education Network), and an Ambassador of the AMEE (Association of Medical Education in Europe) in Japan. His recent publications include a paper on doctors intrinsic motivation to work for patients.

Chapter 5
How Medical Students in the United Kingdom Think: About Anthropology, for Example

Lisa Dikomitis

Introduction

The title of this chapter has been modelled on Marshal Sahlins's well-known book *How Natives Think: About Captain Cook, For Example* (1995)—itself modelled on the French philosopher-cum-anthropologist Levy-Bruhl's book *How Natives Think* (2018). My 'natives' however are not Sahlins's Hawaiians, and what concerns me about their thinking is not a person, but an academic discipline. I am concerned with how medical students think about anthropology. There is a long tradition of social scientists studying medical students. The classics include *The Student-Physician* (Merton et al. 1957), *Boys in White* (Becker et al. 1961), and *Making Doctors* (Sinclair 1997). The majority of these studies focussed on the student culture in medical schools: how do medical students experience their training and what are their socialisation patterns? There are two other related, but distinct, bodies of social scientific research on medical education. Firstly, social scientists turned their attention to the *medical curriculum* itself (e.g., Atkinson 1984; Brosnan 2009; Forrest 2017; Good and Good 1993; Hafferty 1998; Taylor 2003) and secondly, to literature on cultural competence curricula within medical education (Betancourt 2006; Fox 2005; Seeleman et al. 2009).

When I moved from a social science department to a medical school in the United Kingdom, I started teaching anthropology to medical students. They showed great enthusiasm, but simultaneously expressed concern and unease with the material and 'the way anthropologists think', as one student put it. Their worry revolved mainly around the usefulness and applicability of this learning content to their future clinical practice. Students found it interesting, but questioned if it was really necessary to devote precious study time to anthropology. Although, in a certain sense, it is more

L. Dikomitis (✉)
School of Medicine, Keele University, Keele, UK
e-mail: l.a.dikomitis@keele.ac.uk

I. L. Martinez, D. W. Wiedman (eds.), *Anthropology in Medical Education*,
https://doi.org/10.1007/978-3-030-62277-0_5

challenging to teach medical students (as I need to 'explain' and 'defend' anthropology) in comparison to teaching social science students, I loved it so much that I subsequently chose to further develop my academic career in medicine and took up a permanent appointment in a medical school. These observations and experiences were the main impetus for a long-term ethnographic study to: (1) obtain views from medical students about the social scientific learning content, with a special focus on anthropology; (2) examine the challenges, barriers and opportunities in bringing approaches and insights from anthropology into the medical classroom; and (3) make suggestions as to how anthropology can be better integrated into mainstream medical education.

In this chapter, I examine the social science component in UK medical education. In doing so, I specifically explore the perceptions, beliefs, understandings and attitudes medical students hold on anthropological learning content that they receive during their years at medical school. I also include an autoethnographic perspective on my experiences of working as an anthropologist in medical education. I use qualitative data from that study—ethnographic vignettes, quotes from interview transcripts, excerpts from my field diary and students' written accounts—to explore how anthropologists might have a continued and sustained engagement in medical education.

First, I will briefly trace the inclusion of anthropology in medical education in the UK. This is followed by details on how I conducted ethnographic fieldwork in two UK medical schools. From there, I present my findings addressing the study objectives and include suggestions on how anthropological knowledge can be more robustly incorporated in a medical curriculum. My main contention in this chapter is that although the social sciences are officially a core component of medical education, social science knowledge is often still considered peripheral learning content by medical students as well as by clinical and bioscience educators. This, in turn, reinforces misunderstandings and misconceptions held by medical students, biomedical scientists and clinical educators around disciplinary boundaries within the social sciences and the contributions anthropology makes to medical education.

The Place of the 'Alley Cats' in Medical Education in the UK

Although it is only since 1993 that the UK's General Medical Council (GMC) firmly stipulated that a social science component should be core in the undergraduate medical curriculum, the debate about its inclusion has been long going. While earlier engagements have existed as early as the turn of the twentieth century (see Chap. 2), anthropologist Ashley Montagu made a notable recommendation to include his own discipline, social anthropology, as part of standard medical education. Montagu (1963: 579) was convinced that exposure to anthropological ideas would make for 'better doctors':

> Anthropology is the science which asks: What is man? How did he get to be the way he is now in all his remarkable variety? Anthropology, therefore, can supply some of the answers to these questions, and distilling them for the medical student, can offer him an approach to the theories, techniques, and practice of medicine which will make him a far better doctor than he could ever otherwise be.

Montagu (1963: 579) goes on to describe the anthropologist's approach to observe and reflect and that clinicians, just like anthropologists, should 'hang a question mark on the things we take most for granted'. He ended with the proclamation that medical schools should 'make the anthropologist part of the medical environment' (Montagu 1963: 583). Almost 20 years later, a 1980 editorial in the *British Medical Journal*, entitled '*More anthropology and less sleep for medical students*', reflects on such a possible place of anthropology in medical education (BMJ 1980: 1162). The unnamed author divides the subjects in the medical curriculum into two distinct categories: the 'alley cats' (psychology, sociology, epidemiology, statistics, anthropology, communication studies, etc.) and the 'lions and tigers' (surgery, anatomy and physiology). The author lists some reasons why medical students should be exposed to anthropological thinking and ethnographies, noting that many medical schools resist the less traditional disciplines. The rationale is that there is no time to teach about values and attitudes because the curriculum is already overloaded with "facts", with 'great battles fought' over which subjects should be included. The author concludes with the suggestion that medical students could perhaps read more novels (with Dickens, Steinbeck and Dostoevsky as examples) in order to have an understanding of how others see the world! As I will explain below, this is echoed in my own study findings: medical students and medical educators recognise the value of anthropology, but if there is no time to do it properly (and there rarely is), there are "ways around" studying it, in comparison to the biomedical science that cannot be learned, in students' opinions, at one's leisure. The debate on the overloaded medical curriculum has been ongoing (Kadambari et al. 2018; Morrison 2015; Weatherall 2011). Although beyond the scope of this chapter, an investigation as to what extent this overload (GMC 1993) affects the robust inclusion of anthropology medical education deserves further attention.

Anno 2019 it is still unusual to find (medical) anthropology as a stand-alone *core* subject in a UK undergraduate medical curriculum, but considerable progress has been made and many of the 'alley cats' as identified above are now fully incorporated in medical curricula. These 'alley cats' are often grouped together under one umbrella-term with widely used acronyms 'SBS' (Social and Behavioural Sciences) or 'BSS' (Behavioural and Social Sciences). Let us first have a closer look at how these are now integrated in UK medical education.

In the UK, the GMC sets the knowledge, skills and behaviours that medical students learn at UK medical schools: these are the outcomes that new UK graduates must be able to demonstrate. These standards were first laid down in *Tomorrow's Doctors* (1993), its flagship document. In 1993, the GMC included the social and behavioural sciences as core and vital areas of medical education. In the most recent version, renamed to *Outcomes for Graduates* (GMC 2018), there continues to be an

Newly qualified doctors must be able to apply social science principles, methods and knowledge to medical practice and integrate these into patient care. They must be able to:
a recognise how society influences and determines the behaviour of individuals and groups and apply this to the care of patients
b review the sociological concepts of health, illness and disease and apply these to the care of patients
c apply theoretical frameworks of sociology to explain the varied responses of individuals, groups and societies to disease
d recognise sociological factors that contribute to illness, the course of the disease and the success of treatment and apply these to the care of patients – including issues relating to health inequalities and the social determinants of health, the links between occupation and health, and the effects of poverty and affluence
e explain the sociological aspects of behavioural change and treatment concordance and compliance, and apply these models to the care of patients as part of person-centred decision making.

Fig. 5.1 'Outcomes 3—Professional knowledge' (GMC 2018: 22)

explicit commitment required from UK medical schools to integrate social sciences in their undergraduate curricula (Fig. 5.1).

(a) recognise how society influences and determines the behaviour of individuals and groups and apply this to the care of patients
(b) review the sociological concepts of health, illness and disease and apply these to the care of patients
(c) apply theoretical frameworks of sociology to explain the varied responses of individuals, groups and societies to disease
(d) recognise sociological factors that contribute to illness, the course of the disease and the success of treatment and apply these to the care of patients—including issues relating to health inequalities and the social

(continued)

determinants of health, the links between occupation and health, and the effects of poverty and affluence
(e) explain the sociological aspects of behavioural change and treatment concordance and compliance, and apply these models to the care of patients as part of person-centred decision making.

As the socio-cultural aspects of health and the biopsychosocial approach have become ever more prominent in UK medical education, the role of anthropology in educating the future clinical workforce should equally become more pronounced in medical education. But is this really the case? Although the inclusion of social science is now standardised in medical education, the position and status of social science as applied to medicine still varies greatly between different medical schools in the UK. There are vast differences in contents, teaching methods, assessment, and scope (Benbassat et al. 2003; Russell et al. 2002, 2004; Satterfield et al. 2010; Forrest 2017). Indeed, researchers have identified a number of themes that need further investigation, including medical students' perceptions (Gallagher et al. 2015; Thompson et al. 2010), students' attitudes with regards to social and behavioural science (Beagan 2003; de Visser 2009), teachers' and stakeholders' perceptions (Dogra 2007; Peeraer et al. 2011) and the institutional culture of medical education (Taylor 2003). With my research, I aim to contribute to our understanding of how medical students and educators perceive anthropology and how we can more robustly integrate anthropological insights in medical education.

Ethnographic Research in Two UK Medical Schools

My study consisted of two fieldwork streams: (1) ethnographic fieldwork at the North England Medical School (NEMS)—a pseudonym (2014–2016) and (2) autoethnographic research at Keele's School of Medicine, where I have been teaching medical students since 2016.

Context and Field Sites

It is important to provide some context around the training provided at the two medical schools where I conducted fieldwork, as the schools' pedagogical approach hugely influences how much exposure medical students have to anthropology. In general, there are a number of approaches to medical education in the UK, but the main distinction is between the 'traditional courses' and the 'integrated' or 'systems-based' courses'. A traditional medical course typically consists of two 'pre-clinical' years where students are taught in separate discipline-specific modules (such as physiology, anatomy, etc.) followed by three 'clinical years'. The integrated courses are the GMC's recommended approach to medicine where students take a bodily system (e.g., the circulatory system) and consider disciplinary knowledge in an integrated fashion. Regardless of whether the medical school offers a traditional or a system-based course, the social science learning content is usually frontloaded in the first 2 years of undergraduate medical education in UK medical schools. Students on integrated courses often have early patient contact and are expected to do a lot of self-directed learning. One popular learning and teaching style of integrated courses is Problem-Based Learning (PBL). PBL is a philosophical approach that underpins many medical curricula, characterized by a focus on structured learning through a problem, rather than on disciplinary knowledge acquisition in isolation (Maudsley 1999; Boud and Feletti 2013). PBL, as a practical teaching method, consists of small-group work, backed by individual study, around PBL cases which are always clinically realistic scenarios. A PBL group, guided by an experienced medical educator (the facilitator) and a student chair and scribe, 'opens' the PBL case with a first structured session in which knowledge gaps are identified and learning objectives for that week are set. In a second session, the PBL group 'closes' the case: students explain to each other and to the facilitator what they learned. During the week students attend lectures, clinical placements, lab and skills sessions focused on topics associated with that week's PBL topic. The set of learning objectives usually includes one or more social science objectives, as I will illustrate below.

The medical schools where I conducted fieldwork are relatively young medical schools, both were established less than 20 years ago, and offer a 5-year integrated PBL-based medical course. Both schools are of a similar size with an annual intake of 150–200 medical students, including students for whom medicine is their first university degree as well as graduate students. The pedagogical model of both schools was similar: an integrated course with a blended learning approach that combines PBL, lectures, workshops, practical classes and student-selected components (SSCs). These are optional modules in the undergraduate medical curriculum that were introduced on the GMC's recommendation in 2002 in order to increase student's choice (Richardson 2009). Both medical schools offered early clinical experience, students had placements in primary and secondary care from the very beginning of their medical education. In practical terms this means that the medical students I observed worked in the same small 'PBL group' of about 8–12 students every week throughout the academic year. Each group is assigned a PBL-facilitator (also called PBL-tutor): at NEMS these were all experienced primary or secondary care clinicians, while at Keele PBL-tutors were a mix of clinicians, teaching and research faculty. This is an important distinction as Keele medical students might have additional engagement with anthropology if their PBL tutor was a social scientist. Most PBL tutors, in both schools, were actively involved in training of medical students, beyond their role in PBL. Many were permanent staff members who delivered a substantial number of lectures in the first 2 years of the curriculum. At the time of fieldwork, NEMS had one sociologist and one psychologist as permanent staff member while Keele's School of Medicine had an entire Behavioural and Social Science team of four staff members as part of the larger

'Medical Science' team that delivered the learning content in the first 2 years of the course. The social science content is taught in the first instance via the facilitated discussions on the social context of the virtual patient cases in the PBL sessions. The medical sociologist (NEMS) and the two anthropologists (Keele) deliver a set of plenary lectures in the first two years of the course on social science topics. These are known, among students and staff, as 'sociology' lectures, although some lectures rely almost entirely on anthropological work. Examples of lecture titles where insights from anthropology are covered, include 'Cultures of biomedicine', 'Social inequalities in health', 'The doctor-patient relationship' and 'Critical perspectives of lifestyle and health'. In addition, students could engage with anthropology via the SSCs, which are taught by those social scientists as well as other researchers.

Ethnographic Fieldwork at NEMS

Atkinson powerfully demonstrates in '*For Ethnography*' that fieldwork does not have a single method for collecting or analysing data. Instead it "refers to a collection of possible methods, used singly or in combination. At its heart, however, is some form of participation in the everyday life of the social world under investigation." (Atkinson 2015: 25) My fieldwork at NEMS was indeed composed of several data collection methods: participant-observation, semi-structured interviews and focus groups with medical students, collecting student reflections on anthropology teaching and keeping a field diary. At the start of my fieldwork I was employed at NEMS where I taught two SSCs: 'Health Inequalities' and 'Introduction to Medical Anthropology'. I taught a total of 63 NEMS students, whom I got to know very well as teaching took place in small groups (ranging from 6 to 19 students) with intensive interactive sessions that lasted between 1.5 to 3 h. Mid-way through the first data-collection phase I took up a position at the social science department at the same university but continued my fieldwork at NEMS.

Participant-observation took place inside the classroom during teaching sessions and during informal contacts outside the classroom. I observed students during PBL sessions, on placements, I attended skills labs, clinical, social science and biomedical lectures, OSCE exams and mock OSLER exams. Ethnographers researching educational settings have long argued that it is paramount to look *beyond* the activities in the classroom (see, for instance, Becker et al. 1968; Dikomitis and Kelly 2018; Tuchman 2009; Willis 1978). Accordingly, my participant-observation did not finish when the teaching ended. There were many occasions when I met NEMS students outside the scheduled teaching sessions. Some of the students kept in touch and would come and see me during office hours, some joined me at local conferences and got involved in extracurricular activities (e.g., debate evenings and fundraising events) to which they would invite me to. There were three students who considered seriously studying anthropology as an intercalated degree and we had a series of meetings around that. One student intercalated after her second year to study Global Health and another student enrolled in a master's degree in Infectious Diseases

- When did you feel **most engaged** in the session? Why?
- At what point did you feel **most distanced** from what was happening? Why?
- What action/activity that anyone (teacher or student) took during the session did you find **most affirming or helpful**? Why?
- What action that anyone took did you find **most puzzling, confusing or most surprising**? This could be about your own reactions to what went on, something that someone did, or anything else that occurred. Please explain.
- What information/insight/discussion will help you **most effectively in your daily activities as a doctor**? Why?

Fig. 5.2 The CIQ I used after teaching sessions, adapted from Brookfield (1995)

undertaking ethnographic fieldwork for his dissertation. Several NEMS students enthusiastically cultivated an 'ethnographic imagination' (Willis 2000) and would email me with stories of incidents and encounters during their clinical placements. After I left NEMS, we started meeting regularly as a group and these students became my key informants. In addition to these regular catch-ups, we would call, email and text in which the conversation would inevitably turn to anthropology and its position in medical education. One evening, for instance, we heavily debated cultural relativism in connection to the first female genital mutilation prosecution in the UK. At the time of writing this chapter, these NEMS students had completed 2 years of working as junior doctors in the UK's National Health Service (NHS) and embarked on different clinical careers, four students have become good friends and still take a professional interest in medical anthropology.

One of my study's objectives was to suggest changes to practice. In that sense, I was keen to collect individual feedback on anthropology teaching sessions, especially about those in which I tried new interventions. I adapted the Critical Incident Questionnaire (CIQ), developed by Stephen Brookfield (1995). Each CIQ had the session title and date in the header and contained the same five questions. Medical students were asked to complete the CIQ at the end of the session before they left the classroom. They would typically write two-three lines per question. I collected a total of 184 CIQs at NEMS (Fig. 5.2).

- When did you feel *most engaged* in the session? Why?
- At what point did you feel *most distanced* from what was happening? Why?
- What action/activity that anyone (teacher or student) took during the session did you find *most affirming or helpful*? Why?

(continued)

- What action that anyone took did you find *most puzzling, confusing or most surprising*? This could be about your own reactions to what went on, something that someone did, or anything else that occurred. Please explain.
- What information/insight/discussion will help you *most effectively in your daily activities as a doctor*? Why?

I have used these CIQs as a way to be informed about my students' learning and engagement with the session content and about the (non-)impact of my teaching strategies: what works and what does not work? For the purpose of this study I wanted to identify 'critical incidents' during my teaching. These are not dramatic or unusual episodes in the classroom, but common, everyday events that 'are rendered critical through analysis' (Tripp 1993: 24–25). I also asked one cohort of 19 students who took the 'Medical Anthropology' SSC to write a reflective text at the beginning (about the reasons they chose to study medicine) and at the end of the 2-week intensive module (about their perceptions of anthropology in medical education). Some students have also sent me (unsolicited) lengthy emails during and after the module. With the students' explicit permission, I have also added these anonymised writings to my data set. The NEMS students really became critical partners in exploring the research questions I set out to answer. It was in that light that the 11 students who had taken the Health Inequalities SSC proposed themselves that we should hold a focus group in the last session. I agreed but left the choice for students to drop out and not attend the session if they felt they did not want to contribute. They all participated. The session was recorded and later ad verbatim transcribed.

The second phase in the ethnographic fieldwork at NEMS was an interview study. This was important, as I wanted to triangulate findings from my participant-observation and wanted to explore the views and perceptions of NEMS students whom I had not met. I contacted 34 students who had indicated they would be interested to participate in the interview study and 12 students I had not taught whose contact details were provided by the medical sociologist at NEMS. Students were approached via a personalised email with the study information and consent form. A total of 11 students agreed to take part in the study: 6 students I taught and 5 students I did not know. Of these, 7 were female and 4 were male. Students' ages varied between 19 and 26 with a mean age of 22 years. Single, face-to-face semi-structured interviews were conducted in the winter of 2014. The average length of the interviews was 46 min. All interviews took place in my University office, often during the weekend when medical students were available. The themes I explored in the interviews were derived from my ongoing analysis of the ethnographic data. The topic guide was comprised of the following broad headings: (1) student background and profile; (2) views on medical students and other students; (3) views on medical education; (4) Teaching (PBL, lectures, and SSCs) and assessment; (4) social sciences in the medical curriculum.

Autoethnography at Keele's School of Medicine

That first intensive fieldwork phase came to a close at NEMS when I took up a senior position at the School of Medicine at Keele University. In addition to conducting anthropological research, I lead the Behavioural and Social Science (BSS) team and I teach medical students social science and qualitative research methods lectures, am a PBL-tutor and teach SSCs around medical anthropology and global health. I also lead staff development sessions in Keele's School of Medicine and deliver training on how to incorporate social science learning content in PBL-sessions in other UK medical schools.

In order to further my own understanding of how social science is integrated in medical education and to develop and improve my own teaching I continued to engage with this research project when I joined Keele's School of Medicine. I kept a field diary in which I jotted, on a regular basis, short scenes I observed in the classroom and the staffroom, my own reflections on encounters with students and colleagues, and suggestions of what I could do differently. Such autoethnographic engagement allowed me to reflect on my educational practice, and how my teaching was perceived by students and colleagues (Farrell et al. 2015). Ellis and Bochner (2000: 739) describe autoethnography as a genre of writing that 'displays multiple layers of consciousness connecting the personal to the cultural'. One important objective was to reflect on my own disciplinary position—a social anthropologist teaching medical students—but also on how different social sciences relate to each other in medical education.

Ethics

This ethnographic study was low-risk and the main ethical challenges revolved around the power relationships in doing ethnography while protecting and safeguarding the participants' privacy. These are concerns of all ethnographic studies, but conducting ethnographic fieldwork in an educational institution where the ethnographer is an 'insider' might bring with it specific ethical and political consequences (see, for instance, Nathan 2005; Tuchman 2009). I was a member of staff in the medical schools where I conducted the research. This included participant observation in my own classes at NEMS, where I was, as the educator, in a position of power and authority over my students. Students were also reassured that their (non) participation in my study would have no influence on their marks. At NEMS I taught two optional SSC modules, groups ranging from 6 to 19 students. I taught each SSC several times. Students did not receive a mark for their SSC assignments, these became part of their undergraduate coursework portfolio. I was not involved, at NEMS, in marking any exam papers, nor did I have any knowledge about the academic performance of the students in my SSC modules, unless students explicitly told me.

During my auto-ethnographic fieldwork at Keele, I was a PBL tutor to a group of 12 students and taught a range of sociology and research methods lectures to groups of 140 students. A PBL tutor does not provide marks to the students in their PBL group. All exam questions are first marked and second marked by two different staff members. Exams are anonymous in that students write a number on the cover sheet and not their names. Although I was in no position to (consciously or unconsciously) influence students' grade, I ensured that students taking part in my study were aware of this and reassured them at regular intervals throughout the study.

All NEMS medical students were provided with detailed information about my research at the beginning of each SSC module I taught. I introduced the concepts of 'ethnographic fieldwork' and 'participant-observation' and showed the students my field diary and illustrated with examples what type of notes I might jot down during and after teaching sessions. The students were given assurance that their real names would not be used and that any identifying factors would be changed or eliminated in the research outputs. Verbal informed consent was acquired at the start of each module and was obtained regularly throughout the teaching. Additional consent was sought when I wanted to use students' anonymous written material, such as email communications, written session feedback and short essays produced for the medical anthropology module. The students who participated in the focus group and the interviews received written study information and provided informed, written consent prior to the focus group or interview. Research participants chose their own pseudonyms, which I also use in this chapter, so they can recognize themselves in the research outputs. The ethnographic study at NEMS gained formal ethical approval from the Research Ethics Committees at the University's Department of Education and the School of Social Sciences. The study was not funded externally, I obtained a small budget for transcription costs from internal university funding.

The Invisibility of Anthropology

The first key theme I identified after analysis revolves around understanding of disciplinary knowledge and how conversant medical students are with regard to anthropology and the discipline's contributions to medical education.

Institutional Slang

There was absolute consensus among all stakeholders—medical students, educators and clinicians—that their medical school was putting a lot of emphasis on the social side of medicine:

> I think the social stuff is themed across the year, I think. It is a big part [of the curriculum], especially for this medical school, because I have friends at other medical schools and they do not have anywhere near as much emphasis on social stuff. (Focus group participant)

That 'social stuff' was officially named 'Theme X' (a pseudonym) at NEMS which brought together all the health, social and population sciences learning content. Students would rarely refer to 'Theme X' and would commonly use the term 'fluffy stuff'. My data reveals that students get to know and use this specific term very early on in the course. Some pick it up from a fellow student, as was the case with Ashak: '*The first time I've heard 'fluffy stuff' was from a second year [student] during Fresher's week, when we just started going out and just talking about the courses and things.*' Others learned the term from their PBL tutor. A focus group participant explained: '*Our own lecturer even says it as well*'. Another participant added: '*Our PBL tutor was like "Oh, we've got quite a lot of fluffy stuff this week"*'. The term was mostly used in a negative manner, indicating a lower level of importance and relevance in comparison to other core material. But what exactly is the 'fluffy stuff'? Here is how Charlotte explained it:

> Fluffy stuff: the aspect of medicine that is repetitive and easily understood using common sense. For instance, a patient has been diagnosed with cancer—how does that make them feel? Obviously awful. Or what are the social effects on an elderly lady who has broken her hip and is now not as mobile as she was before? She is not as independent at home so she may need help doing things she used to do, which might make her depressed and even embarrass her or she may even need to go into a home and lose all independence etc. These are very easy to understand, obvious and often self-explanatory topics.

At Keele, students referred to exactly the same learning content with the shorthand 'the psychosocial' or, less often, 'BSS' which in itself is a reference to the 'BSS staff team'. When I met other UK medical educators in the United Kingdom, at conferences or when I delivered training, it became clear that school-specific lingo for the social sciences is widely used. Examples included: 'the non-science', 'the fluf', 'wishy-washy', 'the soft science', 'the waffley' or 'the wooly' stuff. The 'fluffy stuff', according to NEMS students, includes learning content from anthropology, medical humanities, sociology, psychology, professionalism, ethics and public health. In UK medical schools, such learning content is often grouped together under school-specific umbrella terms ('fluffy' or 'psychosocial'), very similar to the umbrella term 'alley cat subjects' used in the 1980 editorial (BMJ 1980). Institutional slang is one of the areas through which a hidden curriculum can be ascertained. I argue that the terms employed locally in each medical school—'fluffy stuff', 'psychosocial' or 'soft sciences'—are part and parcel of that school's hidden curriculum and the uses, understandings, and interpretations of such umbrella terms are reiterated by each new student cohort and teaching faculty. Medical students, biomedical teaching staff and clinicians do not understand the disciplinary boundaries in the social sciences and are not aware of the distinct contributions of sociology and anthropology to medical education.

Topics Versus Disciplines

It was striking that during the PBL-sessions I observed no students would explicitly refer to anthropology or sociology or social sciences when they were discussing learning objectives. Only occasionally was 'psychology' named as a discipline. This was in stark contrast to the explicit and constant mentioning of biomedical disciplines such as physiology, anatomy, immunology and biology. Anthropology as a discipline was not known to medical students. Only those students who had an anthropologist as PBL-tutor or chose an optional SSC in Anthropology had some understanding of the discipline. At the end of one such SSC, I asked the students to write a reflective statement- their honest texts were revelatory. I identified two threads. Firstly, the extent of the invisibility of anthropology as a discipline. Here is what some medical students wrote: '*If I am honest I did not even know the meaning of anthropology*', '*I really had no clue what anthropology was*' and '*I had no idea what medical anthropology was or how it could be useful*'.

This last quote brings me to the second thread: medical students did not understand the distinct contribution of anthropology, its relevance and the usefulness of disciplinary knowledge to them as medical students and their future selves, as clinicians. The widespread assumption that anthropology had '*no applicability to clinical practice*', to use a student's phrase, changed for many students after intensive exposure to anthropological thought in my SSC. This was emphasized in their final texts: '*It wasn't until our session on witchcraft that I learnt exactly how anthropology could be useful*' and '*I believe it [anthropology] is something that can and should play a big part in the medical field*'. Brookfield (1995: 84) defines a critical incident as 'any unplanned and unanticipated event' in or outside the classroom. The realization that anthropology was, after all, relevant and provided students with '*beneficial tools*', as one interviewee put it, was such a critical incident. Judging from the SSC evaluation forms this was the main take-home message. One comment read: '*having completed the SCC I understand how crucial it is to the medical profession*'. Analysis of the answers to the final question on the CIQs ('What will be most effective in your daily activities as a doctor?') provided me with concrete examples of how I could build clinical relevance of social science into my plenary lectures and specialist options. The answers to that CIQ question mirrored the learning objectives I formulated for the course: students wrote about learning content around patient perspectives, awareness of cultural backgrounds, critical perspectives on global health and power structures. The topics I selected for my Anthropology SSC, in turn, reflected the core curriculum for sociology in UK undergraduate medical education designed by the Behavioural and Social Science teaching in Medicine network and endorsed by the British Sociological Association (BeSST 2016).

My field notes highlight that it is not only among students that anthropology is largely unknown, but also among many medical educators. I had just started teaching in NEMS when I met a colorectal surgeon affiliated with the medical school. When I tried to explain what exactly I taught, using the terms 'anthropology' and 'social science', he interrupted me enthusiastically and stated: '*It is very important our students are taught by somebody like you. Nowadays, it is very important that students know how to communicate to patients*'. A fellow anthropologist teaching in medical education had a similar experience when a bioscientist summarized her role as '*she teaches students how to be nice people*'.

On the whole, students named social science *topics*, rather than disciplines. 'Health inequalities', 'disability', 'poverty' and 'impact of disease on patients' lives' always topped the list. During my encounters with colleagues in other UK medical schools, I observed that compartmentalisation of social science learning content into topics is common in medical education. Focussing on separate issues silences the contributions of specific social science disciplines and runs the risk that 'theoretical content may be easily lost or indeed absent from the start' (Forrest 2017: 285).

In a certain sense, the invisibility of anthropology should not be surprising as it is linked to the broader invisibility of the discipline at the national level by the UK's medical profession's regulator. Anthropology is not mentioned in the GMC's *Outcomes for graduates*, which specifies the 'professional knowledge' newly qualified doctors should have acquired during their undergraduate medical education. Medical students must 'recognise biomedical, psychological and social science principles of health and disease, and integrate and apply scholarly principles to the care of patients' (GMC 2018: 20). In the overarching 'social science' learning outcome I cited above, only *1* social science discipline, sociology, is mentioned (GMC 2018: 22). In sharp contrast, in the section 'Applying biomedical scientific principles', *14* biomedical disciplines are explicitly named, including anatomy, microbiology, pharmacology, physiology, immunology and pathology (GMC 2018: 21).

The Hidden Curriculum: 'Fluffy' Versus 'Real' Medicine

The second key theme I identified during my analysis relates to learning, teaching and assessment of social science content in the medical curriculum. Here, I focus on the different ways, in addition to institutional slang, the hidden curriculum manifests and reproduces itself in educational practices around social scientific, and in particular anthropological, learning content.

Hafferty (1998: 404) defines the 'hidden curriculum' as 'a set of influences that function at the level of organizational structure and culture'. In Hafferty's conception, the hidden curriculum refers to what is being taught and learned beyond the official curriculum. In my study, medical students perceived the social science component in a paradoxical manner. On one hand, students were very aware that it is part of the core medical curriculum and they agree that this should be the case. On the other hand, students made a clear distinction between 'fluffy' and 'real' medicine and only the latter was systematically prioritized. 'Fluffy' learning content for students was, as expressed in interviews and focus groups, 'vague' or 'common sense' that you could 'sort of talk about without researching it', which one 'can

Google'. In the medical schools I conducted fieldwork, social science was frontloaded in the first two of the 5-year curriculum. As Forrest (2017: 286) notes, those 'pre-clinical phases' are precisely where the curriculum is at risk of being 'over-populated' and where science tends to be 'squeezed in'. There was very little dedicated social science teaching time in the 'clinical' phase of the medical curriculum.

Social Science Teaching

Social science content was taught, in each school, through PBL and a set of dedicated plenary lectures, delivered by one sociologist (at NEMS) and two anthropologists (at Keele). These lectures, on average 6 in the first and 8 in the second year, were timetabled to link with that week's PBL case. Many PBL cases included cues to social science content (which was made explicit in the handbook for PBL-tutors). Although the PBL-cases in both schools contained a lot of social science focus it was not perceived as essential learning:

> I think most of the social science teaching seem to be part of the PBL thing, like it, like we have an outcome, say on health inequalities, (...) which I think is really vague and I think that's kind of how the social science teaching has kind of been at [NEMS]. It's been quite vague and quite like a, almost like a second thought. (Angela)

I observed that PBL learning outcomes coined as 'fluffy' or 'psychosocial' were routinely left to last, in the students' own preparation time and often in the actual PBL-sessions. The biomedical content would typically be tackled first and more time was dedicated to those. Claudia was laughing shyly when she illustrated how she ranked learning content:

> What the lungs do and what goes wrong with the lungs would be my top priority, but what the impact of lung disease has on the patient? That goes a bit lower down, I don't really have to know much about this now, it seems too far in the future [that she would treat a patient with a lung problem]. I'll do it when I've made sure I've done everything else I need to do, so it can end up being quite a quick job.

It is a study on itself to explore why the PBL experience varied greatly for students in different groups, but it is worth considering this student's quote about PBL group dynamics:

> I was in two PBL groups over the first two years. In my first year, my group was very interested, engaged, talkative, and happy to contribute with opinions and suggestions but also very very diplomatic. In my group in the second year, out of the eight students in it, six were probably some of the quietest members of the year. And it had a very strong impact on the group and I would say the group learning.

The phrase '*very very diplomatic*' is important here. It is my experience too that medical students, certainly in comparison to social science students, are more reserved in their discussions or, in the words of a focus group participant, [medical students] 'tend to keep quiet out of fear of saying the wrong thing'. This was corroborated in my conversations with teaching faculty at both schools. One NEMS clinician, an experienced PBL facilitator, confirmed that students prefer to talk about subjects they are familiar with:

> Students are not comfortable with learning objectives to which there is no wrong answer. My PBL groups tend to latch on to facts and concrete information.

This ties in with my own engagements with medical students; they are often afraid about giving incorrect information saying something socially unacceptable or offensive. Discussions of social inequality, race, class, and health inequities are often emotionally fraught, and many medical students fear engaging in them (see Willen et al. 2010).

Another important finding, a critical incident for me, is that medical students shared the widespread perception that what they considered 'fluffy' is not 'science'. When I explicitly asked why the 'fluffy' learning outcomes in PBL are left until the end and, as a result, are not seriously discussed or not covered at all, James replied: '*I think it's because we are all scientists*'. NEMS students who participated in the study were adamant about this: medical students are scientists and the main focus should be on sciences. One SSC student wrote she was surprised I started one teaching session, in her words, '*with a bold statement, that anthropology is a science, a social science*'. Another student wrote: '*I feel ashamed now that in the past I overlooked anthropology as a robust science but admittedly I did*'. Tom chose the optional module in anthropology because [he] '*thought it might be fun to try something different from the more strictly science SSCs*'. The CIQ responses on the question 'what was most surprising' included the statement: '*Science is not just biology, chemistry and physics*'. This constitutes a paradox. On the one hand, students perceive social sciences as commonsensical, easy, vague, less important and not a real science. This also applied to anthropology, many of my SSC students assumed it would be easy. On the other hand, they find it difficult to initiate or sustain a good discussion around a social science topic in PBL sessions.

Plenary lectures were considered very useful when it came to what was perceived as 'real medicine', but were often regarded as of no value with regards to the social science component. As my fieldwork progressed, I realized that attendance in the NEMS social science lectures, taught by a medical sociologist, were extremely low. Lecture attendance was not monitored and students would instead use the time 'more efficient' to revise the 'sciences'. Angela explained:

> If it was a lecture on anatomy the lecture hall would be packed, like from front to back, nearly every single person in the year would be there in the lecture theatre, but then on something, like I know we've used this term before, like, it's not a term that I like, the 'fluffy stuff' they use, erm, which incorporates quite a lot of the 'social sciencey' sort of things, erm, I think the lecture hall would probably be like forty per cent full.

Social science lectures were known in both schools as 'sociology lectures', even when anthropological learning content was taught by an anthropologist and were, on the whole, perceived as '*problematic*', '*boring*' and '*a waste of time*'. One student in the focus group described social science teaching as '*somebody fluffing away all the time*'. The choice of words is in itself an indication of the low status of social science contents. Indeed, students felt that social science learning lectures were not put sufficiently into context:

> Yeah, someone goes in the lecture hall and just tells you this, this and this, then it doesn't have any meaning, like it's just, I suppose the social, the context.

Again, the CIQs on my SSC sessions indicated that when social science topics which were related to real-life clinical context, they were appraised by students as more relevant to medicine.

Social Science Learning

How do medical students prepare social science learning objectives for PBL sessions or revise it for exams? After data analysis I identified three main learning resources students use: their own lecture notes, Internet search results, and study notes compiled by fellow students. Even though students received, at both schools, detailed reading lists, tutorials on search academic literature in databases and strong discouragement to use online sources (such as Wikipedia), they seem to lack the skill or were not bothered to engage with the social science evidence-base. In contrast to biomedical disciplines, students did not consult textbooks or specialist academic literature when preparing PBL or studying social science content. At NEMS, a 'revision guide' for Theme X circulated. Tom emailed me this guide: two PDF files full of colourful boxes and figures, all in bullet points. These had once been compiled by a student, now long graduated, and were passed down over the years. One page, for instance, was entitled 'Teenage pregnancy and abortion'. This topic consisted of three separate colourful boxes with bullet points. The first box gave five points around the Abortion Act. The next box contained four 'anti-abortion arguments' and the final box summed up the 'social factors that lead to teenage pregnancy' in six keywords: poverty, children or teenage mothers, low educational achievement, low expectations, mental health problems and crime. Medical students learn social science content as a 'list of facts'. Even the first- and second-year students participating in the study were fully aware how students in the higher years prepared for the big final 'Theme X' exam. Here is how Beckie summed it up how social science is studied, showing an understanding that it was part and parcel of the school's hidden curriculum:

> No one actually sits down, not everyone actually sits down and goes through it every single week, they just cram at the end, so you just learn. They put more, as we're learning it, they put more emphasis on the science.

Over the years, backed up by my ethnographic data, I came to realize that medical students definitely engage in 'fact learning', and not in 'deeper learning', when it comes to social science. Medical students learn facts and not how to think about social issues and how to interpret how social factors impact on health. Let me give you an example of an exam question around gender and health, that was designed by myself and a fellow anthropologist at Keele. We expected students to answer the question with a short free-text answer identifying and explaining the concept of 'masculine hegemony'. It was clear that students knew we were expecting them to write about that particular concept, but they did not understand it and had learned a definition by heart. That became abundantly clear when we encountered over 20 different spellings of the word 'hegemony' which we, the BSS team marking that question, wrote (out of sheer frustration) on the whiteboard in the marking room (incorrect spellings included haemonegic, heterogenic, hegemonic, hedgemonic and even congentric). Medical students in the higher years were only engaged with social science in as far as they needed to study that material for their final exams:

> I think we just put them [social science learning outcomes] to the side and so I remember them a lot less. I didn't really do flashcards for everything else but I did have a set of flashcards for my fluffy stuff. I find having discussions about it interesting, but to study it's just, it's an, *a bit of a nuisance* (laughs). The exam is very much, you have to say the right thing, so it becomes a chore to learn all the facts and *it doesn't test you on your understanding*. (. . .) I just need to learn all these facts so I can regurgitate them in the [Theme X] exam. (Claudia, my emphasis)

This approach to studying social science is shared by many, if not most, medical students I engaged with. Social science knowledge is reduced to a list of facts, whereas other learning content '*needed to be understood*'. Students in one of the focus groups also added that they are aware that 'more people fail the social stuff than the science stuff'. The critical incident here is that when students do not see the value of the assessment and the relevance of learning content is not clear, students will '*regurgitate*' a '*list of facts*' only to pass the exam. This resonates with an anthropologist's experience of teaching anthropology to Human Science students at the University of Oxford. His experience was that these students are 'surface learners' who had little interest in anthropology which was not a central component of their curriculum. His students were not able to distinguish anthropology's guiding principles and would passively accept ideas and information and focus strategically on that which was necessary for the exams (Bastide 2011). This points to another critical incident: we need to be conscious about the assessment format we use to examine students on social science content. I have used, for SSCs, different assessment types (including a conference presentation, a portfolio, a research pitch to a funding body) which were welcomed by the students and routinely demonstrated a deeper engagement with the material.

Professional Status of Social Scientists in Medical Education

Forrest (2017: 285) explains how medical schools replicate hierarchies in medicine and that, in turn, reinforces the status of disciplinary knowledge: 'clinicians' knowledge is seen to rank above that of other health professionals and all of these above the knowledge and expertise of social scientists'. My study findings and experience support the argument that teaching social science is a 'specialty skill' and should be delivered by social scientists (Litva and Peters 2008: 310). That is in contrast to a widely held assumption that social sciences can be taught by anyone. This reflects the perception in the hidden curriculum that social sciences, including anthropology, is 'common sense'. BSS learning content is often taught by scholars from a range of disciplines in the UK. Russell et al. (2002: 11–12) reported that SBS teachers in UK medical schools included seven sociologists, four social anthropologists, three health psychologists and a number of academics from other disciplines (economics, demography and public health). At NEMS, students all knew the cardiologist and neurosurgeon by name, although these clinicians would deliver only one lecture in Phase 1. Except for two students who did a sociology SSC, none of the interviewees could name the medical sociologist at NEMS, even though that sociologist delivered the 12 plenary social science lectures.

It is different at Keele's School of Medicine where there is a dedicated BSS team that is highly visible in the larger 'medical science team' that delivers social, behavioural and biomedical science teaching to first-and second-year medical students. This may go a long way to explain why Keele medical students refer to 'psychosocial' and 'BSS' and do not use more derogative umbrella terms like 'fluffy stuff'. Although I need to add that Keele students and colleagues are not always able to distinguish the two psychologists from the two anthropologists in the BSS team, our professional identity is perceived as 'BSS'.

Sustained Engagement with Anthropology in Medical Education

> The tools of 21st century medicine include anatomy, physiology, pharmacology, genomics, proteomics, and the related sciences, but it is only when social science is added to the tool box that medicine gains the ability to understand and respond to the wants and needs of individual patients, social networks, and whole communities. (Kottke 2011: 931)

Although UK medical schools emphasize the biopsychosocial model (Engel 1977), throughout the training of the future clinical workforce, many UK curricula still reflect the dominance of the biomedical model in their educational approach. As a consequence, and although it is now institutionalised as a 'core' component of the formal medical curriculum, social science still remains peripheral in the hidden curriculum.

The dominant, often unconsciously held view that medicine, and more broadly natural science, is objective and exists independently of society is problematic. Medicine is part and parcel of society and constitutes a specific social, cultural and historical way of perceiving the world. It is paramount that all stakeholders (students, educators, professional regulators) accept that medical education itself is a social construct and does not exist independently of social conventions. What is selected from a possible range of things to be studied during medical education, reflects a hierarchy of disciplinary knowledge and an understanding of what is worthy of focussed attention. Far from being objective, what our students consider 'facts' to be studied, are a selection we made. This, I believe, goes a long way to explain why anthropology remains largely invisible in medical education.

But there is another problem: the social is understood mainly through personal experience and therefore what social science has to offer is often perceived as 'common sense'. 'Common sense' is not enough to understand society and to see the relationship between individual lives and the effects of larger social forces. Our medical graduates should be able to conceptualize the personal problems they encounter in clinical practice as part of wider societal processes. They should be able to understand that the personal is social. It is therefore high time that medical education takes the hidden curriculum with regards to social science, and in particular anthropology, seriously. Our objective should be to cultivate a 'sociological imagination' in our future doctors: the ability to see the relationship between individual experiences of health and illness and the wider society (Mills 1959).

In order to bring social science, and specifically anthropology, from the margins to the centre in medical education we need to ensure that all key stakeholder groups (medical students, medical educators and clinicians) understand the relevance of social sciences as applied to medicine and are aware of the specific disciplinary contributions of sociology versus anthropology. I have learned over the years that my biomedical and clinical colleagues ask what they can do, in practical terms, when I present them with the challenges I outlined above. Therefore, I end this chapter with some recommendations, based on my ethnography and the critical incidents I identified. I am fully aware that the feasibility of implementing these largely depend on institutional structures, available staff budgets and, indeed, the influences of each school's hidden curriculum. I formulate my suggestions for changing educational practice in the favourite—bullet point—style of our medical students:

- For UK medical schools: recruit, integrate and involve social scientists, including anthropologists, fully in all educational aspects: curriculum development, educational delivery and assessments and reconsider how anthropology is integrated in the school's curriculum. Many UK medical schools do not have social scientists as permanent staff members in the medical school, colleagues from other departments provide 'service teaching' and are not fully integrated in the culture of medical education.
- For PBL courses: ensure PBL tutors receive tailored training on how to integrate social science learning objectives and raise awareness of institutional slang and the tendency to de-prioritise social science learning content. This should be delivered by an experienced social scientist in medical education.
- For anthropologists: recognize that anthropology feels less directly into clinical practice than other core components and make anthropology teaching useful and relevant to medical education. Anthropologists should tailor their material and teaching style to the curriculum's overarching learning outcomes and to clinical practice.
- For all stakeholders in medical education: be aware of the formal and hidden curriculum and take appropriate action. Engage with medical students through focus groups, town hall meetings, teaching evaluations and take students' reflections seriously

Acknowledgments I would like to thank all the medical students and medical educators who participated in this study. Special thanks to Dr. Sophie Wellum, Dr. Matthew Eggleston and Dr. Andrew Ghobrial for sharing their insights on anthropology during their medical education and becoming good friends over the years. I am especially grateful to the fantastic BSS team at Keele's School of Medicine for their support and collegiality: Dr. Karen Adams, Dr. Penny List and Dr. Eva Luksaite. With special thanks to Professor Andrew Hassell for his support and encouragement for my medical education research. Finally, my gratitude goes to the BeSST Co-Chairs and all colleagues involved in this network (see www.besst.info).

References

Atkinson, Paul. 1984. Training for certainty. *Social Science & Medicine* 19 (9): 949–956.

———. 2015. *For ethnography*. London: Sage.

Bastide, Hubert. 2011. Three challenges in teaching anthropology. *Teaching Anthropology* 1 (2): 56–67.

Beagan, Brenda. 2003. Teaching social and cultural awareness to medical students: "it's all very nice to talk about it in theory, but ultimately it makes no difference". *Academic Medicine* 78 (6): 605–614.

Becker, Howard, Blanche Geer, Everett C. Hughes, and Anselm L. Strauss. 1961. *Boys in white: Student culture in medical school*. Chicago: Chicago University Press.

Becker, Howard, Blanche Geer, and Everett C. Hughes. 1968. *Making the grade: The academic side of college life*. New York: Wiley.

Benbassat, Jochanan, Reuben Baumal, Jeffrey M. Borkan, and Rosalie Ber. 2003. Overcoming barriers to teaching the behavioral and social sciences to medical students. *Academic Medicine* 78 (4): 372–380.

BeSST. 2016. *Behavourial and social science teaching in medicine*. http://www.besst.info. Accessed 20 Jan 2020.

Betancourt, Joseph. 2006. Cultural competence and medical education: Many names, many perspectives, one goal. *Academic Medicine* 81 (6): 499–501.

BMJ. 1980. More anthropology and less sleep for medical students. *British Medical Journal* 281: 1662.

Boud, David, and Grahame Feletti. 2013. *The challenge of problem-based learning*. New York: Routledge.

Brookfield, Stephen. 1995. *Becoming a critically reflective teacher*. New York: Wiley.

Brosnan, Caragh. 2009. Pierre Bourdieu and the theory of medical education: Thinking "relationally" about medical students and medical curricula. In *Handbook of the sociology of medical education*, ed. Caragh Brosnan and Bryan Turner, 65–82. Oxon: Routledge.

De Visser, Richard. 2009. Psychology in medical curricula: "Need to know" or "nice to know". *The European Health Psychologist* 11 (2): 20–23.

Dikomitis, Lisa, and Emma Kelly. 2018. Enquiry into learning and teaching in the social sciences: Engaging with Ethnographic research. In *Teaching and learning in higher education: Disciplinary approaches to educational enquiry*, ed. Elizabeth Cleaver, Maxine Lintern, and Mike McLinden, 253–265. London: Sage.

Dogra, Nisha. 2007. The views of medical education stakeholders on guidelines for cultural diversity teaching. *Medical Teacher* 29: e41–e46.

Ellis, Carolyn, and Arthur P. Bochner. 2000. Auto-ethnography, personal narrative, reflexivity. In *The handbook of qualitative research*, ed. Normal K. Denzin and Yvonna S. Lincoln, 733–767. California: Sage.

Engel, George. 1977. The need for a new medical model: A challenge for biomedicine. *Science* 196 (4286): 129–136.

Farrell, Laura, Gisele Bourgeois-Law, Glenn Regehr, and Rola Ajjawi. 2015. Autoethnography: Introducing 'I' into medical education research. *Medical Education* 49 (10): 974–982.
Forrest, Simon. 2017. Teaching social science research methods to undergraduate medical students: The state of the art and opportunities for practice and curriculum development. *Teaching Public Administration* 35 (3): 80–300.
Fox, Renée C. 2005. Cultural competence and the culture of medicine. *The New England Journal of Medicine* 353 (13): 1316–1319.
Gallagher, Stephan, Sarah Wallace, Yoga Nathan, and Deirdre McGrath. 2015. 'Soft and fluffy': Medical students' attitudes towards psychology in medical education. *Journal of Health Psychology* 20 (1): 91–101.
GMC. 1993. *Tomorrow's doctors*. Recommendations on Undergraduate Medical Education. https://www.gmc-uk.org/education/standards-guidance-and-curricula/standards-and-outcomes/outcomes-for-graduates. Accessed 26 Aug 2019.
———. 2018. *Outcome for graduates*. https://www.gmc-uk.org/education/standards-guidance-and-curricula/standards-and-outcomes/outcomes-for-graduates. Accessed 26 Aug 2019.
Good, Byron, and Mary-Jo DelVecchio Good. 1993. Learning medicine. The construction of medical knowledge at Harvard medical School. In *Knowledge, power, and practice: The anthropology of medicine and everyday*, ed. Shirley Lindenbaum and Margaret Lock, 81–107. Berkeley: University of California Press.
Hafferty, Frederic W. 1998. Beyond curriculum reform: Confronting medicine's hidden curriculum. *Academic Medicine* 73: 403–407.
Kadambari, Dharanipragada, Kumar Santosh, Z. Zayapragassarazan, and Subhash C. Parija. 2018. *Improving discipline-based undergraduate medical curriculum: An evidence informed approach*. Singapore: Springer Nature.
Kottke, Thomas E. 2011. Medicine is a social science in its very bone and marrow. *Mayo Clinic Proceedings* 86 (10): 930–932.
Lévy-Bruhl, Lucien. 2018. *Revival: How natives think (1926)*, Revival series. Abingdon-on-Thames: Routledge.
Litva, Andrea, and Sarah Peters. 2008. Exploring barriers to teaching behavioural and social sciences in medical education. *Medical Education* 42: 309–314.
Maudsley, Gillian. 1999. Do we all mean the same thing by "problem-based learning"? A review of the concepts and a formulation of the ground rules. *Academic Medicine: Journal of the Association of American Medical Colleges 74* (2): 178–185.
Merton, Robert K., George G. Reader, and Patricia Kendall, eds. 1957. *The student-physician: Introductory studies in the sociology of medical education*. Cambridge, MA: Harvard University Press.
Mills, C. W. (1959). *The sociological imagination*. New York: Oxford University Press.
Montagu, Ashley. 1963. Anthropology and medical education. *JAMA* 183 (7): 577–583.
Morrison, Jill. 2015. Undergraduate medical education: Looking back, looking forward. *Scottish Medical Journal* 60 (4): 149–151.
Nathan, Rebekah. 2005. *My freshman year: What a professor learned by becoming a student*. Ithaca: Cornell University Press.
Peeraer, Griet, Vincent Donche, Benedicte Y. De Winter, Arno Muijtjens, Roy Remmen, Peter Van Petegem, Leo Bossaert, and A.J.J.A. Scherpbier. 2011. Teaching conceptions and approaches to teaching of medical school faculty: The difference between how medical school teachers *think* about teaching and how they say that they *do* teach. *Medical Teacher* 33: e382–e387.
Richardson, Jane. 2009. Factors that influence first year medical students' choice of student selected component. *Medical Teacher* 31 (9): e418–e424.
Russell, A.J., van Teijlingen, E., Lambert, H. & Stacy, R. 2002. *Social and behavioural sciences in medical education*. Report on a Workshop held on 27–28 June 2002. University of Durham, Department of Anthropology.

Russell, A.J., E. van Teijlingen, H. Lambert, and R. Stacy. 2004. Social and behavioural science education in UK medical schools: Current practice and future directions. *Medical Education* 38 (4): 409–417.

Sahlins, Marshall. 1995. *How "natives" think: About Captain Cook, for example*. Chicago: University of Chicago Press.

Satterfield, Jason M., Shelly R. Adler, H. Carrie Chen, Karen E. Hauer, George W. Saba, and Rene Salazar. 2010. Creating an ideal social and behavioural sciences curriculum for medical students. *Medical Education* 44: 1194–1202.

Seeleman, Conny, Jeanine Suurmond, and Karien Stronks. 2009. Cultural competence: A conceptual framework for teaching and learning. *Medical Education* 43 (3): 229–237.

Sinclair, Simon. 1997. *Making doctor: An institutional apprenticeship*. Oxford: Berg.

Taylor, Janelle. 2003. Confronting "culture" in medicine's "culture of no culture". *Academic Medicine* 78 (6): 555–559.

Thompson, Britta M., Paul Haidet, Robert Casanova, Rey P. Vivo, Arthur G. Gomez, Arleen F. Brown, Regina A. Richter, and Sonia J. Crandall. 2010. Medical students' perceptions of their teachers' and their own cultural competency: Implications for education. *Journal of General Internal Medicine* 25 (Suppl. 2): S91–S94.

Tripp, David. 1993. *Critical incidents in teaching: Developing professional judgement*. London: Routledge.

Tuchman, Gaye. 2009. *Wannabe U: Inside the corporate university*. Chicago: University of Chicago Press.

Weatherall, David. 2011. Science and medical education: Is it time to revisit Flexner? *Medical Education* 45 (1): 44–50.

Willen, Sarah S., Antonio Bullon, and Mary-Jo D. Good. 2010. Opening up a huge can of worms: Reflections on a "cultural sensitivity" course for psychiatry residents. *Harvard Review of Psychiatry* 18 (4): 247–253.

Willis, Paul. 1978. *Learning to labour: Why working class kids get working class jobs*. Farnborough: Saxon House.

———. 2000. *The ethnographic imagination*. Oxford: Polity Press.

Lisa Dikomitis, PhD is a social anthropologist and works in the School of Medicine at Keele University. She is Director of Research at Keele's School of Medicine and Academic Lead of Keele's Institute for Global Health. Professor Dikomitis also leads the team that delivers the behavioural and social science teaching to Keele's medical students. Her research is situated at the intersection of social sciences, arts, humanities, and medicine. An experienced ethnographer, she conducted fieldwork in a mountainous Cypriot village and in several healthcare contexts, including in a Flemish psychiatric hospital and primary care settings in the United Kingdom. Professor Lisa Dikomitis is internationally recognised for her work on Cypriot refugees. She is the author of *Cyprus and Its Places of Desire: Cultures of Displacement among Greek and Turkish Cypriot Refugees* (IB Tauris, 2012) and co-editor of *When God Comes to Town: Religious Traditions in Urban Contexts* (Berghahn Books, 2009). In recent years, her research has focused on global health, she currently leads a number of large, interdisciplinary teams carrying out anthropological work in the Philippines, Brazil, Ethiopia, and Sri Lanka.

Chapter 6
Anthropologist as University Strategic Planner Envisioning a New Medical School with a Focus on Community-Based Care

Dennis W. Wiedman

Introduction

One may ask, what kind of background prepared an anthropologist for a leading role in planning the future of an entire university with a vision for a new medical school training physicians focused on community care? Reflecting on factors shaping anthropology and medicine over the past 50 years, this story highlights an anthropologist purposefully directing organizational culture change. Teaching courses and conducting research are important. However, administrative roles in the University are also important for the anthropology profession to influence an organization's mission, goals and policies. Policies and procedures structure beliefs and practices for generations to come. While a university administrator, by innovatively inserting anthropology topics, values and perspectives into plans for a future of medical school, this anthropologist purposefully and consciously influenced the culture of medicine at FIU.

A reflexive, autoethnographic and life history approach illustrates the training, research, applied and practicing experiences that provided a foundation for a medical anthropologist to be a university strategic planner envisioning a future medical school at Florida International University (FIU). Autoethnography, a qualitative research methodology, emphasizes reflexivity, deep and careful self-reflection to interrogate the intersections between self and experiences connecting wider social, cultural, political, economic, meanings and understandings. This relatively new method of writing portrays people in the process of figuring out what to do, the meaning of their actions, and often on how to make life better (Adams et al. 2014: 2). In this case, autoethnography provides an understanding of how key leadership roles

D. W. Wiedman (✉)
Department Global and Sociocultural Studies, School of International and Public Affairs, Florida International University, Miami, FL, USA
e-mail: wiedmand@fiu.edu

I. L. Martinez, D. W. Wiedman (eds.), *Anthropology in Medical Education*,
https://doi.org/10.1007/978-3-030-62277-0_6

with unprecedented power as a practicing anthropologist literally shaped a new medical school. From the perspective as a Past-President of the National Association for the Practice of Anthropology (NAPA), and Executive Board Member of the American Anthropological Association (AAA), this story reflects on anthropology as a valuable and important professional career, not only in teaching and administration within medical education, but also in the planning process for medical schools.

Anthropological theory, methods, and practices enabled this anthropologist as an strategic planner and helped shape this twenty-first century university and medical school. From 1990 to 1996, as an applied and practicing medical anthropologist, I was the lead academic planner coordinating the university-wide strategic planning efforts. In this role, I worked to identify strengths, weaknesses, opportunities, and threats based on extensive research. When strategic planning formally began in 1990, FIU was a regional university of approximately 23,000 students with an emphasis on teaching and service, offering mostly undergraduate degrees and a few masters and doctoral degrees. As the university's strategic planner, we brought together hundreds of people, dozens of committees, and every administrative unit in the University to contribute to envisioning a future for the university. Over these 6 years, several major University plans were issued, discussed, revised, and refined, leading to the 1996 public release of "Reaching for the Top", which portrayed a vision for a top, public, urban, research university (Wiedman 2013, 2016). Within this planning document was a conceptualization of a new medical school with a vision of training culturally responsive physicians to meet the health needs of the diverse multicultural community in South Florida.

It took university leaders 10 years of political and economic challenges at the local, state, and national levels to gain approval in 2006 by the State of Florida, for what was to become the Herbert Wertheim College of Medicine (Breslin and Roller 2016). In 2007, one of the first medical school faculty hired was anthropologist, Dr. Iveris L. Martinez, who developed and implemented the social and cultural curriculum serving as the Chief of the Division of Medicine and Society (Martinez 2015). In 2009, the first students enrolled, to be graduated in 2013. Over the 20 years, the university doubled its number of students from 25,000 in 1996 to over 54,000 in 2015. Incredibly in 2015, FIU joined the top tier of research universities in the United States by achieving the Carnegie rank of R1: Doctoral Universities for Highest Research Activity. As Miami's only public research university, FIU is now among the top 10 largest universities in the nation, graduating more than 200,000 alumni, 115,000 of whom live and work in South Florida. In 2015, the medical school finalized its own "Strategic Plan: 2015–2020," envisioning the school's priorities and goals for the next 5 years (HWCOM 2015).

To assess the influence of the role of anthropology in strategic planning for a new medical school emphasizing community care, Dr. Martinez and I (2017) used NVivo, a qualitative data analysis software to compare the 1996 university strategic plan, "Reaching for the Top," which contained the first details of the proposed medical school, with the 2015 medical school plan. Our goal was to evaluate how this new organization was initially conceptualized and eventually fully operationalized. In this process, we developed a methodology for cultural theme longitudinal analysis, contributing to anthropological theory on cultural themes, directed organizational culture change, and strategic planning. The overwhelming majority of the cultural themes formulated in 1996, were recurrent narratives in 2015, thereby, continuing to shape the goals, faculty hires, curricula, community programs, and organizational structure. This longitudinal analysis demonstrated the influence of the 1996 planning on the emergence and continuation of this new organization. Community care continued as the dominant emphasis, while there were few new themes indicating that the 2015 medical school did not deviate from the original conceptualizations, intentions, and meanings. This emphasis continues in the current 2020 mission: "Herbert Wertheim College of Medicine prepares socially accountable, community-based physicians, scientists, and health professionals who are uniquely qualified to transform the health of patients and communities" (HWCOM 2020).

This autoethnography encapsulates an important time period in the history of anthropology beginning in the 1970s when medical anthropology was just emerging as a subdiscipline and professional career choice. It portrays a time when the initial key concepts, theories, and approaches of medical anthropology were being debated and solidified, then over the next decades how these were refined and operationalized in applied medical anthropology research and practical applications. Briefly stated, brought up in Miami, Florida, my family interests in Native Americans, led me to an anthropology Bachelor of Arts degree at the University of Florida. Having an interest in Native American health and healing led me to enroll in the University of Oklahoma anthropology doctoral program. My medical anthropology research and training at the University of Oklahoma College of Medicine and my employment at the University of Miami School of Medicine, provided the experience and perspective that led me to believe that an FIU medical school with a community focus was needed and feasible.

Planning for a new medical school reveals much about the changing times, places, and politics of medical education. Placed within the South Florida multicultural and political economic context, this story illustrates my engagements with traditional healing, individual clinical care, social group processes, community health systems, academic institutions, and the culture of biomedicine. These career experiences empowered me with political and academic authority at a critical time where decisions were being made for a new medical school uniquely suited for pioneering community-oriented medical education.

This career trajectory reflects a time period in the history of anthropology and medicine. In the 1970s, there was a call for biomedical services concentrated in urban hospitals to be dispersed to community clinics and centers (Chap. 2). It was also during the 1970s when medical anthropology was just beginning to be formalized as a sub-discipline within anthropology, and when departments of anthropology were beginning to offer tracks in this new emphasis. Each of my career experiences, research projects, applied or practicing employment positions illustrate the coming of age of applied medical anthropology, led to the authority of a medical anthropologist to envision a medical school in the 1990s, and then the ready acceptance of the voice and authority of an anthropologist to initially plan the foundation for the new medical school. Placed within this historical, chronological and longitudinal narrative, the social, cultural, economic, and political context of this work speaks to the factors shaping anthropology's shifting authority in the medical educational setting and the relative value of anthropology's emphasis on "culture" and "community" in medical training.

Career Experiences

Native American Health and Healing

With a Bachelor's degree in anthropology from the University of Florida, I moved to Oklahoma with my wife to be among Native American peoples, intertribal pow-wows, and ways of life. While living in northeastern Oklahoma among Lenape (also known as the Delaware), Pawnee, Shawnee and Comanche Peyotists, I learned traditional Native American healing. My experiences over 5 years with Peyotists and the Native American Church deeply engaged me with local lived experiences striving for health and well-being. It was due to the influence of Allen and Grace Dale that I pursued graduate training in anthropology. Allen was President of the Native American Church of the United States for 10 years from 1946 to 1956. Though peyote meetings were commonly viewed as a religion and church, I documented that two-thirds of the purposes for peyote meetings were specifically for the healing of physical health issues. In the journal *Medical Anthropology,* I described Peyotism as a traditional health care system that is complementary to the services of the allopathic medicine provided at the Indian Health Service hospital (Wiedman 1990a). This extensive participant-observation grounded me in the value of recognizing local alternative and complementary healing systems in the provision of health care. My later ethnohistorical research found that during the imposition of Federal and State laws in the formation of the State of Oklahoma in 1905–1907, Native American public discourse shifted from portraying peyote as a medicine to a religion instead of a healing system. The governance structure of the new state could recognize this way of life as a religion, but not as a medicine or health care delivery system. This research reinforces the importance of an understanding of medical pluralism and culturally sensitive health care (Wiedman 2012b).

University of Oklahoma: Anthropology Department

The Department of Anthropology at the University Oklahoma (OU), one of the oldest anthropology departments in the US following Columbia University, trained me in the four anthropology subdisciplines of linguistics, archeology, physical, and cultural anthropology at the Master's degree level before proceeding to the specialized Ph.D. Among the faculty was Professor Morris Opler, known as a leader in Culture and Personality studies, who was one of the earliest anthropologists to document the psychotherapeutic value of Mescalero Apache peyote use. His guidance provided me a way to conceptualize my Northeast Oklahoma peyote fieldwork within a health care and psychotherapeutic system. His articulation of "Culture Themes" as powerful social forces, is the basis for my purposeful use of specifying five "themes" in the 1996 FIU Strategic Plan to focus, motivate and guide university development. The explanatory power of this theoretical paradigm was verified in our evaluation of the organizational culture themes of the FIU medical school (Wiedman and Martinez 2017).

University of Oklahoma Medical School: Interdisciplinary Social Scientists

Medical Anthropology was just being formalized as a specialization for anthropologists in 1972 when I started my graduate training. Since there were no specific courses, I began independent studies with Dr. Robert Hill, who had just been hired at the University of Oklahoma Health Sciences Center in Oklahoma City, Department of Family Practice, Community Medicine and Dentistry. Reading what are now the classic medical anthropology publications, grounded me in this new specialty and familiarized me with its founders and key concepts that were being debated by this new professional specialty at the American Anthropological Association conferences. Many of these readings are incorporated in the Wiedman and Martinez history Chap. 2 in this volume.

While taking classes in the OU anthropology program in Norman, I would travel to Oklahoma City to build relationships with medical anthropologists and social scientists at the OU Health Sciences Center and Medical School. Among these was medical anthropologist Howard Stein, and medical sociologist Thomas May, a key person in the Society for Applied Anthropology. Over time, under their guidance, I engaged in many health-related research projects and enjoyed access to OU Medical School faculty, resources and programs, particularly family medicine, psychiatry, epidemiology, and the physician associate program.

Howard Stein's publications on the culture of medicine were influential for me, as he interpreted doctor/patient discourse and relations from a psychoanalytical perspective while emphasizing the overall culture of the clinic, hospital and profession of medicine. Howard Stein and Robert Hill published their book *Ethnic Imperative*, which gave me insights into the powerful influence of culture, ethnic identity, and ethnicity (Stein and Hill 1978). Rather than accepting the current assimilation model of the US as a melting pot, they documented how ethnicity and cultural pride resurges after several immigrant generations. Not only was this important for my strategic planning, and my understanding of the diverse multicultural communities of South Florida, but for my guidance that a new medical school focused on providing culturally sensitive care would be a long-lasting endeavor and necessity for new physicians.

University of Oklahoma Medical School: Urban Indian Clinic

With my years of experience among Oklahoma Native Americans, Native health, and healing, I desired to learn more about how western medicine provided care to Native Americans. Under Dr. Robert Hill's guidance, I interned at the Oklahoma City Indian Clinic, a community clinic affiliated with the OU Medical School that served urban Native Americans. During the 1800s, tribes signed treaties with the Federal government that took their lands and moved them to Oklahoma; entitling tribal members to receive free health care. Now, six Indian Health Service hospitals serve over 40 tribal nations in Oklahoma.

I had already experienced Delaware people's long car rides, access and biomedical care at Claremore Indian Hospital in northeast Oklahoma. As an ethnographer and participant-observer of the Oklahoma City Indian clinic, I was able to directly observe physician/patient relations in the examination room, on-site laboratory procedures, pharmaceutical and food issuances, as well as the flow of patient welcomes, check-in and discharge processes. Mothers with young children and elders were the most frequent patients. Interactions with advisory board members and clinic managers provided insights into the administrative and funding challenges.

Here I recognized the benefits of community-based primary care staffed by health professionals from the same ethnic group being served. Considering the historical traumas suffered by Native Americans, there is a longstanding distrust of the government and medical institutions. Having clinic staff composed mainly of Native American health professionals along with non-native physicians, taught me how community-level health care fostered better understanding and communications.

For my first applied medical anthropology initiative, at the urging of clinic administrators, I was asked to compile demographic characteristics of the patients served. Native Americans who moved to Oklahoma City needed to travel great distances to their respective rural hospitals. The most frequent users of the Oklahoma City Indian Clinic were Cheyenne and Arapaho of western Oklahoma, who had to travel over 80 miles to the Clinton Indian Hospital. Identifying Cheyenne and Arapaho as the most frequent users of the Indian Clinic, I was asked to develop a motion addressed to the Cheyenne and Arapaho Tribal Council specifying the number of tribal members, types of care provided, and a request for funding from the tribe to support the clinical services. This was approved by the Tribal Council on the first attempt! Subsequently, I was told, the text of the motion modified with tribal-specific patient statistics continued to be used by clinic administrators in requesting funding from various Oklahoma tribal nations sustaining the Indian clinic for years to come. This internship and training experience provided me a holistic view of a community clinic in its relationships with the OU Medical School and tribal governments. Observing the high prevalence of elders with foot ulcers and amputations impressed upon me the need for Native American health research, especially to understand Type II diabetes.

University of Oklahoma Medical School: Department of Psychiatry

An opportunity arose to be part of an interprofessional team in a research project at the OU School of Medicine, Department of Psychiatry. We investigated psychosocial stress and on-the-job accidents among Oklahoma City Fire Department firefighters. Over 30 stations serve the Oklahoma City area with community-based emergency care. I worked with the lead psychiatrist, a medical anthropologist, a medical sociologist, and a biostatistician. In this research project I administered a printed psychosocial survey to hundreds of firefighters in their firehouses. Participant-observation of life in the firehouse profiled their highly-scheduled daily lives, and the strict lines of authority and communications. I then worked to computerize and analyze the data. Although trained in SPSS statistical software on a large mainframe computer with punch-cards entry, the latest computer system used keyboard data entry into a computer about six, by five, by two feet wide. Use of standardized questionnaires measuring social and psychological stress and daily living experiences taught me how psychologists and psychiatrists attempt to correlate mental status, stress, and injuries (Rush et al. 1977).

Important for my later employment in the Department of Psychiatry at the University of Miami School of Medicine, I learned psychiatric categories and interpretations of mental health symptoms detailed in the *Diagnostic and Statistical Manual of Mental Disorders.* This experience provided valuable insights into the institutional lives of firefighters who are front line medical personnel in community health care. Computer data management prepared me for my university strategic planner role in coordinating team research, large-scale data collection and analysis in a large institution with very structured roles and statuses.

University of Oklahoma Medical School: Epidemiology Department

A major disease among Oklahoma Native Americans was Type II diabetes. This became obvious while among the Delaware, and reinforced again at the Oklahoma City Clinic. Physician and epidemiologist Dr. Kelly West at the OU Medical School, had been conducting diabetes research for years among Oklahoma Native Americans. Combined with his study of 12 different countries, he proposed that "Adiposity" or obesity was the commonality and this occurred as populations modernized.

His publications proposed that diabetes symptoms were rare among Native Americans prior to the 1940s (West 1974).

This became the research question for my doctoral dissertation. I was the project ethnologist working with OU archaeologists on the Parris Mound Project in Lee Creek of eastern Oklahoma. I documented the historic Cherokee land use and demography over the past 150 years using historic archeology, ethnography, oral histories, mapping, and historic documents (Wiedman 1986). From this demographic land use data, I identified that between the 1930s and the 1940s a major demographic shift occurred as the Cherokee transitioned from subsistence farming to working at cattle ranching for cash. They moved their scattered homesteads from the hilltops and valleys to a new gravel road that connected to distant towns outside the valley. With a cash economy, they increasingly began purchasing processed foods, cars, trucks, and labor-saving household appliances (Wiedman 1979, 1987). This economic and technological transition correlated with the beginning of the Native American diabetes epidemic. More recently, I formulated the "Chronicities of Modernity Theory" for the global epidemic of obesity, diabetes and the metabolic syndrome that is unfolding among developing populations around the world today (Wiedman 2010, 2012a, 2014).

This land use and populations experience enhanced my abilities as a strategic planner of a university medical school with a broad health ecology theoretical perspective, a view that communities change over time with historic shifts in environmental resources, subsistence economies, demography, political systems, disease frequencies, and health care systems.

Plains Apache Tribe: OU Stovall Museum of Science and History

Continuing my work with tribal communities, my first professional planning experience was with the Plains Apache of southwest Oklahoma to develop a traveling exhibit in collaboration with the OU Stovall Museum, now known as the Sam Noble Museum of Natural History. With funding from the National Endowment for the Arts, we inventoried material culture items in museums such as the Smithsonian Institution. Working closely with tribal leaders we designed a way to tell the Plains Apache story to the general public. The exhibit traveled for years throughout the Plains states. This planning experience taught me the intricacies of working closely with community representatives to express their history, perspectives and core values (Baugh et al. 1982).

University of Miami Medical School: Department of Psychiatry, Office of Transcultural Education and Research

Concluding my training as a medical anthropologist in Oklahoma, I returned to my hometown of Miami in 1981, joining the University of Miami Miller School of Medicine in the Department of Psychiatry, Office of Transcultural Education and Research. I became Director of Neighborhood Family Services, a community mental health unit of the Department of Psychiatry. Here I joined an interdisciplinary group of social scientists led by anthropologist Dr. Hazel Weidman, a founder of the Society for Medical Anthropology (Although our last names are similar, we are not kin related). The Office of Transcultural Education and Research, within the Department of Psychiatry, formed the core location for anthropologists in the medical school involved in health research, education and services. Multi-disciplinary social scientists consulted with physicians in providing culturally sensitive care and trained a wide array of health professionals (Lefley and Bestman 1991).

Beginning a decade earlier in the early 1970s, Dr. Hazel Weidman had received federal funding for research using anthropological methods to document the health decisions, beliefs, and practices of ethnic groups in neighborhoods surrounding Jackson Memorial/UM hospital with the goal of increasing use of health services. This first large-scale federally funded medical anthropology research, reported in the "Miami Health Ecology Project," led to further federal funding for the UM Department of Psychiatry to establish out-patient clinics in each of the ethnic communities: Bahamian, Cuban, Puerto Rican, Southern Black, and Haitian (Weidman and Egeland 1978). With these clinics, and the addition of two already established Neighborhood Family Services to non-Hispanic White and American Black geriatric communities, Dr. Weidman implemented her concept of a "professional culture broker" by staffing the clinics primarily with persons from the cultural group being served and with the Director being a professional knowledgeable of the cultural group and the biomedical health system.

In a special issue of *Psychiatric Annals*, Dr. Weidman and her team of social scientists each presented their findings (Sussex and Weidman 1975). Her published concepts of "co-culture," "health culture," and "transcultural health care," are at the foundation of my work. A major pursuit of Dr. Weidman was to professionalize the role of "clinical anthropologists" in medicine. She honored me with a printed "Clinical Anthropologist" certificate acknowledging my skills. The influence of Dr. Weidman and the Office of Transcultural Education and Research on medical school education is detailed in Chap. 2 of this volume by Wiedman and Martinez.

University of Miami Department of Psychiatry: Neighborhood Family Services

Joining the Department of Psychiatry in 1981, I became the Director of Neighborhood Family Services, which served the white non-Hispanic (Anglo) geriatric population in northwest Miami with health, nutrition, and social programs (Wiedman 1984). This "culture broker" role provided me the perspectives and management skills to engage in community-based care as it was happening. This facility in one of the first shopping malls in northwest Miami was within walking distance to numerous trailer home parks where northern US retirees expected to live out their years. Now aging in place, their community infrastructure and housing had declined in quality. Neighborhood Family Services was conceptually founded with a self-help model by psychologist Hilda Ross.

When I arrived as Director this was a fully-functioning and well-developed community institution. Over 200 elders used this facility, many in specific volunteer roles. I supervised the full-time nurse, social worker, receptionist, and the weekly visits of psychiatrists from the UM Department of Psychiatry and other specialists. Open Monday through Friday, this was a focal point in the social lives of members. On entry a person was greeted by a volunteer in a welcoming sitting area with couches and chairs. Led and managed by volunteer members, nearly 100 people could receive a daily hot lunch from a county food program. In the clinic examining room, the full-time nurse would evaluate and assess individuals. A meeting room held special events, therapy groups, and meetings. As this was an out-patient clinic of the UM Medical School Department of Psychiatry, individuals would schedule appointments with the psychiatrist for prescriptions and medications.

For prior decades, the mentally ill in the US were institutionalized in residential psychiatric hospitals. With the development and use of psychotropic medicines, individuals were being released into the community under doctor's supervision. Neighborhood Family Services provided this type of community mental health care. As Director I was engaged with the doctors, nurse and social worker in providing the most appropriate care given the person's history, culture and background. Most were independently living, well-elders who found this program to be a safe place, with social friendships, nutritional and psychological support. Volunteering gave them a purpose and a daily feeling of accomplishment. For persons with severe mental issues, it was their connection to doctor supervision, prescriptions, hospital and social support services.

An important learning experience for me was working with our interprofessional team to stabilize a middle-aged man who was living in very poor home conditions, threatening to hurt himself and others. Against his will, the psychiatrist "Baker Acted" him to the psychiatric ward of Jackson Memorial/UM hospital. The Florida "Baker Act" empowers physicians and mental health professionals to initiate involuntary institutionalization and examination of an individual. This immersed me in the power of biomedical physicians, psychiatric intervention and treatments with psychotropic medicines, as well as the psychiatric hospital conditions for those institutionalized for mental issues. Being part of the Office of Transcultural Education and Research provided me relevant comparative perspectives on the health care for each of the ethnic specific clinics. This comparative experience revealed that for best health care outcomes the "one size fits all" approach of biomedicine, needed to be more culturally sensitive and appropriate.

Dramatic change was underway in Miami. A major riot burned a portion of the inner city in 1980, and the same year the Mariel Boat lift brought over 100,000 Cubans to Miami in a few months' time. Many were released from prisons and mental institutions in Cuba. Jackson Memorial Hospital/UM was greatly impacted, and the clinics needed to quickly adjust services. This was a crisis time for all of Miami and South Florida. The UM psychiatric out-patient clinics were overwhelmed by this rapid demographic change with the arrival of Cubans with pre-existing psychological issues and new immigrant stresses. As the new immigrants settled in the surrounding community and trailer parks, Spanish-only speaking elders began to regularly attend Neighborhood Family Services. Spanish speaking elders quickly volunteered to serve as interpreters for monolingual English speaking nurse, psychiatrists, and myself. UM/Jackson community clinic funding increased dramatically generating many new hires to address the crisis. Given the great need for Spanish speaking health professionals at all levels, we struggled to hire a Spanish speaking professionally trained social worker.

Republican US President Ronald Regan decreased federally funded social and health programs. When Hazel Weidman retired to Maine in 1990, the Office of Transcultural Education and Research dissolved, with faculty dispersing applying these experiences in their respective ways. As federal community health care policies and funding changed, these UM clinics emerged as New Horizons Community Mental Health System which continues today (Mas 2019: 297–299).

Florida International University: Sociology/Anthropology Department, and Southeast Florida Center on Aging

While practicing anthropology at the UM Medical School, I usually taught one anthropology course each semester at FIU, the regional public university that opened to students in 1972. Teaching "Racial and Cultural Minorities," for the Department of Sociology and Anthropology, I was able to directly share my practicing, research, and knowledge of South Florida and the Miami Health Ecology Project with students. At FIU, I engaged with the Elders Institute and the Southeast Florida Center on Aging on the Biscayne Bay campus. Here I worked with interdisciplinary faculty to write research grants. I became an expert in the new use of desktop microcomputers and database management software for enrollment and budgeting. Very important skills for compiling and analyzing the enormous amount of information for being a university planner. By 1984, I was a visiting professor teaching courses in the Department of Sociology and Anthropology. These roles familiarized me even more with the community of retired elders living seasonally in northeast Dade County condominiums and the importance of community institutions that facilitate social group formation supportive of health and wellness.

Florida International University: Accreditation

Recognizing my abilities to organize faculty and programs, in 1986 the Vice President for Graduate Studies recruited me to finalize the accreditation of Florida International University's transition from a regional comprehensive university with undergraduate and a few graduate programs to a doctoral-degree granting university. Following this successful administrative experience engaged with the Southern Association for Colleges and Schools (SACS), I was then asked to be Associate Director of Accreditation for the 10-year self-study of the entire university. From 1988 to 1990 we coordinated hundreds of academic and administrative organizational units using the new SACS institutional effectiveness accreditation criteria requiring on-going planning and evaluation procedures to conduct the self-study (Kravitz et al. 1990). Few schools had conducted self-studies under this new requirement. As a result of the SACS site visit to validate our self-study, SACS recommended that the University begin strategic planning and evaluation on a regular basis.

This role provided me the opportunity to direct culture change—to shift the organization's members from present to future thinking, from crisis management to strategic management, and from oral to written traditions (Wiedman 1990b, 1992). I became very familiar with the power of regional and discipline-specific accrediting agencies to homogenize academic culture, limiting professional schools such as medicine to the accrediting association's ideal management structures, curriculum, and degree standards.

After successfully leading the reaccreditation in 1990, my organizational and analytical skills were recognized when I was asked by the Vice President for Academic Affairs to join the Provost's Office to help manage the Division of Academic Affairs, as Assistant to the Provost. I worked in the Provost's Office for more than a decade from 1990 to 2004, leading academic planning, policy development, accreditation, program evaluation, among others. A decade later (1998–2000), I was again the Associate Director of the SACS self-study for reaccreditation (Himburg et al. 1999). For a decade, from 1990 to 2000, I was the University Accreditation Officer representing the President and university to SACS. From 2000 to 2004, I was the first Director of Program Review establishing the evaluation and accountability system for all the academic degrees and programs. It is from this program evaluation perspective that I comment in this book on how anthropologists can better contribute in positive ways to medical school education.

Over this time FIU developed from a comprehensive college of 17,000 students in 1982 to a research-extensive university of 33,000 students in 1996, serving one of the most culturally diverse student bodies in the country (Wiedman 1999). During these years of rapid growth in student enrollments, accrediting agencies and the state legislature mandated the implementation of ongoing planning and evaluation that increased accountability with the formulation of written plans, goals, measurable outcomes, policies and procedures. From 2000 to 2009, FIU attained Carnegie I Research University status, lost it, and regained it again in 2019. By this time, it grew to 54,000 students placing it among the top 10 largest universities in the nation.

These teaching, training, research, administrative, applied and practicing medical anthropology experiences empowered me with the professional confidence to envision a future medical school with the mission to train physicians to work in local communities with culturally diverse populations.

Florida International University: Academic Policies and Procedures

Ethnographic skills were invaluable in documenting behaviors, beliefs, practices and the organization's priorities. FIU, being a relatively young university, primarily communicated orally without university written plans or policies. My ethnographic skills of recording behaviors, compiling historical documents, and interviewing people about how things worked, empowered me to become the compiler and editor of the first set of undergraduate and graduate policy manuals (Wiedman 1993). My training as a participant-observer enabled me to move among the various administrative divisions and academic units inquiring about how things were done and if they had written policies. Good human relation skills facilitated the approval of these policies by the faculty, the Faculty Senate, the Deans, and the Provost. This was a time when the internet was just beginning, and I designed the first university web pages. Approved academic policies posted on the web page facilitated communication of these standardized forms of behavior to students, faculty and staff. By facilitating this transition from oral traditions to written traditions impressed upon me the power of written policies and plans in influencing organizational culture and behavior (Wiedman 1992).

Florida International University: Strategic Planner

Strategic planning was new for universities in the early 1990s. Its purpose was to refine the university's vision, identify strengths within the external environment, assess the opportunities and challenges facing it during the remainder of the twentieth century, and recommend actions to address them. It was during the final stages of 6 years of strategic planning that the goal of a new public medical school that trained local physicians to address the needs of the local community, emerged from faculty, student, staff and community discussions led by the President.

Building upon the university-wide information accumulated for self-study for reaffirmation of accreditation, working with the President and Vice- Presidents, we began to implement SWOT analysis: strengths, weaknesses, opportunities and threats. In 1991 we issued the "1991–1996 Academic Affairs Strategic Plan" which detailed the future of the academic programs. By 1994, the 257 page "Florida International University in the Year 2001: Opportunities and Challenges", compiled detailed future goals and needs of units throughout the University. This was refined in the 1994 "Florida International University on the Threshold of the 21st Century." By 1996, the 54 page "Florida International University: Reaching for the Top," published by the Office of the President, communicated to the public in a succinct format, the strategic vision and future directions of FIU (Wiedman 1994a, b, 1996b). From this foundation of strategic management, every 5 years a planning initative produced another 5-year strategic plan guiding the university unit's goals and behaviors into the future (See https://president.fiu.edu/12694-2/).

My efforts were facilitated by key decision makers. President Modesto Maidique, Ph.D. in electrical engineering and a Professor of Business Management, led the overall strategic planning initiative (Burgelman et al. 2001). Provost and Vice President for Academic Affairs, Professor James A. Mau, had co-edited a book on the Sociology of the Future (Bell and Mau 1971). Historian and Professor of International Relations, Thomas A. Breslin, Vice Provost for Research and Graduate Studies, had years of academic program development experience with health programs (Breslin and Roller 2016). Steven Sauls, Vice President for Community Relations, in the final years communicated the planning details to the Executive Board, community stakeholders, and state politicians. Historical trend information about aspects of the university, faculty, students and community was compiled with the support of the Office of Institutional Research. Each administrative unit projected its goals and needs for years to come.

Through numerous focus group sessions led by the President, we heard from various internal and external stakeholders. As I organized, recorded, and computerized these dialogs, recurrent concerns and visions emerged. Being a public regional university, the vision emerged to become a research university. What academic programs, faculty expertise, staffing, buildings and budgets would be needed to do this? With the Office of Institutional Research, we generated many different scenarios. Identifying public urban research universities that we strove to be like, we gathered benchmark institutional characteristics that led to their success. Over this 6-year process the vision was succinctly communicated in five words: Top, Public, Urban, Research University.

As we neared completion we widely circulated a draft of the strategic plan. Four themes identified the directions for the future of the university: International, Urban, Environment, and Information. In several more presidential focus groups we heard ways to improve and refine the future vision. At this time there was a strong voice from the health faculty in our many allied health disciplines for the addition of health as a strategic theme. This was supported by institutional evidence: each of the benchmarked universities had a medical school.

Following the series of forums, my summary report to the Provost and President contained this justification for the elevation of "Health" to the major academic themes:

> Prevention of disease and wellness is a major national focus now, not traditional medicine. Emphasis is on care of the chronically ill in home and community, outside of institutions and hospitals. Health and medicine are different issues. With strong nursing and public health programs we can successfully excel in community health issues. A Medical School could develop with distributed training of M.D.s in various facilities, not necessarily in the traditional teaching hospital. We already have a large number of faculty and resources devoted to health. (Wiedman 1996a)

It was at this point that my background as a medical anthropologist became very influential. By compiling, then circulating the concept paper and text section of "Reaching for the Top", the vision of what the future medical school could become famous for was accepted. This vision for a medical school could have been excluded from consideration at this point. Other scenarios were being discussed for the future medical school such as "Tropical Health" which was removed from consideration since it was already a well developed area of study, and other universities were leaders in the topic. FIU wanted to be best at new cutting edge academic programs.

My years of experience at the community level of health care from Native American traditional healing and urban Indian clinic, to directing culturally appropriate health care using the Hazel Weidman culture broker model, gave me the confidence to use my authoritative role to influence the selection of community-based care as the strategic foundation for the establishment of a medical school that trained physicians with this community perspective and level of care.

The "Health Theme" section specifically noted the characteristics of a future medical school that would not adopt a traditional model of a teaching hospital, but rather would develop clinical training through a network of hospitals and community-based settings in order to train culturally responsive physicians. Historically, since the 1940s, medical schools increasingly followed the Johns Hopkins' model of medical students being trained in a teaching and research hospital. Often these are many miles from the main university campus, thus isolating the medical school faculty from the breadth of academic engagement.

FIU Medical School's emphasis on training minority students and culturally competent medicine fit well with *Reaching for the Top*'s management philosophy of "Diversity;" where differences among all people are celebrated as a source of rich creativity and innovation (Wiedman 1996b). The resulting university strategic plan, "Reaching for the Top," expressed it this way:

> In building upon these disciplines FIU can take advantage of the surrounding urban community to prepare the next generation of health care professionals and primary care physicians for practice in diverse community settings. With the national de-emphasis on highly technical specialty training, and reemphasis on prevention and primary care at the community level, FIU has the opportunity to be a unique innovator of curricula and interdisciplinary programs which groom health professionals and physicians to focus on the general health and primary care needs of people, especially those in the under-served urban community. In addressing this trend, rather than adopting a traditional model of a teaching hospital, FIU has the opportunity to develop clinical training through a network of

hospitals and other community-based settings. FIU is located in a diverse multicultural community comprised of persons of a variety of ethnic backgrounds and countries of origin. (Wiedman 1996b: 11)

Knowing anthropology theory I was able to direct organizational culture change by organizing information, symbols, and people in ways that influenced the allocation of resources and facilitated change in directions consistent with the goal of the organization. For example, applying cultural theme theory (Opler 1945), I purposefully worked to build a consensus around specific words and phrases that would clearly communicate shared meanings and motivate future behaviors (Wiedman 2000b). Five academic themes guided the development of academic teaching, research, and service programs; two management philosophies led the ways in which administrative units strived to excel. Working with the health faculty, we formulated the "health" academic theme and a vision for the university's future health programs, including a new medical school.

Recognizing the similarities and differences between organizational and management cultures can be effective in solving human problems by influencing decision—making, planning, and policy development. These can be viewed as sociocultural adaptations to a changing environment. The strategic planning initiative that led to the medical school came at a time when the invention and diffusion of electronic information technology was revolutionizing the communication patterns, decision-making, and authority structures of the workplace and of organizations. Strategic planning is a conscious, purposeful effort to influence the future. To be successful at these efforts, we must consider the organization's external environment, especially the political, economic, and demographic context. The holistic perspective enables the anthropologist practitioner to excel at identifying and assessing the importance of these macro influences as well as the micro processes of human interactions and beliefs (Wiedman 2013).

Florida International University: Medical School Concept Committee

To conceptualize a new medical school is just the beginning, to have it approved, funded and initiated is another. Recruiting faculty to build the foundation for the new medical school began at this time in 1996. In the years following the publication of *Reaching for the Top*, division, unit, and academic department directors began to align their budgets and new personnel hires with the university's strategic initiatives. The Medical School Concept Committee met occasionally for years detailing the various parts of the university that would need to be enhanced and expanded in order for a medical school to be established. Led by Dr. Thomas A. Breslin, Vice President for Research, I continued to represent Academic Affairs on this committee as we met with representatives from health-related academic disciplines and local hospitals that had an interest in affiliating with FIU. We strengthened the information necessary to convincingly state the viability and need for a new medical school. By reviewing the staffing of the academic programs required for a medical school, we focused on such things as where to add and strengthen faculty, laboratories, and library resources. Additions and strengthening were to be accomplished incrementally over the years so that at a future time when the medical school was publicly requested, we would already have much of the health-related faculty and program infrastructure in place.

Primary among these planning discussions in the Medical School Concept Committee was the need for physicians to serve the culturally diverse populations of South Florida. This need could be best met by focusing the curriculum on training community-based physicians, not specialists, and by recruiting and graduating a diverse array of minority students. FIU was already a national leader in graduating minority students. Data indicated that the nearing-retirement age of South Florida physicians would soon create a critical shortage and that a large percentage of physicians were trained elsewhere, especially at Caribbean medical schools. This kind of data further refined the goal to recruit students who would more likely stay in the area to serve the South Florida health needs. This helped justify the FIU Medical School and differentiate the FIU Medical School from the University of Miami Medical School and Nova Southeastern College of Osteopathic Medicine. The Medical School Concept Committee continued for years until a professional medical school planner was hired to coordinate the effort.

It took 10 years to initiate the medical school after the 1996 initial plan. FIU's President and administrators needed to convince the Florida Board of Regents that a new medical school was needed in Florida, and most challenging was the medical school accrediting body that had not approved a new medical school in some years. The public announcement to initiate the Wertheim College of Medicine came before the Board of Regents in July 2004; approval was received in 2006.

Among the first faculty to be hired was anthropologist Dr. Iveris Martinez who initiated and led the "Medicine and Society" curriculum and programs. Inviting her as a guest speaker in my medical anthropology course, we began to share our experiences with planning and implementing the medical school resulting in this edited book. Her Chap. 13 on the implementation of the medical school complements this chapter on the envisioning and planning of the medical school (Wiedman and Martinez 2017). A fuller discussion and interviews with key medical school founders is presented in the 2016 book: *Anatomy of a Dream: The Making of the FIU Herbert Wertheim College of Medicine,* edited by Thomas A. Breslin and Barbra A. Roller (Breslin and Roller 2016; Wiedman 2016).

It is important for anthropology practitioners to maintain their "anthropologist" identities by being active in professional organizations. It is easy to identify yourself to others with the job title and role, diminishing or hiding the anthropologist. For good mental health, networking, and career longevity, I purposefully brought my research, planning and administrative skills to the benefit of anthropology professional organizations. These experiences benefited my university employer, my publications on directing organizational culture change, and recognition as an applied and practicing anthropologist. As treasurer of the Society for Applied Anthropology, I worked to refine the SfAA vision and goals (Bennett et al. 1999).

In 2001, I was elected to the practicing and professional seat on the Executive Board of the American Anthropological Association (AAA). This was a time when practicing anthropology was being recognized by the AAA, and I successfully proposed a number of organizational changes that would promote practitioners' inclusion in AAA conferences and membership. The Career Expo at annual conferences is one example where faculty and students can speak face-to-face with experienced practitioners in a multitude of employment areas. This 3-year term was followed by my 2006–2008 term as President of the National Association for the Practice of Anthropology. NAPA, a section of the AAA, supports anthropologists employed in professional positions outside of academic departments. As NAPA President, I strived for inclusion of anthropologists employed in practicing anthropology professions. The establishment of the Ethnographic Praxis in Industry Conference (EPIC), affiliated anthropologists employed in industrial, design and engineering corporations. Anthropologists in occupational health collaborated to initiate the NAPA/OT Fieldschool in Guatemala that is AAA sponsored. Both EPIC and the NAPA/OT Fieldschool continue today. In both leadership positions, on the AAA Executive Board and NAPA Presidency, I used the directing-culture-change lessons learned in university planning, policy development, program evaluation and leadership.

After moving from central FIU administration in 2004, to a faculty position as a clinical associate professor in the Anthropology/Sociology Department, I shared these applied and practicing career experiences with Ph.D. students and by regularly teaching undergraduate medical anthropology to predominantly pre-med and health majors. With the merging of cultural geographers, the department transformed to the Department of Global and Sociocultural Studies offering Ph.D. tracks in Sociology, Anthropology or Geography. Rarely do practicing anthropologists move to a full-time faculty position in a Ph.D. granting department later in their career. I am honored to have been part of the team that planned the future of public higher education and research in my hometown of Miami and Southeast Florida.

Lessons from the Perspective of a Planner

Biomedical Hegemony

Biomedical hegemony continues to be a challenge for anthropologists working in medical schools, even one with a strong mission for change, such as that of the FIU Medical School. From my view as a medical anthropologist, who helped conceptualize this new medical school focused on training community-based, culturally sensitive physicians, I am aware of the threat of a shift back to the traditional medical school curriculum with an emphasis on the biomedical model of disease, emphasizing biology and disease. This is especially challenging when student outcomes must be assessed with certification, licensing, and accrediting standards. Questions repeatedly arise of what must be taught in the curriculum for medical students to pass these assessment standards. Every time the curriculum is questioned by faculty, and by the students, the social and cultural aspects of the curriculum are threatened. For the health of our multicultural community, it would be disappointing to see a de-emphasis on the sociocultural dimensions of health. Patient-centered curriculum instilling cultural humility enables FIU trained physicians to effectively communicate, build trusting relationships, improve patient compliance, and health outcomes. There is also the risk of physicians assuming that they can adequately train medical students on matters of culture and cross-cultural communication and that anthropologists are not necessary. Ultimately, the success and longevity of anthropological engagement in any medical school will depend on broader engagement of the discipline of anthropology with medicine.

Value of Ethnography and Methods

Ethnographic skills are invaluable in documenting behaviors, beliefs, practices and an organization's priorities. FIU, being a relatively young university at the beginning of the Internet, primarily communicated orally without university written plans or policies. In this young university the accreditation requirements forced academic subcultures to develop written traditions, thus making explicit what was implicit when orally communicated (Wiedman 1992). My ethnographic skills of recording behaviors, compiling historical documents, and interviewing people about how things work, empowered me to become the compiler and editor of the first set of undergraduate and graduate policy manuals. Good human relations skills, an understanding of social structure, social organization, and culture change facilitated the building of a consensus for approval of the various sections of the university strategic plan. For example, engaging, listening, recording, and synthesizing the narratives, concerns, and future visions expressed by the health-related faculty in diverse disciplines was key to envisioning a new medical school. Understanding linguistic and cognitive processes facilitated the creation of words and symbols for prioritizing contested values for portraying a shared future vision built on acceptable cultural themes (Wiedman 1990b; Wiedman and Martinez 2017).

Maintaining an Anthropologist Professional Role and Identity

Often anthropologists lose their identities as anthropologists and begin to identify with their job title. I experienced this conundrum. During the 14 years I worked in the Provost's Office, while I was considered an administrator, I consciously maintained my professional identity by consistently introducing myself as an anthropologist—a practicing anthropologist, and by continuing to be engaged in anthropology professional organizations and conferences. Describing this experience in the *Anthropology Newsletter* in 1994 (republished in 2001), I described the value of anthropology in this way: "If one views anthropology as the study of humans in all their complexities throughout time and in all places, then anthropological theories and methods should be replicable and useful in any human situation, not only among exotic and distant peoples, but in our own society and institutions as well" (Wiedman 2000b: 99).

A major challenge to maintaining a professional role is the ability to thrive in ambiguous roles and to sacrifice one's individual recognition to the good of the organization. Most of what is produced by a staff member will not have your name on it. It will be disseminated under either your boss's name or that of the unit as a whole, often with no acknowledgment of authorship at all. For example, the Office of the President is noted as the author of the university strategic plan: "Reaching for the Top". This is counter to the emphasis that academic faculty place on the authorship of publications, journal articles, and books. In a unit staff position, you will be paid for your contribution to the university and unit; individual recognition comes only with continued employment, career advancement opportunities, occasional employee recognition awards, and most importantly, salary merit increases.

To maintain an identity as an anthropologist, for long-term career development, and mental wellbeing, it is wise to attend the yearly conference associated with a professional group, to be a presenter at the conference, and to be an active committee member or elected officer. This enables you to keep abreast of the state of the art in the field, to bring back best practice information to your job, and to build networks of experts you can call upon for advice. By being active and engaged in the professional organization related to your job title, you can bring recognition to your university, improve your understanding of the common issues facing those in your career, and enhance the quality of your own organization. By attending conferences, making presentations, and serving on committees you become nationally recognized, enhancing your employability within your university and also increasing your opportunities for moving to another university for career advancement. Some professionals build a reputation in a specific area, enabling them to be asked to come to a university to improve operations quickly. As consultants, or as full time employees, these change agents do not have the historical baggage that sometimes prevents tough decisions from being made.

Applying Anthropological Theory and Directing Organizational Culture

Knowing anthropology theory we can organize information, symbols, and people in ways that influence the allocation of resources and facilitate change in directions consistent with the goal of the organization (Wiedman 1990b, 1998, 2000b). For example, applying cultural theme theory (Opler 1945), I purposefully refined specific words and phrases that would clearly communicate shared meanings and motivate future behaviors. Five academic themes guided the development of academic teaching, research, and service programs; two management philosophies led the ways in which administrative units strived to excel. To provide an example: working with the health faculty, we formulated the "health" academic theme and a vision for the university's future health programs, including a new medical school.

Anthropologists can succeed in influential positions of authority and power. Anthropologists who recognize the similarities and differences between organizational and management cultures can be effective in solving human problems by influencing decision—making, planning, and policy development. These can be viewed as sociocultural adaptations to a changing environment (Wiedman 2000a). The strategic planning initiative that led to the medical school came at a time when the invention and diffusion of electronic information technology was revolutionizing the communication patterns, decision-making, and authority structures of the workplace and of organizations. Strategic planning is a conscious, purposeful effort to influence the future. To be successful at these efforts, we must consider the organization's external environment, especially the political, economic, and demographic context. The holistic perspective enables the anthropologist practitioner to excel at identifying and assessing the importance of these macro influences as well as the micro processes of human interactions and beliefs (Wiedman 2013).

Anthropologists have a holistic perspective that allows us to conceptualize the role of an organizational unit within the overall social institution and to understand the changing demands placed upon it and the changing environments within which it must operate. Our understanding of "culture" and human diversity as anthropologists enables us to conceptualize, observe, and explain how diverse people in a workplace can enhance quality while adapting to social processes and changing environments. As experts in human behavior, we can work with a wide array of people and even take the proactive role of culture change agents. Our ability to observe people and systems enables us to make good observations, and to write up our recommendations for systems improvements and enhanced efficiencies. These reports are most important in relation to program improvements and justifications for funding. A proactive way for a practicing anthropologist to influence organizational change is to be the President, Provost, Vice President, Dean, Faculty Senate and Union leader. Become involved, lead university committees, task forces, and special projects that address critical issues. These are often positions of power within an organization where social structures are changed and cultural themes modified, resulting in new plans, policies, procedures, organizational units, and employment roles. By continually demonstrating the usefulness of our anthropological skills, we can be given further responsibilities with opportunities for leadership and power within medical schools and universities.

Conclusion

This autoethnography highlights key professional experiences that empowered an anthropologist with political and academic authority to influence decisions and plans for a new medical school uniquely suited for pioneering community-oriented medical education. Brought up in Miami, I was very familiar with Southeast Florida history, peoples, and issues. Having conducted applied social science research on critical Southeast Florida issues, and directing UM Department of Psychiatry community clinical care provided first-hand knowledge to envision a medical school focused on multicultural South Florida.

At the individual level, this story demonstrates a variety of skills, perspectives, and values useful for practicing anthropology in a wide array of employment roles. They include a holistic theoretical perspective using systems and culture theme theory, expertise in social and culture change processes, leadership and management skills, ability to move among very different cultural groups and social hierarchies, while thriving in ambiguous and tense social roles. Skills involved using a wide array of research methods from classic ethnography, participant-observation, surveys, focus groups, applications of computer technologies, big data management and analysis. A well rounded and integrated theoretical understanding of cognitive, social, and material theory enables predictions at multiple levels of human behavior. Of importance is the ability to gather and integrate complex social, cultural and psychological data/theory into succinct and brief concepts that could be easily understood in written, spoken, policy, and visual presentations. At the personal level, good interpersonal relations, a positive attitude, and a strong value for inclusion of marginal groups and minorities were necessary. Most importantly, among these include the value of ethnographic writing and analysis, the holistic perspective, surviving in ambiguous social roles, and maintaining one's identity as an "anthropologist" while practicing anthropology in medical settings and university administration.

One must view these institutional and personal career trajectories as part of larger cultural changes in medicine and health. By the 1960s and 1970s, the growing disillusionment and dissatisfaction with the mainstream medical profession, a shift to community health emerged, along with re-valuing the importance of general and primary care practice in medical schools. New departments for the medical behavioral sciences formed in medical schools across the country to address the humanistic communication gaps between medical institutions, patients, and the communities they targeted for health provision and research. FIU's medical school espoused these values of community-oriented health care from the very start.

Acknowledgements External reader of the initial manuscript, Dr. Catherine Mas, greatly improved the focus and larger historical contexts. A final review by Dr. Thomas A. Breslin verified historical accuracy, and my wife Felicia made the text much more readable.

References

Adams, Tony E., Stacy Holman Jones, and Carolyn Ellis. 2014. *Autoethnography: autoethnography*. Oxford: Oxford University Press.

Baugh, Timothy, Julia Jordon, Dennis Wiedman, et al. 1982. *From generation to generation: The Plains Apache way. Museum Exhibit which toured the central United States 1982–1990+.* Norman, OK: Plains Apache Tribe and Stovall Museum of Science and History.

Bell, Wendell A., and James A. Mau, eds. 1971. *The sociology of the future: Theory, cases, and annotated bibliography*. New York: Russell Sage.

Bennett, Linda, Dennis Wiedman, and Linda Whiteford. 1999. *Society for Applied Anthropology mission, vision and goals*. www.sfaa.net/sfaagoal.html

Breslin, Thomas A., and Barbra A. Roller, eds. 2016. *Anatomy of a dream: The making of the FIU Herbert Wertheim College of Medicine, 2006–2016*. Gainesville: University of Florida Press.

Burgelman, Robert, Modesto Maidique, and Steven Wheelwright. 2001. *Strategic management of technology and innovation*. Boston: McGraw-Hill/Irwin.

Herbert Wertheim College of Medicine (HWCOM). 2015. *Herbert Wertheim college of medicine strategic plan 2015–2020: collaborate, act, transform*. Miami, Florida International University.

——— 2020. *Herbert Wertheim college of medicine mission, vision, and values*. https://medicine.fiu.edu/about/mission-vision-values/index.html. Accessed Nov 18, 2020.

Himburg, Susan, Tom Syracuse, Mary Free and Dennis Wiedman, comps. and eds. 1999. *Florida International University: 1998–2000 self-study for reaffirmation of Accreditation by the Southern Association of Colleges and Schools*. Miami: Florida International University. December 1, 1999. 493 pages plus appendices.

Kravitz, Sanford, Dennis Wiedman, and Scott Kass, eds. 1990. *Excellence and diversity. Ten-year reaffirmation of accreditation self-study*, 423 pages. Miami, FL: Florida International University.

Lefley, Harriet P., and Evalina W. Bestman. 1991. Public-academic linkages for culturally sensitive community mental health. *Community Mental Health Journal* 27 (6): 473–488.

Martinez, Iveris L. 2015. Integrating anthropology in medical education: Opportunities, challenges and lessons. *Practicing Anthropology* 37 (1): 35–39.

Mas, Catherine. 2019. *The culture brokers: medicine and anthropology in global Miami.* Doctoral Dissertation. Department of history, program in the history of science and medicine, Yale University.

Opler, Morris. 1945. Themes as dynamic forces in culture. *American Journal of Sociology* 51 (3): 198–206.

Rush, John, Robert Hill, William Stanhope, Paul Costiloe, and Dennis Wiedman. 1977. *Psychosocial assessment of firefighters injuries and disabilities: A pilot study*. Submitted to the Oklahoma City Fire Department and Firefighters Union.

Stein, Howard, and Robert Hill. 1978. *Ethnic imperative: Examining the new white ethnic movement*. University Park, PA: Pennsylvania State University Press.

Sussex, James, and Hazel H. Weidman. 1975. Toward responsiveness in mental health care. *Psychiatric Annals* 5 (8): 8–9.

Weidman, Hazel, and Janice Egeland. 1978. *Miami health ecology project report, parts I and II*. Miami: University of Miami.

West, Kelly. 1974. Diabetes in American Indians and other native populations of the new world. *Diabetes* 23: 841–855.

Wiedman, Dennis. 1979. *Diabetes mellitus and Oklahoma native Americans: A case study of culture change in Oklahoma Cherokee*. Ph.D. Dissertation, University of Oklahoma. Ann Arbor: University Microfilms International.

———. 1984. Directing geriatric health care: Some practical issues. *Practicing Anthropology* 6 (3): 7–8.

———, ed. 1986. *Ethnohistory: A researcher's guide. Studies in third world societies* (Vol. 35). Williamsburg, VA: College of William and Mary.

———. 1987. Type II diabetes mellitus, technological development and the Oklahoma Cherokee. In *Encounters with biomedicine: Case studies in medical anthropology*, ed. Hans Baer, 43–71. New York: Gordon and Breech Science.

———. 1990a. Big and little moon peyotism as health care delivery systems. *Medical Anthropology* 12 (4): 371–387.

———. 1990b. University accreditation: Academic subcultural and organizational responses to directed change. In *Crosscultural management and organizational culture*, ed. Tomoka Hamada and Ann Jordan, 227–246, 42 pages. Williamsburg, VA: Studies in Third World Societies.

———, ed. and comp. 1991. *1991–1996 academic affairs strategic plan*. Miami, FL: Florida International University.

———. 1992. Effects on academic culture of shifts from oral to written traditions: The case of university accreditation. *Human Organization* 51 (4): 398–407.

———, ed. and comp. 1993. *Academic affairs policies and procedures: Division of academic affairs, Florida International University*, 380 pages.

———, ed. and comp. 1994a. *Florida International University in the year 2001: Opportunities and challenges*. 2nd, 257 pages. Miami: Florida International University. (University Strategic Plan).

———, ed. and comp. 1994b. *Florida International University on the threshold of the 21st century*, 109 pages. Miami: Florida International University. Dennis Wiedman, ed. and comp. (University Strategic Planning Document).

——— 1996a. *Questions or suggested refinements from the presidential forums on FIU reaching for the top. February 13, 1996*. Four-page summary by Dennis Wiedman for review by Provost James Mau. Unpublished notes. Miami.

———, ed. and comp. 1996b. *Reaching for the top: Florida International University*. Miami: Florida International University. (University Strategic Plan).

———. 1998. Effective strategic planning roles for anthropologists. *Practicing Anthropology* 20 (1): 36–39.

———. 1999. Celebrating diversity at FIU: A role model for the future of U.S. higher education. *Journal for the Art of Teaching. Special Issue: Diversity in Education* 6 (1): 37–46.

———. 2000a. "Best practices" compared to strategic management and total quality management: A new paradigm or an incremental change in management culture. *High Plains Applied Anthropologist* 20 (2): 146–152. (Now known as "*The Applied Anthropologist*.").

———. 2000b. Directing organizational culture change through strategic planning and leadership. In *Careers in anthropology: Profiles of practitioner anthropologists*, ed. Paula Sabloff. *NAPA Bulletin* 20: 99–103. (Now known as "*Annals of anthropological practice*"). Washington, DC: American Anthropological Association.

———. 2010. Globalizing the chronicities of modernity: Diabetes and the metabolic syndrome. In *Chronic conditions, fluid states: Chronicity and the anthropology of illness*, ed. L. Manderson and C. Smith-Morris, 38–53. New Brunswick: Rutgers University Press.

———. 2012a. Native American embodiment of the chronicities of modernity: Reservation food, diabetes and the metabolic syndrome among the Kiowa, Comanche and Apache. *Medical Anthropology Quarterly* 26 (4): 595–612.

———. 2012b. Upholding Indigenous freedoms of religion and medicine: Peyotists at the 1906–1908 Oklahoma constitutional convention and first legislature. *American Indian Quarterly* 36 (2): 215–246.

———. 2013. Anthropologists working in higher education. In *Handbook of practicing anthropology*, ed. Riall Nolan, 184–195. New York: Wiley/Blackwell.

———. 2014. Chronicities of modernity and the contained body as an explanation for the global pandemic of obesity, diabetes and the metabolic syndrome. In *Controversies in obesity*, ed. Haslam David, Arya M. Sharma, and Carel W. le Roux, 109–115. London: Springer.

———. 2016. Strategic planning. In *History of the Florida International University Medical School*, ed. Thomas Breslin and Barbra Roller. Gainesville: University of Florida Press.

Wiedman, Dennis, and Iveris L. Martinez. 2017. Organizational cultural theme theory and analysis of the strategic planning for a new medical school. *Human Organization 76* (3): 264–274.

Dennis W. Wiedman, PhD, is Professor of Anthropology, Department of Global and Sociocultural Studies. Florida International University. Miami, Florida. He received his Ph.D. in Anthropology from the University of Oklahoma in 1979 where he trained in medical anthropology at the University of Oklahoma College of Medicine. Employment in the Department of Psychiatry at the University of Miami School of Medicine in the Office of Transcultural Education and Research grounded him in clinical anthropology as Director of a Department of Psychiatry community mental health unit. He is the Founding Director of the FIU Global Indigenous Forum with the mission to bring the Indigenous voice to FIU, South Florida, and the world. His research interests include Native American health, organizational culture, applying anthropology, and directing culture change. He specializes in social and cultural factors for the global pandemic of Type II diabetes and metabolic syndrome. He teaches courses in medical anthropology, anthropological theory, and ethnohistorical research methods. During more than a decade in the FIU Provost Office he was the Assistant to the Provost, University Accreditation Officer and first Director of Program Review. As lead strategic planner for the university's first major strategic plan he had a key role in planning and envisioning the new FIU Medical school incorporating medical anthropology principles and a community focus. He served on the Executive Board of the American Anthropological Association (AAA) in the practicing/professional seat, and was President of the National Association for the Practice of Anthropology (NAPA). Throughout these academic, applied, and practicing leadership experiences, he consistently published on organizational culture theory and analysis in leading journals and book chapters.

Part II
Beyond Cultural Competency

Chapter 7
Participatory Anthropology for Teaching Behavioral Sciences at a Medical School in Zambia

Mutale Chileshe

Introduction

Worldwide increases in global migration and trade have made communicable diseases a concern throughout the world. In addition, the increase in diseases with behavioral or social components is staggering and have highlighted the connections in health and medicine among and between continents. Heart disease, stroke, cancer, and other chronic Non-communicable Diseases (NCDs) kill 41 million people each year, equivalent to 71% of all deaths, globally (WHO 2018). In response to the increasing diversity of social problems and communicable and non-communicable diseases around the world, present and future doctors need to be fully equipped and trained not only in biological problems, but in the behavioral model of health care (Nilambar et al. 2005; Foucault 1994). This model of care expects the doctor to be an effective communicator and an ethical practitioner of the art and science of medicine, (Ha et al. 2010) who trains himself or herself, in the study of the cultural, economic, political and psychosocial aspects alongside the biological determinants of health and disease (Farmer 2003; Foucault 1994). This doctor should be able to extend healthcare beyond the patient to include the family and community and emphasize as much on the prevention of illness and promotion of health as on the treatment of disease (Alsan et al. 2011; Institute of Medicine 2003; WHO 1996). To achieve this, anthropologists need to play a critical role in the changing world of medicine (Ashraf 2009) because health does not depend on medical knowledge alone (Farmer 2003). There are other important factors such as impact of socioeconomic and cultural factors and lifestyle characteristics on health and illness.

Anthropology, Psychology, Sociology and the Humanities in general provide good tools to assess, understand, and appreciate the role of these factors in health and

---

M. Chileshe (✉)
Public Health Unit, Copperbelt University, Michael Chilufya Sata School of Medicine, Ndola, Zambia
e-mail: chileshe.chibangula@gmail.com

I. L. Martinez, D. W. Wiedman (eds.), *Anthropology in Medical Education*,
https://doi.org/10.1007/978-3-030-62277-0_7

disease. This has resulted, over the years, in the formal incorporation of Behavioral Science (BS) teaching in medical school curricula worldwide. In developing nations, however, except for a few instances, many medical schools lack even awareness of the importance of fully incorporating BS. This chapter is based on my experience as an anthropologist teaching BS for the past 4 years in a medical school in Ndola in the Copperbelt Province of Zambia called the Copperbelt University, Michael Chilufya Sata School of Medicine. The purpose of the chapter is twofold. First, to describe as an anthropologist my role, place, pedagogical approaches and strategies implemented in teaching BS, including the challenges faced and overcome. Second, to reflect on the perceptions of medical students regarding BS learning in order to highlight the important contributions that anthropologists make to medical training. Anthropologists can use both the contributions and challenges faced as another stepping stone to foster a positive continuation of the field in medical education. In addition, the chapter can contribute to the literature on BS with the view to start a discussion so that medical education and practice in Zambia, Africa and worldwide can become even more holistic and humane. It is also my hope that my work provides useful insight and positively influences the future careers of anthropologists who are currently engaged or considering a career in medical education.

The Place and Role of an Anthropologist in a School of Medicine

Copperbelt University, Michael Chilufya Sata School of Medicine (CBU SOM) has an integrated curriculum, and was the first medical school in Zambia to introduce a dedicated behavioral sciences component into its curriculum, which runs throughout the medical training.[1] The school started in October 2011 and is one of the three public medical schools in Zambia. There are three other privately run medical schools in Zambia. CBU SOM is the only medical school in Copperbelt Province. The school offers four key undergraduate programs and ten post-graduate programs. The undergraduate programs are Bachelors of Dental Surgery (BDS), Bachelors of Medicine and Surgery (MBChB), Biomedical Sciences (Biomed), and Clinical Medicine (CM). The training duration is 5 years for all degree programs except for CM.[2] The BS course or Society and Medicine as it is popularly known at CBU SOM, is taught longitudinally to all students in the four degree programs though the levels and intensity of the course varies for some programs. For example, BS (hereon

[1]Other medical schools in Zambia have what they call community medicine but this is taught only to preclinical students.

[2]CBU SOM is one of ten schools under the Copperbelt University which is the Parent University located in Kitwe on Jumbo Drive in Riverside. Ninety percent of the students enrolled at CBU SOM are selected from a cohort of the best students at the parent university who have spent 1 or 2 years studying natural sciences. The other 10% is selected from the best of students who have a 2 year study of A levels in Zambia or abroad, the best Diploma holders of dental/clinical medicine and individuals with degrees in any of the sciences.

society and medicine) is taught only in the third year of the Biomed program. BDS and CM students stop learning society and medicine after the fourth year of their training while MBChB students learn society and medicine throughout their sixth year of medical training except in fifth year. Therefore, this means that the MBChB program society and medicine is taught to both preclinical and clinical students. Presently, like many other universities (Rajapakse et al. 2014; Humayun and Herbert 2011; Dogra and Karnik 2003) that offer behavioral sciences, the term is an all-inclusive term for a wide spectrum of diverse topics. However, the topics covered by the Society and Medicine course at CBU SOM are summarized as follows:

Basic behavioral sciences I and II: the students learn about mind-body interactions which focuses on the interaction between biological, behavioral, psychological, and social factors which contribute to health issues. Students also learn about personality, memory and intelligence, learning, good medical practice, and relationship dynamics. This module helps students to understand behaviors that put patients at risk and offers them the ability to think about developing interventions for behavior change and to discriminate between technically possible and morally permissible interventions.

Communication skills: offers students skills to effectively communicate not only with patients but with communities, families, colleagues, and friends. It teaches students proper assessment of scenarios focusing on effective implementation of communication, while promoting the student's expressive skills.

Personal development: promotes identification, development, and application of skills to optimize learning not only in class, but outside class so that the student can have a productive medical career. Management and basic entrepreneurship skills are taught in this module with the aim of impacting good leadership and management skills and behaviors necessary for interaction with colleagues and as health professionals. The module also works at improving personal well-being while promoting good attitudes and thinking skills.

Medical ethics: creates awareness about ethical issues and the application of principles of medical ethics with special emphasis on cultural issues. The module offers students the ability to analyze ethical issues and possible ways to successfully resolve such issues while promoting ethical behavior.

Social and cultural issues in health care: provides appropriate care to patients with differing social, cultural, and economic backgrounds. The module also encourages students to think about their own personal background, beliefs and attitudes and how these can influence patient care.

Basic health information technology: keeps up with new technologies knowledge for effective health care and for their whole life (Fig. 7.1).

Generally, the society and medicine course provides a framework for considering the important questions of health in a thoughtful and evidence-based manner such that students are be able to critically analyze and understand how biological, behavioral, cognitive, socio-cultural, and environmental issues influence health care; and how other factors, such as personal background, health policy and economics, affect physicians' ability to provide optimal care for their patients. The

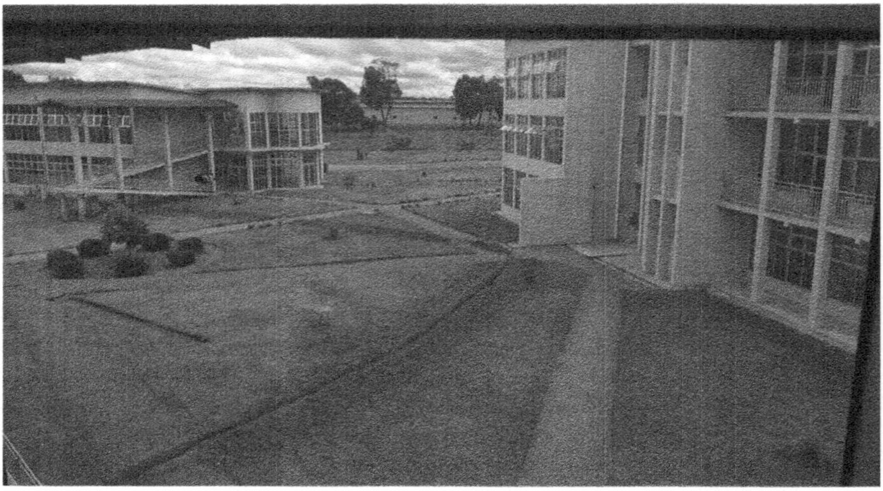

Fig. 7.1 Copperbelt University, Michael Chilufya Sata School of Medicine

course takes an interdisciplinary approach with staff from different disciplines, but I am the only anthropologist. It is important to note that there are very few anthropologists in Zambia and this is due to a number of reasons. One of the main reasons is that no university offers anthropology as a course whether at undergraduate or postgraduate level. The second reason is that "Anthropology as a discipline was considered colonial, something that was used to colonize the continent" (Nkwi 2006: 160). This was because anthropology emerged from the colonial expansion of Europe, thus, colonialism in a negative way structured the development of anthropology as a field in Zambia and some parts of Africa. After independence, African and Africanist anthropologists found it difficult to practice anthropology openly therefore, the discipline was slowly incorporated into sociology.

Anthropology not being offered in universities around Zambia means that it isn't an option for students attending universities in Zambia. In fact, many are unfamiliar with the discipline. This was exactly my experience. Before going to university, I was unfamiliar with anthropology and what exactly it entailed. Throughout my undergraduate studies at the University of Zambia, anthropology was rarely discussed. When discussed, anthropology was concomitant to sociology. All the subjects on kinship, African political and social institutions, ethnography, participant observations, and other subjects with anthropological content were all taught in the department of sociology. In South Africa, anthropology continued to function as a formal discipline at the University of Cape Town and the University of Witswatersrand, as well as at Rhodes and Natal Universities (Nkwi 2006). Today, due to many social problems that developing countries continue to face, the stigma that anthropology suffered has since disappeared. There is an increasing demand (from private and public institutions and non-governmental organizations) for anthropologists to help solve some of the problems Africa is facing. Over the years, anthropologists have made great contributions with research on social economic issues (Chileshe 2008, 2014; Colson 1962), AIDS and sexuality (Hunleth 2011; Chileshe and Bond 2010; Bond 1998, 2006, Bond et al. 2003), and children's health (Hunleth 2011, 2013, 2017). They continue to make contributions and are on high demand.

I first came into contact with 'real' anthropology after my undergraduate training at my first job at ZAMBART Project—a research organization that grew out of a collaboration between the University of Zambia's School of Medicine and the London School of Hygiene and Tropical Medicine established in 1988. ZAMBART conducts multidisciplinary research in the areas of epidemiology, clinical research, social science, laboratory, operations research, health policy analysis, health economics, development communications, counselling, and community based research in TB, HIV and other areas of public health importance. At ZAMBART, I worked under the supervision of an anthropologist, Dr. Virginia Bond. Through my contact with Dr. Bond, I became familiar with anthropology scholars who worked in Zambia, such as Audrey Richards, Henrietta Moore, Megan Vaughan, and Thayer Scudder. Through my association with Dr. Bond, I also met and became inspired by Deborah Crooks, Elizabeth Colson, Jean Hunleth, Lisa Cliggett, Owen Sichone, Pauline Peters and Sandra Wallman. Under the supervision of Dr. Bond, I worked closely with households in rural, peri-urban, and urban areas as well as staff and patients in hospitals and clinics in Zambia. Generally, I worked a lot with vulnerable communities and though I did not know it at that time, I was carrying out ethnographic research and utilising ethnographic techniques in the communities we visited. Through this journey and career progression, I was motivated to become an anthropologist. I studied anthropology at the University of Cape Town in South Africa where I obtained my Masters and Doctorate degrees. Since then, I have worked as a researcher in and outside Zambia using a range of qualitative, ethnographic, and community-based participatory research methods at the individual, family, community, and clinic levels. In 2013, I ventured into teaching and eventually found myself at CBU SOM.

At CBU SOM with various strengths from an interdisciplinary team, we work together as a team to train physicians in a manner that provides students with the skills to be successful practitioners in the modern changing environment. Typically, a behavioral science team includes fields like sociology, economics, public health, anthropology, law and ethics, demography, and political science. For better utilization of resources, the society and medicine team was comprised of two psychologist, a pastor, a lawyer,[3] and an anthropologist. Economic, public health and demography related issues are covered by the public health team. Overall, we encourage a shift from episodic care of individuals in hospitals to a continuous and comprehensive care that incorporates a biopsychosocial mode (Kleinman et al. 2006; Kleinman 1983) in the prevention and promotion of health in the community (Jones et al.

[3]Lawyer, Ms. Kateule Chitupila, from the legal aid volunteers to teach studies law and medicine and ethics.

2001). One of our aims is to have a course that is more "student centered, with an emphasis on active learning rather than on the passive acquisition of knowledge" (ibid: 700) and to achieve that we encourage a type of learning that focuses on problem solving rather than transmission of information without context.

As an anthropologist, I play a number of roles at CBU SOM and some of them are research, administrative duties, and teaching both undergraduate and postgraduate students. At CBU SOM, society and medicine falls under Public Health. As head of the Public Health Unit and coordinator of the society and medicine course, my role is to ensure that the courses in all the degree programs run smoothly. My role in undergraduate education is to teach society and medicine, and educate socially responsible and culturally competent medical practitioners to serve and practice in underserved and multicultural communities (Martinez 2015; Tervalon and Murray-Garcia 1998). My major contributions in teaching society and medicine are in communication skills (especially communicating with communities), medical ethics, social and cultural issues in health care. Apart from the three listed areas of contribution, I also try in some way to allow students to see the connection between food insecurity and health. Food insecurity is associated with poor health outcomes, yet is not routinely addressed in health care (Smith et al. 2017).

The Structure of Modern Medical Education

In order to discuss my teaching role as an anthropologist at CBU SOM, preliminary background is required to understand the structure of modern medical education as a whole and the organization of the society and medicine course. Training in modern medical education is usually done in two phases, the theoretical phase and the clinical phase. During the first 2 years at CBU SOM, students are taught within the university classroom where theoretical and experimental training is provided. The last 3 years focus on clinical medicine, or the practical part of training as a doctor or a dentist. It involves working in different hospitals in Copperbelt Province with a team of qualified doctors. Through this method, students learn medicine by apprenticeship- by watching and doing under instruction. During this period, students receive morning lecturers, tutorials and seminars in medical science, dental science, and review the materials taught in the first 2 years. The two phases correspond to different educational needs that have to be met when teaching communication skills, medical ethics, or social and cultural issues in health care. The first 2 years as stated, happen in the classroom and involve theory. The clinical phase is mainly done in a hospital setting.

Students are taught communication and the different "tribes" (i.e. nurses versus doctors) that exist in a hospital and how the tribes can be embraced for the best interest of the patient. According to global estimates from the World Health Organization (2019), millions of patients die in hospitals because of injuries in their care and as many as 4 in 10 patients are harmed in primary and outpatient health care. Around two-thirds of all adverse events resulting from unsafe care, and the years lost to disability and death occur in low- and middle-income countries (LMICs). The most detrimental errors are related to diagnosis, prescription and the use of medicines. Up to 80% of harm is preventable as it is usually caused by a breakdown in doctor-patient or physician-to-physician communication.

Studying hospital culture through the lens of anthropology offers a way for students to understand, know and think about the best way to prevent medical errors resulting from communication breakdown. Furthermore, hospitals are places of intensity, of life-and-death drama, creating moments of truth, self-discovery and rites of passage not only for the patient but the doctor (Long et al. 2008; van der Geest and Finkler 2004; Wind 2008) and are good sources for students to learn about doctor-patient relationships and components of communication, such as breaking bad news. Overall, even though I use the hospital to teach students, the hospital is only an institution for the practice of medicine and a central agency through which the study of disease is pursued, the boundaries of medicine science widened and skill increased and does not offer many opportunities to teach a holistic approach to health care.

Therefore, to teach clinical students requires a lot of creativity and this is where I play a critical role as an anthropologist. By using various anthropology tools and methods, I create an environment for creative learning, as later explained in this chapter, that helps provide students with the necessary skills for them to function in diverse communities and settings. Unlike other disciplines on the society and medicine team, anthropology brings to the table ethnography which—after many years of research within and outside the hospital—I have found, is especially useful for medical education. This is because simply walking the wards might not be adequate to provide students with the opportunity to effectively practice communication skills and develop cultural competence and neither can it offer an opportunity to develop "a critical consciousness—which places medicine in a social, cultural, and historical context and which is coupled with an active recognition of societal problems and a search for appropriate solutions" (Kumagai and Lypson 2009: 782). Preparing students with skills they need to engage diverse populations in Zambia, Africa, or in the world, generally requires that we provide opportunities for them to completely immerse themselves in settings that are socially, culturally, ethically, and economically diverse (Dao et al. 2017; Hitchins et al. 2014). This is important because the biological human body, as explained by Scheper-Huges and Lock (1987), is also a social and political entity that symbolizes, and is affected by, the inequalities, and power structures of the larger society. Thus, exposing students to different settings provides an opportunity for them to appreciate the fact that human illness occurs in a wider context other than just the doctor's surgery. For the rest of the section, I will show how I use anthropology to contribute to medical education in both the preclinical (in class) and clinical (in the hospital) levels.

In the clinical years through rotations, students are introduced to clinical clerkships in internal medicine, paediatrics, obstetrics and gynaecology, surgery and surgical sub-specialties. The courses are a continuation of the fundamentals of the practice of medicine introduced earlier and a progression from basic science knowledge to application of basic sciences in clinical practice. At this level, students learn

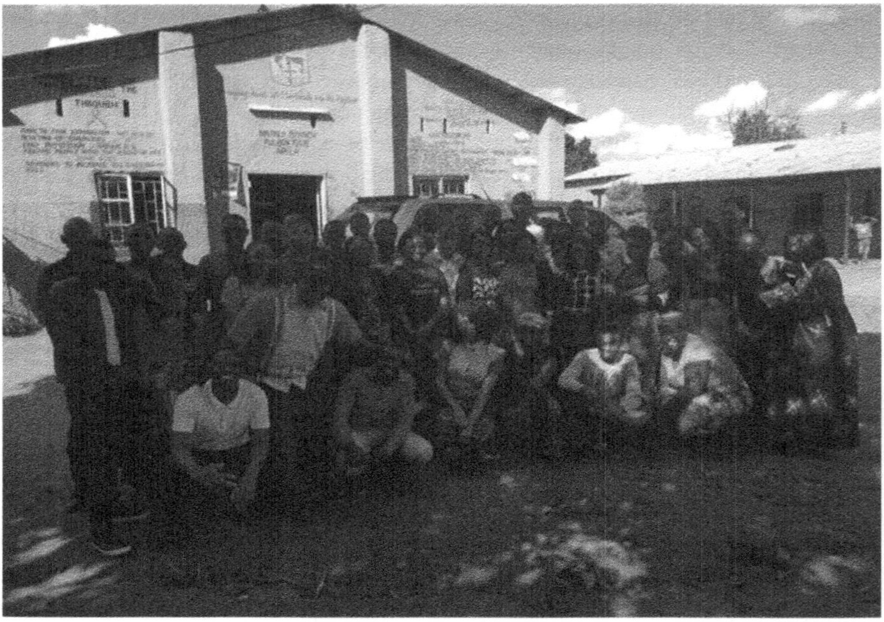

Fig. 7.2 Fourth year students during fieldwork in Mapalo community, Ndola

society and medicine through a rotation by spending one full week with the society and medicine team every term—there are four terms for clinical students in the school calendar. As a team we plan how to teach and effectively utilise the week during our rotation. During this planning, I am given an opportunity as an anthropologist to plan several activities for students. Such activities, for example, can include 2 full days in the hospital doing ethnography or any other creative ways we think may provide an opportunity for students to put the theory learned from the first 2 years of medical training into practice.

Through experience, I have learned that as an anthropologist, one important creative way of teaching medical students is by incorporating field work. It is an exciting and important part of learning for the clinical students. Fieldwork is among the most distinctive practices anthropologists bring to the study of human life in society and this is one of the unique contributions I bring to medical education (Bernard 2006; Atkinson and Hammersley 2004) and to the society and medicine team. Through fieldwork, the anthropologist and the students can seek a detailed and intimate understanding (Strang 2009; Bernard 2006; Spradley 1980) of the science of human behaviour, social actions and relations within the context of illness, health and disease. Through the fieldwork my students get to see different factors (social, cultural, biological and economic) at play in a patient's everyday life. To do this, I provide them with an "embedded" experience, in which they engage with the patient and family members within the hospital walls and with local communities and the families within a particular community (Fig. 7.2).

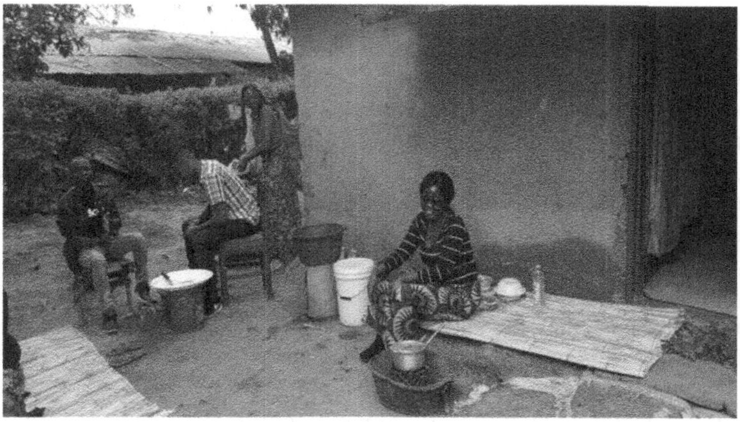

Fig. 7.3 Students taking part in household activities during fieldwork

Communities that we visit with the students are, in most instances, in resource-poor settings. This is because resource-poor areas face numerous health challenges such as, high rates of undernutrition, poor sanitation, high prevalence TB/HIV, diarrheal disease, and malaria (UNICEF 2019; Chileshe 2016). As poverty increases, so do the chances of poor health. Poor health, in turn, traps communities in poverty. It further denies people access to reliable health services and affordable medicines, and causes children to miss out on routine vaccinations.

Ethnography is carried out in local resource-poor communities with students splitting into small groups of three to four. During the first visit, which takes place at the home of the family,[4] students listen to families various stories of life and illness as they unfold during the conversation. The students carry out participant observations by taking part in the families activities from morning until late afternoon and are encouraged to observe and pay attention to the families' social and economic situation and how that might affect the patient's everyday life, including the families' cultural practices (Fig. 7.3).

The participant observation is done under the supervision of faculty and local collaborating home-based caregivers and health practitioners. Students are also encouraged to find answers to the following: *What is unique, different, or interesting about the household visited? Have the meetings between you and the family made any change, and to whom? What is different between the patient visited and the patients you see in the hospital? What have you learned from the family? Reflect on*

[4]I work with different clinics, community members and home based caregivers to identify families where the students can spend time and learn. I visit the homes prior to the student visits to get consent, help build rapport and establish that the home is safe and a good learning ground for my students. Identifying and approaching the communities has over the years become easy because I have worked with them for many years. However, students still get to practice communication skills when introduced to the households as they need to build rapport to make it easy for them to work with the family for a full day or two.

the time you were sick—How is the patient's illness experience similar or different from yours? What have you learned from the interaction? What have you learned about yourself? Are there challenges observed in the households? If so, how do these challenges affect the patient? What are the possible solutions?

At the end of the week, students are required to make a presentation to the class and faculty where the patient's and families' stories are recounted, and the student's own involvement reflected upon. To appraise the extent to which students had obtained the required knowledge from the field, in addition to the presentation, all students write an essay at the end of the rotation. During the presentation, students also discuss the types of communication issues that occurred when interacting with the families and how they felt about the process. They describe what happened and explain how the difficulties made them feel. During the discussions, students also reconsider what they have learned.

The presentations and essays by students reveal that students' appreciation towards the fieldwork and active learning through experiencing and involvement rather than the classroom learning. In response to the questions, "*What is unique, different, or interesting about the household visited?*" and "*What is different between the patient visited and the patients you see in the hospital?*", many students clearly explain that by spending time with the patient in the local community, they improve their skill and ability to see the disease in the context of the patient, the family, and society. Students become familiar with the patient's social and economic networks, their culture, and understand how these influence the illness experience. They also get to see that in some cases, patients miss a doctor's appointment due to limited or lack of economic resources. Households in resource-poor areas not only face illness, but are faced with increasingly difficult choices between essentials and competing expenses such as, food versus healthcare or schooling versus rent (Chileshe 2014; UNAIDS 2006). Thus field work offers a holistic analysis of a patient's illness journey unlike observing a patient in a hospital.

In addition most students, some of whom reluctant to participate in the fieldwork at the beginning, reported to have enjoyed the rewarding interactions/friendships with patients and their families. The learning process helps students to improve their communication skills. Students often report having challenges in communication i.e. language, dress code, and in most cases are unease because they are unsure of how to relate with the family however, by the end of the fieldwork, they are relaxed and easily communicate with the families. Some students request for personal visits to the families' months after fieldwork has ended. Students also report taking many aspects of their lives for granted such as eating three meals in a day, a parent to care for them while sick, being able to have friends, and able to afford medical care. They appreciate and report that they did not realize that they had a lot to be grateful for. Through the field activities, discussions, and presentations, students learn about themselves and about health and illness in practical terms.

The field activities expose students to patients' realities, which in most cases, are different from the students realities. I have come to learn over the years that resource-poor settings are good learning environments for the medical students. Students are usually unaware of the magnitude of the challenges faced by individuals or households in resource-poor settings. Thus, most students experience "cultural shock" when exposed to the realities of the communities. Through this exercise, students get an opportunity to see and learn about causes of poor health, not only for people in Zambia, but for millions of people globally who are rooted in political, social and economic injustices (Sorsha 2018; World Bank 2005; Farmer 2003; Naraya et al. 2000). Ethnography as a powerful teaching tool, helps students to observe these processes play out and map their effects on people.

Another important role as an anthropologist is to ensure that students understand and appreciate that cultural factors play a role in medical practice. Cultural factors, for example, are crucial to diagnosis, treatment, and care in that they shape health-related beliefs, behaviours, and values (Kleinman 1981, 2004). Culture influences the experience of symptoms, the idioms used to report them, decisions about treatment, doctor–patient interactions and much more. To demonstrate, I will give an example of a case experienced in the field.

Sample Case Study: Participant Observation and the Importance of Context

In anthropology most cases are not as simple as what meets the eye. Every case is unique and requires in-depth analysis for better understanding and creating a divide between first glance and prevailing situation. One such example is the case of Judith, who I met in 2017 in Chipulukusu, one of the communities where I work with community health workers and home based caregivers. Judith was a single parent with six children, earning a living by selling vegetables in the streets of Ndola for a commission. One of her six children, Mwansa, was sickly and required assistance to do practically everything. Due to Judith's work, she was unable to provide Mwansa the care she needed. With the other children away at school, Judith used to leave Mwansa locked outside with a plate of food and relied on the neighbors to keep an eye on her while she went around the streets vending. After having made prior arrangements with Judith, who was out vending, I introduced Mwansa to my students in early 2018 (Fig. 7.4).

As earlier stated, on the field the situation is not always as it seems. When I first met Mwansa, I was shocked to learn that she was 18 years-old. When my students met her and learned of her real age, they were equally shocked because to them, Mwansa looked like a 9 year-old child. During our debriefing sessions, students explained that they were concerned about Mwansa's condition. Mwansa was once taken to the hospital but did not return for further investigations and treatment because her mother was busy making a living for her family as the money she earned (about $5) per day from selling vegetables, was not enough to pay for food and transportation to the hospital.

In efforts to help Mwansa, students started a fundraising venture. During their spare time, they washed cars for faculty members at CBU SOM, who generously

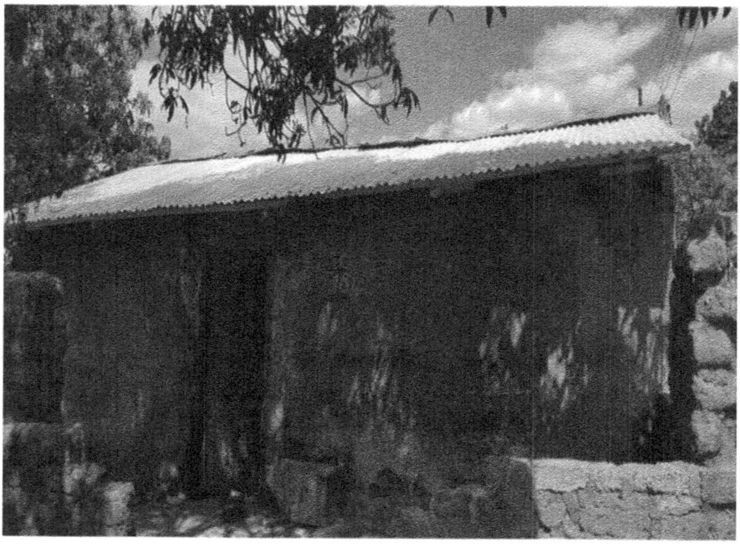

Fig. 7.4 Picture of a typical house in Chipulukusu Community

paid for the service knowing that it was for a good cause. They lobbied local businesses for cash to enable Judith to start a business that allowed her to work from home—selling vegetables, tomatoes, cooking oil, and charcoal from the comfort of her home. Through the local clinic and with the help of my students, Mwansa was referred to the hospital. The idea behind the field visits is not only to learn about a holistic approach to health, but also engage students to think about how best they can use local networks and resources to address local health needs in communities. I encourage my students to have a down-to-earth focus and try to make tangible impacts if they can (of any kind—big or small) that make a difference while learning. After several tests at the hospital, many of students were surprised with the doctor's diagnosis as further explained by one of my students:

> After Mwansa was taken to the hospital, I was surprised at the doctor's diagnosis. I thought she was HIV positive, but discovered she was severely malnourished and was in fact an epileptic patient. Her body wasting was simply due to lack of food and proper care. (female Medical Student 2018)

Understanding the cultural, religious, and social principles of Mwansa's family was also of utmost importance. Judith on the other hand believed her daughter was bewitched. Due to this belief, she heavily invested economically and spiritually in the local Pentecostal pastors (popularly known as prophets) for prayers and healing. Economically, because she had to "sow a seed"—pay the prophet—for a miracle. The visits to the prophet did not yield much in terms of Mwansa's health improvement. Nevertheless, Judith continued to take her daughter to the prophet because she believed "a miracle will happen". This is a common practice in modern Zambia as many patients consult faith healers first before attending to medical treatment.

Her faith in the prophet was in some ways motivated by her religious beliefs. Mwansa's case had many dimensions at play and this was contributing to her recovery or lack of it and her overall well-being as a patient. Taking into account Judith's beliefs and spiritual conviction, the students needed to communicate the diagnosis of Mwansa's illness in a proper manner. A proper manner in this case meant not demeaning Judith's spiritual life but incorporating it in the course of action. This is because religious commitment for Judith was a "way of coping with pain" and family struggles (Peprah et al. 2010). Religious commitment improves stress control by offering better coping mechanisms, richer social support, and the strength of personal values and worldview (Peprah et al. 2010; Akpenpuun 2014; Cohen et al. 1995; Yates et al. 1981). Secondly, spirituality was a dynamic in Judith's understanding of her daughter's disease. To start with, her husband left her for another woman and she explained that she did not have a good relationship with her in-laws. Culturally, women are blamed for broken marriages. In line with this, Mwansa blamed herself for being abandoned by her husband. Furthermore, apart from her neighbours, she had a limited social network. She believed people hated her and the more reason they were bewitching her daughter. Therefore, it was important for her to come to terms with the fact that people did not hate her and no one was trying to harm her or her children. She needed time to work out her own issues of economic struggles, blame, and abandonment before being able to accept her daughter's illness and deal with it. In many patients' lives as observed in this family, cultural, spiritual or religious beliefs may affect the decisions they make about their health and illness and affect the treatment choices they make (Akpenpuun 2014). Mwansa's actual diagnosis by the doctor at Ndola Teaching Hospital was adult malnutrition in a known epileptic. The way forward was physiotherapy to straighten her legs and hopefully get her walking again. There was also a need to correct her nutritional aspect as well as putting her on anti-epileptic drugs.

Educating Judith about Mwansa's disease or the underlying causes of symptoms experienced by Mwansa, caused a bit of conflict. In a nutshell, though Judith knew that the students meant well and the doctors at NTH certainly were trying to do what was best for Mwansa, Judith seemed not to believe that "the doctor had the best solution" in this case. Only God through the prophet knew the "perfect answer" because according to her, the root cause of Mwansa's disease were her enemies. However, after taking into account her religious beliefs and affiliations, her economic situation, and her failure to adequately provide for her daughter and the rest of her household, it led to positive changes in Mwansa's wellbeing. Through well-wishers and student fundraising ventures, Judith was able to start a business of selling charcoal and other goods at her doorstep, in turn spending more time with Mwansa and her other children. I should state not all patients are offered financial help because it is not sustainable however, Mwansa's case was special in that students had spent a lot of time with the family and had come to appreciate the merits of a long-term relationship. The interaction with the family also gave them an opportunity to learn. One of the students wrote:

> I have learned a lot from Mwansa and her family, I have learned how to be a good listener, not to be judgmental and I have also realized that healing a patient requires much more than just medical history. (Fourth year male medical student 2018)

Like many other medical cases, Mwansa's medical case was entangled with the diverse nature of economic, social, religious, and cultural dimensions. In most cases, these diverse dimensions remain invisible in medical training or practice but enthnography helps us reach the complex and complicated dimensions of health and healing. To fulfill this mix of responsibilities and deliver the best care possible students utilized anthropological tools to enable them to be dynamic in their way of thinking, were flexible in the way they treated Mwansa, and were sensitive to the family's situation (Freeman and Hughes 2010). Students learned that by taking into account the impact of socioeconomic and cultural factors, as well as lifestyle characteristics on health and illness, and by engaging different local networks and systems within the community, health and well-being can be achieved.

Participant observations, as seen from the case above, can help to teach medical students "cultural humility," and "cultural sensibility" (Tervalon and Murray-Garcia 1998; Dogra and Karnik 2003). By engaging and participating in household activities, students draw on relational communication skills, an appreciation of differing social positions, and a stance of humility and openness. Ordinarily a medical student, by virtue of being in a medical school, acquires this "superior status," but by venturing into a poor setting with the aim of "fitting in" and "hanging out" with people in their everyday life, allows them to take a step towards cultural humility. Through this, a student comes to appreciate the different strengths of a patient and their everyday struggles as explained by some students:

> Hanging out with patients and their families has taught me to be humble and to treat them with respect. I have learned that patients have a lot of struggles like lack of money that prevents them from getting the medical attention they deserve. (Female student 2018)

> I have learned that there are complex interactions between the social, economic, cultural and medical systems and the family. In fact family context influences the way one copes with health and illness. (Female student 2018)

Overall, the use of fieldwork helps to shift the medical student's perspective, from an individual patient to a family and community orientation, and makes the student more aware of the cultural, economic and social context of his or her ministrations. The field work experience equally raises a critical consciousness for both students and me (Hutchins et al. 2014; Kumagai and Lypson 2009). All these activities are personally enriching and very exciting. However, despite the experience being exciting, it has not been an easy task due to the many challenges I have faced over the years.

The Challenging Experiences at the Medical School: Barriers and then Progress

The following section highlights the challenges I faced before I could find "my feet" as an anthropologist in a medical school. Bearing in mind that literature has documented challenges in fully integrating BS in medical schools (Ouakinin 2016; Rajapakse et al. 2014; Cardell et al. 2008; Dogra and Karnik 2003), this section will focus more on the specific personal challenges that made me question my role at the university as an anthropologist in my first year of joining the university. Overall, and on paper, CBU SOM presents a very good strategy for society and medicine. Despite the fact that society and medicine is important in medical education, it is yet to be fully appreciated. The lack of appreciation for the course can be expressed through a number of challenges faced. Although at inception, the school took a lead in Zambia by including society and medicine in its medical training (from year one to the final year) and allocated it a weight of 100%—full course; within a short space of time, the course was cut and merged with the Public Health with a miserable weight of only 25%. This was done to create more room and time for the "hard sciences". Public health (75%) and society and medicine (25%) were easier to cut and merge because they were not the core components of medical teaching. Before I go into the consequences of this cut, I should state that students especially in the first year of training have difficulties understanding why society and medicine has to be studied as it is not "hard science". At first, not only do medical students at CBU SOM struggle to see the relevance of society and medicine components to their training, but all other undergraduate students do as well. For my students, at times I would see that the inability to see the relevance of the society and medicine course "replicated the negative critical evaluation conveyed by some of the senior role models" (Ouakinin 2016: 872). In turn, students also demonstrated devaluation in relation to my classes.

Thus, the cut in curricular time had a negative impact on the course as a whole. Although the course is mandatory and attendance is taken, students were not motivated to attend class or study. They knew that the course did not impact their aggregate marks at the end of the exams. The lack of motivation was reflected in their non-serious attitude towards class, assignments, or tests. The students presumably calculated that it is wise to spend more time on courses with more weight as one could still pass without the 25%. The low weight of society and medicine relegated the society and medicine course to second class status—a less pressing priority (Rajapakse et al. 2014; de Visser 2009). This in turn promoted rote and cramming rather than an environment conducive for student centered, self-directed learning as evident in students' answers/responses in their assessment. I remember giving an assignment on doctor-patient relations to my students but, more than half copied and pasted their answers from the internet without a care in the world on the consequences of plagiarism. Another example happened in 2015; I only found 10 out of a 130 students in a class. Students had a test in pathology the following day and opted to use the BS class time to study pathology. Although low class attendance is not a rare phenomenon in universities due to several factors such as illness, workloads, or family vacations, (Lukkarinen et al. 2016; Perlman and McCann 2005) the low levels of attendance on that day was extremely alarming. Looking back, I was greatly affected and extremely concerned about the lack of interest for society and medicine among students. The low attendance continued even on days when students did not have tests in "hard sciences". For a while, I grappled with the idea of giving up and moving on but was motivated by Gerhard Gshwandtner's words, "challenges are nothing but wake-up calls for creativity,"—and so I 'woke' up and became creative.

To overcome student participation, through negotiations and presentations to the school administration, we argued for an increase in course marks but only managed to get a 40%. However, negotiations continue and currently society and medicine is not just a course offered to students but has developed into a unit with the hope of growing into a department. It was a plus that the course had gained some value but the most critical part was yet to be tackled, being to stimulate students' participation and engagement in the course. Some students reported they found the lectures too detailed, confusing, and boring. A change in how the course was delivered had to happen, especially for the first phase (pre-clinical), which is rather theoretical in nature. This was important because an amazing course without students to engage and learn is of no value.

I then decided to draw on my strengths as an anthropologist however, this only happened when it dawned on me (after many months of struggle and informal chats with students) that I was going about it the wrong way. Doing participant observation assumes you can become 'one of them' (Strang 2009; Bernard 2006). The biggest problem I came to realise was that when I joined the university, I approached the medical school like one who was doing participant observation without really asking myself what type of participant observation I was engaging in—passive, active, or complete participation? (Spradley 1980). My gaffe, I later realised, was that I was teaching anthropology like an ordinary course at the medical school. I had suspended the 'anthropological identity' in order for me to fully integrate with the medical school. I had abandoned the anthropological tools, perspectives, methods, and way of doing things. This approach, however, did not work. Looking back, I came to understand that at a medical school, the anthropologist assumes no fixed participation but is constantly moving through the different categories of participation. What was important for me then was to keep the 'anthropological identity' in every role. I had to keep and use all the properties—methods, perspectives—anthropologists use, such as fieldwork, participatory approaches, making our field distinct from other disciplines.

I began to see my role at the medical school as an apple bringing spice in a single fruit salad of bananas. I realised that an anthropologist at a medical school needs to maintain the anthropological 'fire' of fun and adventure because in truth, anthropology is one interesting subject. To achieve this, I needed to be original and not be completely consumed by the medical but to maintain anthropological 'authenticity'—continue with anthropological methods and ways of teaching—and in turn bring 'life' to the education of my students. Drawing on over 20 years of working in diverse communities—in and outside Zambia,—(Chileshe 2016) I decided to incorporate not only the fieldwork that I earlier discussed, but more participatory anthropology in my teaching. The participatory approaches use a range of techniques to facilitate learning and sharing.

Overall the teaching of behavioral science in medicine does not involve a passive absorption of didactically-delivered information, but active learning based on curiosity and problem solving, teaching methods involving problem-based learning, small and large group discussions, patient cases, and self-directed learning. The assessments include end of term and end of the course exam, in-course quizzes, short write-ups, reflective writing, extended essays, and project work and class presentations. However, the participatory approaches I describe, go beyond forming a small group for a discussion. It is more action-oriented and focuses more on arousing curiosity and stimulating discussion. Participatory approaches are not new to anthropology. Lassiter (2005) for example, demonstrates that all anthropological research has always involved some degree of participation through 'gatekeepers' of a local community, translators, assistants, and interlocutors way before the eighteenth century. Off course, participatory approaches have evolved over time, (Chambers 1994; Lassiter 2005) but constantly remain a valuable tool for applied anthropology and research. I argue that this is a valuable tool for "hands-on" creative teaching in medical training. Through active participation, it is believed that students understand better and remember more of what they learn by action. Below is an example elaborating how I use the participatory activities in my teaching.

The Dream House: The Importance of Communication

In one lesson, I ask students to pair up and each couple should have one piece of paper and a pen or pencil. The task is to draw what they imagine a modern dream house should look like. Once everyone has settled in, I split the class into two groups, A and B. The pairs in Group A are asked to both hold the same pen or pencil, and draw a house, without any form of communication. In Group B, one person holds the pen and is asked to communicate as they carry out the task of drawing a house. When the time is up, I ask students to compare the drawings from group A and B. We discuss why there are differences (there always are!). Usually, the houses drawn by the group that are not allowed to communicate while both drawing with one pen are funny and show a state of confusion as no houses can be seen on any of the papers presented. However, those drawn by the group that is allowed to communicate might not be perfect due to the student's drawing capacities, but show some form of order and illustrate a 'beautiful' house (see Figs. 7.5 and 7.6).

The discussion points are shaped around the differences between the houses. Was it the communication or lack of it? What about the struggle of holding one pen and trying to draw a common thing (house) but failing to do so? What about the power dynamics? I also ask the students how they felt about the task. Were they frustrated

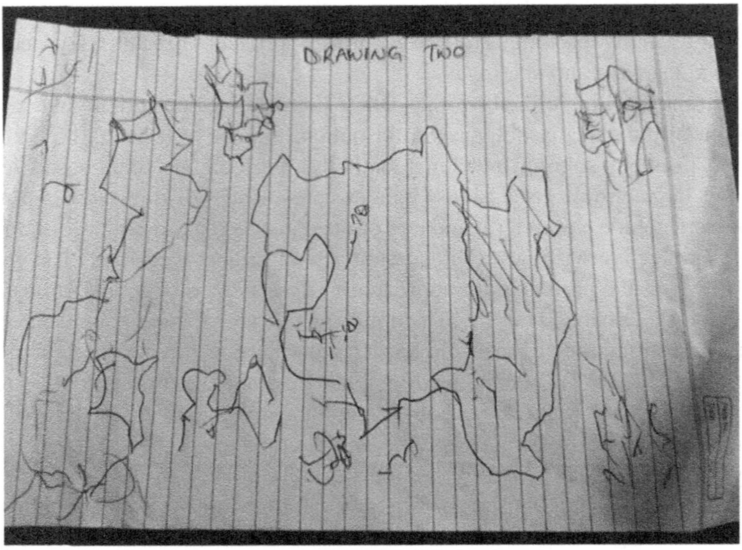

Fig. 7.5 A sample of a dream house by members of Group A third year class 2017

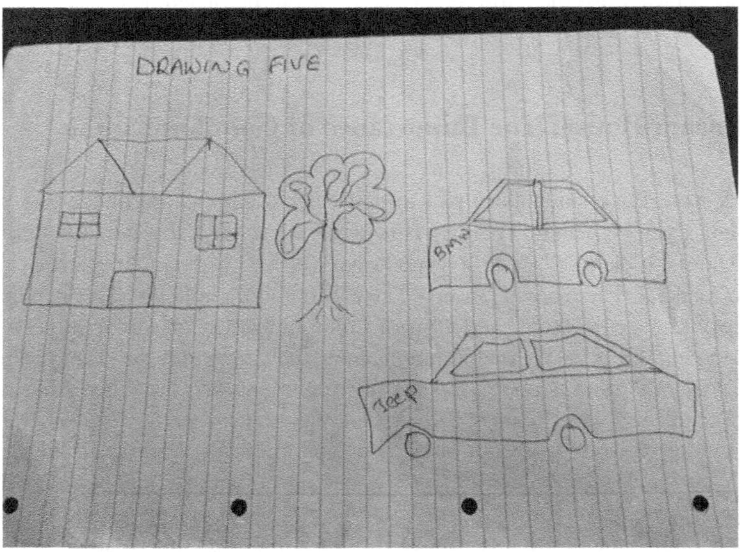

Fig. 7.6 A sample of a dream house by group B third year class 2017

with the inability to draw what they wanted? During the discussion, students usually point out that they found it extremely hard to draw their imagined dream house—the giggles and laughter during the exercise shows clearly that the students are struggling to put their dream across.

Some of the female students express their frustrations about being overpowered by their partner and not being able to draw anything during the exercise, especially when their partner is male as expressed by one female student:

> It was fun doing the exercise but also frustrating. I did not get a chance to draw anything because John overpowered me and stirred the drawing in his own direction throughout the exercise. So what we have here is not my dream house but his. (Third year female student 2017)

The male students tend to have more strength and advantage during the exercise. Most of students expressed that the lack of communication during the exercise makes it hard for two people to hold one pen and perform the exercise. Group B on the other hand shared very little or no complaints and usually report to have enjoyed the exercise. Overall, some of the conclusions that students make during this discussion are that communication is very important, power dynamics are important in any interaction, people have different perspectives on issues, and group activities are a fun way of learning.

There are many lessons to draw from this exercise, but the major lesson is that communication is very important. In the doctor-patient example, while both the doctor and the patient might have a common goal—patient well-being (dream house), if they do not effectively communicate, they will end up with results that look like the houses drawn by Group A. Secondly, our social and cultural background shapes the ideas and perception we have. In the example, although the pair has a task to draw a dream house, there is a difference in both parties of what that dream house looks like, therefore they need to communicate to come to an understanding. The other lesson is that during the exercise, the students in Group A with more physical power (grip) often end up taking control of the whole drawing exercise while dragging their partner along. In addition, the frustrations by the female students over male domination helps to draw lessons on gender issues and challenges that women face in everyday life. Similarly, in the doctor-patient communications, we need to be aware of the power dynamics. If we have the greater power within a relationship, we may be more likely to set the agenda, make assumptions, and be unaware of other people's opinions or feelings. For instance, this sometimes could result in non-compliance to treatment options. Overall, the exercise is and can be used to tackle different components in communication skills, cultural backgrounds, and much more.

Participatory Anthropology as a Strategy

The exercise above shows how participatory anthropology, as a participative act of learning, creates the space for interacting, participating, and imagining. From the exercise, students learned the complete understanding of the topic due to the elaborated and contextualized participatory anthropological perspective, which is made useful for critical thinking and meaningful engagement. The other methods I employ in my classes include role plays, games, videos, and documentaries. Documentaries are frequently used and seen as useful teaching tools in anthropology more commonly than in other disciplines (Bird and Godwin 2006). Internet resources, such as YouTube, also play a role in my teaching. This is important, given today's rapid increase of social media. It is fulfilling to see that with the creative act of teaching and the diverse use of methods, students are constantly looking forward to learning and taking part in that learning. They are more engaging and the low class attendance rate has significantly reduced over the years. Now, students relate well and rarely miss class. Anthropological methods I can safely argue have greatly contributed to the medical education at CBU SOM and these methods continue to inspire and keep students actively involved and interested in society and medicine.

The other challenge, however, in relation to the classroom, is that I struggle with the questions of "what exactly is relevant within anthropology to medical education?" and "how much of that relevant material should the medical student know in order to be a better doctor?" For instance, the topic of cultural competence is wide, but how much of that should the doctor know? These are challenging but very important questions that I struggle with and sometimes feel that I am not answering correctly due to the little time allocated to the course and that it is not deemed as a core course. Therefore, my too much might be too little and vice versa. There is a need for anthropologists in medical schools to constantly engage with each other on the best forms or ways of contributing to medical education.

Apart from challenges experienced in the classroom, anthropologists like myself, working in hospitals, may find themselves experiencing institutional challenges. Though the "hospital offers a really neat laboratory for anthropologists", working in a hospital setting as an anthropologist comes with many barriers (Health Care Blog 2018: 1). One of them is that hospital staff, patients, and family members are often suspicious and as explained by some anthropologists (Long et al. 2008; van der Geest and Finkler 2004) the work of the anthropologist in a hospital often appears trivial. The "hanging around, taking notes and chatting" (van der Geest and Finkler 2004: 83) with patients and caregivers are activities that do not look like work and they definitely do not look like serious academic activities to be taught to a medical student. These activities are seen as "time wasting or even interfering with the real work of the health workers" (ibid: 83).

To overcome the challenges faced in the hospital, I tried to pay attention to some of the questions an anthropologist asks oneself before applying for a job or going into the field. Questions like: what is my place as an anthropologist within the institution/field? What activities will I perform? Are my activities the key activities in this institution? How do I negotiate access to be there? And most importantly, "what do I tell people when they ask me 'what am doing'?" (van der Geest and Finkler 2004; Strang 2009; Spradley 1980) These are important questions that nearly every ethnographer answers when venturing into the field. In answering these important questions, I overcame some of my challenges. For example, knowing that Zambian hospitals do not have neatly defined roles for anthropologists but have clear defined offices and roles for social workers, I use the social worker's office as an entry point to the wards. I should mention that CBU SOM has a number of memorandums of understanding with many of the hospitals in the Copperbelt Province for teaching purposes (Mugala and Kawimbe 2017) and these work very well for medical teaching purposes. The anthropological work on the other hand was and is a "daily on-going negotiation", which sometimes goes well and at other times does not (van der Geest and Finkler 2004: 83). Nevertheless, through personal networks and mainly through the social worker's office and the public relations office, the teaching is achieved. The positive side to having the social worker as one of the "gate keepers" also allows students to appreciate the role a social workers plays in the hospital. For doctors to effectively deal with the complex health problems of the twenty-first century, there is a need for doctors to understand that all hospital staff—nurses, social workers, radiographers, etc.—have a critical role to play in the healthcare system.

In addition, teaching society and medicine and carrying out practical work in a hospital setting is similar to going to a field site. In the field, we constantly find ourselves explaining our research to people in the host community who might be suspicious or curious to know what our presence means. The more we explain, the more people begin to develop rapport and gain acceptance. The same principles have to be applied when we teach anthropology to people who are unfamiliar with our work. The more we explain, the more they begin to understand and know the value of the course.

Other challenges faced include common problems found in many other public universities in developing countries, such as lack of internet and infrastructure. Infrastructure includes lack of tables and chairs, interactive boards, and buses to transport students to the field. In cases where the bus is available, it is usually the fuel that is difficult to access due to lack of funds. Furthermore, the number of students are overwhelming (Mugala and Kawimbe 2017). Presently for example, I teach 377 fully registered students[5] in year-one, 223 in year-two, 145 in year-three, 102 year-four and about 52 year-five. The numbers keep growing each new academic year such that it is increasingly becoming difficult to effectively carry out field activities, ward visits, and exams.

All the above mentioned challenges, including other challenges not outlined here, stimulated the need to assess student perceptions regarding society and medicine learning and see if the course was achieving its objectives in terms of teaching/learning and assessment methods. Below I will critically reflect on this evaluation, highlight the lessons learned, and what they mean to me as an anthropologist, who is trying to contribute to the education of my students in the changing face of medical curricula.

[5]Fully registered students here means that students have paid their tuition fees in full. The numbers listed in fact are under reported and do not totally reflect the true picture and thus should be taken as an estimate. By the end of the academic year, the numbers can rise by 10% in each class because students need to be fully registered to be able to get their results and proceed to the following academic year.

Reflecting on the Evaluation of the BS Course: Lessons Learned and Looking Forward

This reflection is based on an evaluation carried out a year after I joined CBU SOM. The main purpose of the evaluation was to learn about the perceptions of medical students regarding society and medicine learning a year after I started incorporating anthropological methods in my teaching. Perceptions regarding society and medicine learning were evaluated among final year students over two academic years—2016 to 2017—using self-administered questionnaires, six focus group discussions, and informal chats. In relation with the perceived importance of the society and medicine course, 52.4% agreed that society and medicine makes an integral component of the medical curriculum, but only 28.6% of the participants were definite in agreement—strongly agree. On the other hand, 14.3% disagreed and 4.8% strongly disagreed that society and medicine is an integral component of the medical curriculum. When asked to respond to the statement "compared to the applied sciences society and medicine is not that important", 57.1% disagreed, 23.8% agreed, 14.3% strongly agreed and 4.8% were unsure.

The study revealed that if the society and medicine course was to be made optional, none of the students would choose to avoid it completely. Furthermore, 95.2% of students said they found society and medicine to be helpful to them and their medical careers and to becoming better practitioners of medicine, while only 4.8% disagreed. They indicated that practical implementation of certain core components of society and medicine was observed and experienced during the clinical rotations with the medical doctors in the hospital. The listed components during the focus group discussion included communication in doctor-patient relations, ethics (especially informed consent), cultural barriers, delivering bad news, and cultural competence. On cultural competence, one student narrated how he had managed to effectively handle a case he had with a Somali woman. In addition, another student narrated how by building rapport with the patient, he was able to pass his clinical examination.

> I was presented with a patient but jumped right into asking her questions about her health but she proved to be a difficult patient and I got very scared because her lack of cooperation meant I was going to fail my exam. Then after some time, I started asking her general questions about how her family was doing and about her stay in the hospital. In no time the patient opened up and I actually learnt more than I had set out to. (male medical student 2016)

The evaluation of society and medicine course offered useful insight into how some CBU SOM students perceive the course. Looking back from where I started and challenges faced, I was somewhat comforted by the positive feedback from the students:

> Society and Medicine is a great and much needed rotation. It is good for us to interact with the community because that is where health starts from. (Male MBChB student 2017)

> The rotations and field trips of Society and Medicine brought out the meaning of life hence appreciating the art of medicine which transcends prescribing medicine to patients. I loved it

and wished we had been given more time to interact with different communities out there. Maybe then as doctors we would associate with an understanding of patient and caregivers welfare better when we start practicing. (Male MBChB student 2016)

Well it was nice experience and no doubt about it... it opened my mind to be able to understand where various patients we attend to come from and possibly what they go through. (female MBChB student 2017)

Even though the feedback was not always in support of society and medicine as expressed by one student, "*I do not like* society and medicine *because I have to write assignments and tests. To me it is more of a fun course and I feel it is a waste of time*" (male MBChB student 2016); I was still excited to see that students were finally realizing the usefulness of the course and through practical experience, they were able to use some of the core concepts in clinical practice. However, the usefulness of these concepts are yet to be fully practiced by students once they graduate and it would be beneficial to carry out another survey then. With 95.2% of students saying that they found society and medicine to be helpful to them and the medical career, I became convinced of its relevance. As anthropologists, "we are concerned with the various relationships of human beings and their well-being, and no study that throws light on the nature and functioning of any of those relationships is irrelevant" (Hay 1952: 41). It is unfortunate that people in the fields of medicine do not understand the potential role that anthropology could play in the education of future physicians. The students in many other universities worldwide, value the contributions of anthropology and generally BS to medical education, but the rigidity to the course is mainly fostered by a few medical personnel who choose to be blind to the positive contributions and suffer from failure to overcome the inertia for change. This is not to say that anthropology is new to medicine. Anthropologists have been involved in medicine for many years (Campbell 2010; Scheper-Hughes 1990, 2000; Good and Good 1993; Baer 1990; Kleinman 1981), but for an anthropologist to effectively contribute to the education of future medical personnel, they need to be accepted and appreciated. For me, the results from the evaluation are a step in the positive direction.

Sustaining Anthropological Engagement in Medical Education and Way Forward

There are many ways to sustain our engagement as anthropologists in medical education, but I will focus on only two because they relate to me personally and have helped in shaping my career. Reflecting back on my years of teaching, I have come to realize that many of the anthropologists and other social scientists in medical education focus on "bringing change" to medical schools. This approach can be frustrating especially when faced with challenges. The best is to approach medical schools with the "aim that goes beyond the needs of medicine to the needs of anthropology" (Murray 1980: 8) or social science as a whole. We need to understand

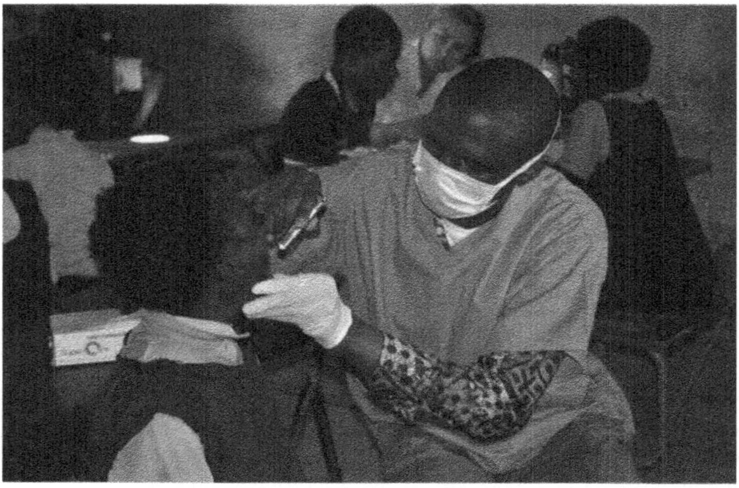

Fig. 7.7 Community dentistry helping vulnerable communities with faculty and students from CBU SOM, University of Mississippi and Nebraska Lincoln

that our work is relevant to our own discipline. This will be a motivation for further engagement and growth.

Furthermore, the work performed in medical schools contributes positively to local communities. For example, by using collaboration with University of Mississippi and Nebraska Lincoln, the CBU SOM medical students through the Public Health Unit, had an opportunity in 2018 to learn and practice community dentistry in six communities— three in Ndola and three in Luanshya in the Copperbelt Province. Students and I had an opportunity to offer free dental services in very poor remote areas. Individuals with "bad teeth" were transported to the CBU SOM Dental Clinic for treatment, sponsored by the two visiting universities. It was enriching for me to see vulnerable children get access to medical treatment that they have failed to gain access to due to economic reasons. While my students are learning, I am constantly honored with opportunities to contribute to change and health care of the less privileged (Fig. 7.7).

Another way to help sustain anthropology is to constantly engage with each other through forums, such as the Society for Applied Anthropology where sessions can allow anthropologists to discuss and learn. The 2016 and 2018 sessions on Sustaining Anthropological Engagement in Medical Schools are such examples. Lastly, as teachers there is a need to constantly engage our students with interesting methods and new ways of teaching in a continuously evolving medical education system.

In conclusion, based on my personal experience of working at a medical school in Zambia, despite challenges faced, anthropologists have a vital role in medical education to ensure the continued production of doctors fit to practice in a rapidly changing society. The overall feedback from students is encouraging, with the majority indicating that the course makes an integral component of the medical curriculum. Informed by my reflective practices and encountered challenges that I have overcome through the years, I conclude that anthropology has a positive contribution to make in medical practice. I reiterate that it offers an opportunity for students to see different factors (social, cultural, biological, and economic) at play in a patient's everyday life. It is also my hope that my work provides useful insight enough to influence the future careers of young anthropologists.

References

Akpenpuun, Joyce Rumun. 2014. Influence of religious beliefs on healthcare practice. *International Journal of Education and Research* 2 (4): 37–48.

Alsan, Marcella, Michael Westerhaus, Michael Herce, Koji Nakashima, and Paul Farmer. 2011. Poverty, global health and infectious disease: Lessons from Haiti and Rwanda. *Infectious Disease Clinics of North America* 25 (3): 611–622.

Ashraf, Ali. 2009. Anthropology and the changing world: How can anthropologists serve humanity? *Management Science and Engineering* 3 (4): 16–26.

Atkinson, Paul, and Martyn Hammersley. 2004. Ethnography and participant observation. In *Handbook of qualitative research*, ed. Norman Denzin and Yvonna Lincoln, 248–261. London: Sage.

Baer, Hans. 1990. The Possibilities and dilemmas of building bridges between critical medical anthropology and clinical anthropology: A discussion. *Social Science of Medicine* 30 (9): 1011–1013.

Bernard, Russell. 2006. *Research methods in anthropology: Qualitative and quantitative approaches*. 4th ed. Oxford: Rowman and Littlefield.

Bird, S. Elizabeth, and Jonathan P. Godwin. 2006. Film in the undergraduate anthropology classroom: Applying audience response research in pedagogical practice. *Anthropology and Education Quarterly* 37 (3): 285–299.

Bond, Virginia. 1998. *Housing capacity and coping up in rural Zambia: Dealing with AIDS, other illness and adversity in Chiawa*. PhD Thesis. Hull: University of Hull.

———. 2006. Stigma when there is no other option: Understanding how poverty fuels discrimination toward people living with HIV in Zambia. In *AIDS, Poverty and Hunger challenges and Responses*, ed. Gillespie, Staurt, 181–197. Highlights of the international conference on HIV/AIDS and food and nutrition security, 14–15 April 2005, Durban, South Africa.

Bond, Virginia, Levy Chilikwela, Sue Clay, Titus Kafuma, Laura Nyblade, and Nadia Bettega. 2003. *Kanayaka—'The light is on': Understanding HIV and AIDS related stigma in urban and rural Zambia*. Working Report, ZAMBART Project, Kara Counseling and ICRW. http://www.icrw.org. Accessed 20 Dec 2017.

Campbell, Dave. 2010. Anthropology's contribution to public health policy development. *McGill Journal of Medicine* 13 (1): 76–83.

Cardell, Wes R., Chad Rowan, and Curt C. Bay. 2008. Dental education from the students' perspective: Curriculum and climate. *Journal of Dental Education* 72 (5): 600–609.

Chambers, Robert. 1994. Participatory Rural Appraisal (PRA): Challenges, potentials and paradigm. *World Development* 22 (10): 1437–1454.

Chileshe, Mutale. 2008. *Tuberculosis, HIV, food insecurity, and poverty in rural Zambia: An ethnographic account of the Southern province*. Thesis collection: University of Cape.

———. 2014. *Economic shocks, poverty and household food insecurity in urban Zambia: An ethnographic account of Chingola*. Cape Town: University of Cape Town.

———. 2016. Emotional reflexivity: Fieldwork among vulnerable and poor populations. *Practicing Anthropology* 38 (4): 49–51.

Chileshe, Mutale, and Virginia Bond. 2010. Barriers and outcomes: TB patients co-infected with HIV accessing antiretroviral therapy in rural Zambia. *AIDS Care* 22 (1): 51–59.

Cohen, S. Robin, Balfour M. Mount, Michael G. Strobel, and France Bui. 1995. The McGill quality of life questionnaire: A measure of quality of life appropriate for people with advanced disease. A preliminary study of validity and acceptability. *Palliative Medicine* 9 (13): 207–219.

Colson, E. 1962. Trade and wealth among the Tonga. In *Markets in Africa*, ed. Paul Bohannan and George Dalton, 601–616. Evanston: North-Western University Press.

Dao, Diane K., Adeline L. Goss, Andrew Hoekzema, Lauren Kelly, Alexander Logan, Sanjiv Mehta, Utpal Sandesara, Michelle Munyikwa, and Horace DeLisser. 2017. Integrating theory, content, and method to foster critical consciousness in medical students: A comprehensive model for cultural competence training. *Academic Medicine* 92 (3): 335–344.

De Visser, Richard. 2009. Psychology in medical curricula: "Need to know" or "Nice to know"? *The European Health Psychologist* 11: 20–23.

Dogra, Nish, and Niranjan Karnik. 2003. First-year medical students' attitudes toward diversity and its teaching: An investigation at one United States medical school. *Academic Medicine* 78: 1191–1200.

Farmer, Paul. 2003. *Pathologies of power: Health, human rights, and the new war on the poor*. Berkeley, CA: University of California Press.

Foucault, Michel. 1994. *The Birth of the clinic: An archaeology of medical perception*. New York, NY: Vintage.

Freeman, George, and Jane Hughes. 2010. *Continuity of care and the patient experience. The ideas that change health care*. The king's fund. https://www.kingsfund.org.uk/sites/default/files/field/field_document/continuity-care-patient-experience-gp-inquiry-research-paper-mar11.pdf. Accessed 20 Jan 2018.

Good, Byron J., and DelVeccio Mary-Jo Good. 1993. Learning medicine: The constructing of medical knowledge at Harvard Medical School. In *Knowledge, power, and practice: The anthropology of everyday life*, ed. Shirley Lindenbaum and Margaret M. Lock, 81–107. Berkeley: University of California Press.

Ha, Fong, Dip Surg Anat Jennifer, and Nancy Longnecker. 2010. Doctor-patient communication: A review. *The Ochsner Journal* 10 (1): 38–43.

Hay, Lorna. 1952. The contribution of social anthropology to social work practice. *Australian Journal of Social Work* 6 (3): 41–53.

Health Care Blog. 2018. *Howard Chiou on the culture of health care*. http://www.nhforhealthcare.com/2018/04/23/howard-chiou-on-the-culture-of-healthcare/

Humayun, Asma, and Michael Herbert. 2011. Towards behavioral sciences in undergraduate training: A core curriculum. *Journal of the Pakistan Medical Association* 61 (8): 800–807.

Hunleth, Jean. 2011. Beyond on or with: Questioning power dynamics and knowledge production in "child-oriented" research methodology. *Childhood 18* (1): 81–93.

———. 2013. "ARVS" as sickness and medicine: Examining children's knowledge and experience in the HIV era in urban Zambia. *AIDS Care* 25 (6): 763–766.

———. 2017. *Children as caregivers: The global fight against tuberculosis and HIV in Zambia*. New Brunswick, NJ: Rutgers University Press.

Hutchins, Frank T., L. DiPrete Brown, and Keith P. Poulsen. 2014. Anthropological approach to teaching health sciences students cultural competency in a field school program. *Academic Medicine* 89 (2): 251–256. https://doi.org/10.1097/ACM.0000000000000088.

Institute of Medicine. 2003. *The future of the public's health in the 21st century*. Washington, DC: The National Academies Press.

Jones, Roger, Roger Higgs, Cathy de Angelis, and David Prideaux. 2001. Changing face of medical curricula. *Lancet* 357 (9257): 699–703.

Kleinman, Arthur. 1981. *Patients and healers in the context of culture: An exploration of the borderland between anthropology, medicine, and psychiatry*. Berkeley, CA: University of California Press.

———. 1983. The cultural meanings and social uses of illness: A role for medical anthropology and clinically oriented social science in the development of primary care theory and research. *The Journal of Family Practice* 16 (3): 539–545.
———. 2004. Culture and depression. *The New England Journal of Medicine* 351 (10): 951–953.
Kleinman, Arthur, Leon Eisenberg, and Bryon Good. 2006. Culture, illness, and care: Clinical lessons from anthropologic and cross-cultural research. *The Journal of Lifelong Learning in Psychiatry* IV (1): 140–149.
Kumagai, K. Arno, and Monica L. Lypson. 2009. Beyond cultural competence: Critical consciousness, social and justice, and multicultural education. *Academic Medicine* 84 (6): 782–787.
Lassiter, Luke Eric. 2005. *The Chicago guide to collaborative ethnography*. Chicago: University of Chicago Press.
Long, Debbi, Cynthia L. Hunter, and Sjaak van der Geest. 2008. When the field is a ward or a clinic: Hospital ethnography. *Anthropology and Medicine* 15 (2): 71–78.
Lukkarinen, Anna, Paula Koivukangas, and Tomi Seppälää. 2016. Relationship between class attendance and student performance. *Social and Behavioral Sciences* 228: 341–347.
Martinez, Iveris L. 2015. Integrating anthropology in medical education: Opportunities, challenges, and lessons. *Practicing Anthropology* 37 (1): 35–39.
Mugala, D. Duncan, and Boniface Kawimbe. 2017. The challenges of training undergraduate clinical surgical students: A study experience after six years in the new school of medicine in Ndola, Zambia. *Advances in Social Science Research Journal* 4 (19): 109–131.
Murray, W. B. (1980). *The relevance of anthropology in medical education a Mexican case study*. Thesis collection: Department of Anthropology, McGill University. Canada National Library of Canada.
Naraya, Deepa, Raj Patel, Kai Schafft, Anne Rademacher, and Sarah Koch-Schulte. 2000. *Voices of the poor: Can anyone hear us?* New York: Oxford University Press.
Nilambar, Jha, K.C. Premarajan, S. Nagesh, S. Khanal, and L.B. Thapa. 2005. Five-star doctors for the 21st century: A bpkihs endeavour for Nepal. *Journal of Health Management* 7 (2): 237–247.
Nkwi, Paul Nchoji. 2006. Anthropology in a postcolonial Africa: The survival debate. In *World anthropologies: Disciplinary transformations within systems of power*, ed. Gustavo Lins Ribeiro and Arturo Escbar, 157–179. Oxford: Berg.
Ouakinin, Silvia. 2016. Teaching psychology in medicine: The context, methodologies and doctor's professional identity. *Acta Medica Portuguesa* 29 (12): 868–874.
Peprah, Prince, Razak M. Gyasi, Prince Osei-Wusu Adjei, Williams Agyemang-Duah, Emmanuel M. Abalo, and Josephine N.A. Kotei. 2010. Religion and health: Exploration of attitudes and health perceptions of faith healing users in urban Ghana. *BMC Public Health* 18: 1358. https://doi.org/10.1186/s12889-018-6277-9.
Perlman, Baron, and Lee I. McCann. 2005. Dealing with students missing exams and in-class graded assignments. *Association for Psychological Science Observer* 8 (6). https://www.psychologicalscience.org/observer/dealing-with-students-missing-exams-and-in-class-graded-assignments/comment-page-1
Rajapakse, Senaka, Mitrakrishnan Navinan, and Dilushi Wijayaratne. 2014. Student perceptions of the behavioral sciences curriculum in a Sri Lankan Medical Faculty. *Education in Medicine Journal* 6: e31–e39.
Scheper-Hughes, Nancy. 1990. Three propositions for a critically applied medical anthropology. *Social Science in Medicine* 30 (2): 189–197.
———. 2000. Coming to our senses: Cultural anthropology in the millennium. *Teaching Anthropology* 7 (2): 8–13.
Scheper-Hughes, Nancy, and Margaret M. Lock. 1987. The mindful body: A prolegomenon to future work in medical anthropology. *Medical Anthropology Quarterly* 1 (1): 6–41.
Smith, Sunny, David Malinak, Jinnie Chang, Amanda Schultz, and Kristin Brownell. 2017. Addressing food insecurity in family medicine and medical education. *Family Medicine* 49 (10): 765–771.

Sorsha, Roberts. 2018. *Key facts: Poverty and poor health*. health poverty action. https://www.healthpovertyaction.org. Accessed 24 Nov 2018.

Spradley, James P. 1980. *Participant observation*. New York: Holt, Rinehart & Winston.

Strang, Veronica. 2009. *What anthropologists do*. Oxford: Berg.

Tervalon, Melanie, and Jann Murray-García. 1998. Cultural humility versus cultural competence: A critical distinction in defining physician training outcomes in multicultural education. *Journal of Health Care Poor Underserved* 9 (2): 117–125.

UNAIDS. 2006. *report on the global AIDS epidemic*. Geneva: UNAIDS.

UNICEF. 2019. *For every child, every right the convention on the rights of the child at a crossroads*. https://www.unicef.org/media/62371/file/Convention-rights-child-at-crossroads-2019.pdf. Accessed 21 Nov 2019.

van der Geest, Sjaak, and Kaja Finkler. 2004. Hospital ethnography: Introduction. *Social Science and Medicine* 59 (10): 1995–2001.

Wind, Gitte. 2008. Negotiated interactive observation: Doing fieldwork in hospital settings. *Anthropology and Medicine* 15 (2): 79–89.

World Bank. 2005. *Dying for change: Poor people's experience of health and ill-health*. Washington, DC: World Bank.

World Health Organisation. 1996. *Doctors for health: A WHO global strategy for changing medical education and medical practice for health for all*. Geneva: World Health Organization (unpublished document WHO/HRH/96.1).

———. 2018. *Non-communicable diseases: Key facts*. Geneva: World Health Organization. http://www.who.int/news-room/fact-sheets/detail/noncommunicable-diseases. Accessed 7 Oct 2018

———. 2019. *Patient safety*. https://www.who.int/news-room/fact-sheets/detail/patient-safety. Accessed 21 Oct 2019.

Yates, Jerome W., Bruce J. Chalmer, Paul St. James, Mark Follansbee, and Patrick F. McKegney. 1981. Religion in patients with advanced cancer. *Medical and Paediatric Oncology* 9: 121–128.

Mutale Chileshe, is the head of the Public Health Unit at the Copperbelt University. She is the holder of BSW degree in social work from the University of Zambia (2004), Masters and Ph.D. degrees in anthropology from the University of Cape Town, South Africa, in 2008 and 2014, respectively. After completing her first degree, she joined Zambart Project, a Zambian research organisation established from a research collaboration between the School of Medicine University of Zambia and the London School of Hygiene and Tropical Medicine (LSHTM). Dr. Chileshe has done extensive work in over 30 communities with diverse and vulnerable populations within and outside Zambia. She has worked hand-in-hand with nurses, doctors and community workers in clinics, hospitals and communities for more than 20 years. Her work explores community barriers that impede access to health care, factors that determine access to health services including how social, economic, and cultural issues influence and shape human development and well-being. Through her work she has contributed to the successful design, development, and implementation of anthropological research in Zambia. She is also a passionate promoter of experiential education. Since 2015, she has been with the school of medicine, Copperbelt University in Zambia.

Chapter 8
From the Patient's Point of View: An Anthropological Response to Medicine's Social Responsibility in Canadian Medical Education

William H. McKellin

Introduction

In 1987, Canadian medical schools embarked on a process of curriculum renewal that kindled a reorientation of educational philosophy and pedagogical practices in medical education in Canada and North America. Though the impact was most evident in new teaching strategies, these changes were based on the assertion that societal needs and expectations should be reflected in the medical curriculum (Neufeld et al. 1991). The proponents described the transformation as a shift from "supply side" education, which presented students with a wide range of medical information from the most basic to the newest research findings in medical science, into a "demand side" curriculum that emphasized information necessary to meet the needs and expectations of patients and their communities (Neufeld et al. 1993).

This curriculum re-orientation brought together two teaching strategies—Problem-Based Learning (PBL) and Evidence Based Medicine (EBM). Replacing the traditional lectures delivered to students, PBL is an inductive approach that presents students with a realistic problem, and working in groups with a tutor, they identify the information that they need to address the issue. In the process, they learn both information for the case and the related medical science. The goal of EBM is to bring epidemiological evidence on the efficacy and effectiveness of treatments to the bedside for patient care. Together these two educational strategies have become conventional approaches in medical education across North America.

The University of British Columbia, after several years of development, implemented a new curriculum in 1997 that incorporated both PBL and EBM. This curriculum renewal reflected both the academic interests of the Faculty of

W. H. McKellin (✉)
Department of Anthropology, University of British Columbia, Vancouver, BC, Canada
e-mail: w.mckellin@ubc.ca

I. L. Martinez, D. W. Wiedman (eds.), *Anthropology in Medical Education*,
https://doi.org/10.1007/978-3-030-62277-0_8

Medicine and British Columbia's provincial health system and health policies. These changes were intended to meet the needs of an expanding population in British Columbia and a declining number of doctors, as many reached retirement age, and the number of new immigrant physicians trained outside of Canada declined. This was coupled with a concentration of physicians in urban areas and a dwindling number of doctors serving people in rural areas. Educational and health policy converged in the medical curriculum because both medical services and education are provincial responsibilities in Canada.

I became involved in curriculum development through my collaboration in an early study of the impact on families of genetic testing for Huntington disease, the first DNA testing for an adult onset genetic disease (Adam et al. 1995; Benjamin et al. 1994; Copley et al. 1995; Cox and McKellin 1999; McKellin 2001). During a break, while recruiting interview participants at the Medical Genetics clinic, the medical geneticist who was heading development of one of the new programs in the curriculum, the Doctor Patient Society courses commented, "The interviewing that you are doing with Huntington Disease families is something that our medical students should learn." This remark began my unanticipated involvement in medical education. I was invited to join the curriculum development team and served as the anthropology/sociology content consultant (1994–2005) and as an Associate Course Director (1998–2005). As a content consultant, I identified the issues that were relevant for the program, designed problem-based case studies, recommended readings for the students, and provided support for the faculty tutors. I also presented some lectures, designed projects, and conducted student evaluations. As an Associate Course Director, I shared responsibility with the Director and another Associate Director for the overall direction of the full-year Doctor, Patient and Society (DPAS) courses for First and Second Year students. This included selecting the topics, writing cases for the PBL format, selecting relevant readings to guide students, recruiting guest speakers, and evaluating students. We were also responsible for selecting, training, and evaluating the faculty tutors for the tutorial groups. These roles enabled me to observe the transformation of educational policy into a new program.

Fortuitously, my anthropological interests in families and kinship fit well with Medical Genetics' focus on families. It was also compatible with the family focus of other members of the committee including a developmental pediatrician, who would later become Course Director, a pediatric psychiatrist, and a pediatric dentist. The core curriculum team also included a medical ethicist and an epidemiologist. Thus, the curriculum development committee was biased towards patient and family issues rather than more systemic and population concerns. This social orientation also lent itself to phenomenological, ethnographic approaches that emphasized the everyday experiences and illness narratives of patients and their families (Kleinman 1988; Mattingly 2000; Garro and Mattingly 2000; Garro 1995), and to the case-based approach of the PBL curriculum.

Many of my new medical colleagues assumed that my fundamental role was to address cross-cultural issues and cultural competence—an experience shared with other anthropologists teaching in medicine (Martinez 2015). Rather than limiting me to this predictable niche, my new colleagues allowed me to include more general anthropological material and provide a more patient and family focussed counterpart to the population-based, epidemiological orientation of EBM. The patient-oriented PBL cases enabled me, in collaboration with other curriculum writers from other disciplines, to weave ethnographically and anthropologically informed issues about topics such as family organization, the malleability of ethnicity, personhood and decision-making, social class, and sociolinguistic code-switching into tutorial topics that were not explicitly anthropological.

Additionally, the PBL format allowed us to shift student evaluations from conventional testing to project-based assessments that often incorporated ethnographic skills. Two examples that I will explain in more detail later are the At Home Interview conducted by students with people who had genetic and chronic conditions in First Year, and the Situation Analysis in Second Year where students identified the social ecology of health issues in a region or community. The goal was not to teach medical students to become anthropologists, but to enable them to use conceptual tools from anthropology to see health, health care, and their patients from new perspectives.

Studies of curriculum revision in medical education have traced the development of formal curriculum though policy documents and curricula (Wiedman and Martinez 2017). Additionally, Hafferty's (1998) reflections on the "hidden curriculum" illuminated less obvious aspects of educational programs that shape learning by setting the pre-conditions for interpersonal interactions among students and between students and instructors. While the formal curriculum—policies, learning objectives, and evaluation, focuses on teaching, the hidden curriculum affects learning and professional socialization. Hafferty identifies four areas to reveal the hidden curriculum: (1) policy development, (2) evaluation, (3) resource allocation, and (4) institutional "slang" or nomenclature. This chapter will examine the intersection of the formal curriculum and the emergence of the hidden curriculum in the implementation of one component of the "new" curriculum introduced in 1997 the undergraduate MD program in the Faculty of Medicine at the University of British Columbia, and the anthropological contributions to this program.

Policy, Healthcare, and Medical Education

The curriculum that we developed and adapted had its genesis in a 1987 confrontation between the Ontario Medical Association that represented Ontario's doctors in fee negotiations, and the Ontario government, which managed health insurance. This resulted in the *Educating Future Physicians for Ontario Project* that included the deans of five Ontario medical schools. The report they produced re-affirmed the social responsibilities of medical education. It served as a guide for a new relationship among medical schools, their curricula, and the public (Hodges and Kuper 2015).

The new curriculum that emerged from this project changed the patterns of faculty-student interaction, and the role of health care data by bringing together Problem-Based Learning (PBL) and Evidence-Based Medicine (EBM) (Servant-Miklos 2018). Problem-Based Learning, which had its roots in McMaster University and University of Toronto in the late 1960s (Servant-Miklos 2018) engages students with a clinical case—a problem to solve, by first asking students to identify the issues and information relevant to the case. Then working together with their faculty instructors in small tutorial groups, students identify and assess the clinically relevant information for a clinical solution. Thus, they move from the specific case to more general medical principles (Albanese and Mitchell 1993; Spaulding and Cochran 1991).

Evidence Based Medicine, which also had its genesis at McMaster University, seeks to apply the best scientific, epidemiologically based evidence, particularly clinical trial results and meta-analyses, to the treatment of patients, bringing data about the effectiveness and efficacy of treatments to decisions at the bedside (Sackett 1991; Sackett et al. 1996; Guyatt et al. 1992). These two educational strategies have proliferated across North America and have become the conventional approaches to medical education in North America. For example, PBL was the basis of Harvard's "new curriculum" described by (Good and Good 1993).

These two educational strategies spread across Canada as the result of successive decisions by individual medical schools. At UBC, the new curriculum met a generally receptive, but apprehensive audience among the medical faculty who had previously taught in the program. Those who had taught in the old lecture-based curriculum discovered that their well-honed presentations of established material were no longer needed, which created apprehension that fundamental knowledge would be missed by the new, less structured approach. Support came from faculty in the Department of Epidemiology, who championed the increased coverage of social determinants of health and Evidence Based Medicine, which they believed would respond to British Columbia's provincial health goals.

There is a general misperception that Canada has a national health service; this is not the case. In Canada, each province is responsible for health services, though federal legislation sets the principles and standards. The Canada Health Act (Canada 1985) states that in each province and territory, health services should be administered publicly, to provide comprehensive services that are publicly administered, universal, portable cross provinces, and accessible. Each province is responsible for providing health insurance, administering hospitals, and delivering public health services. Though health insurance is a single payer system managed by a provincial insurance plan, the vast majority of the doctors, especially primary care family physicians, are private practitioners or physicians in joint practices who are paid on a fee for service basis. A small number of physicians, particularly specialists working in tertiary care centers and rural health public health clinics are salaried employees of hospitals, universities, or public health authorities (Shah 2003; Romanow 2002).

Undergraduate medical education, which results in an MD degree, is offered at 17 medical schools across Canada. Each has its own admission criteria and procedures, and curricula. However, students, at the conclusion of their undergraduate training take the same Medical Council of Canada Qualifying Examinations. Following their undergraduate training and successful examinations, these newly minted doctors find residency "matches" across Canada to complete their training before they are able to practice independently. Residencies in the various specialties, ranging from family practice to internal medicine, radiology, and laboratory science, take place in university-affiliated hospitals. Residents are both trainees and practicing physicians who fill the staffing needs of hospitals and regional health authorities and are paid through provincial funding arrangements with hospitals and university residency programs. Consequently, the number of residents reflects each provincial government's health and educational priorities. At the administrative level, the task of medical schools is to provide not only training for physicians, but also exposure and familiarity with the various communities that health care policy makers target as priorities. Consequently, when medical educators in Canada consider social accountability for medical schools, this refers not only to an attitude of social responsibility cultivated among students and faculty, but also the very real societal expectations and policy implications of training physicians (Bates et al. 2008).

In British Columbia, the University of British Columbia (UBC) is the only university with a medical school. However, in 2005, with encouragement and funding from the provincial government, it entered into an expansion program in collaboration with the University of Victoria, and the University of Northern British Columbia to offer MD and residency programs through four regional sites. The government's intent was to encourage students to return to these communities to practice after they completed their training (Snadden and Bates 2005). Other provinces, such as Quebec employ a variety of strategies, including loans and tuition reductions to encourage students to practice in underserved regions after they are fully accredited.

The Role of Anthropology in the Curriculum Design

The new curriculum dramatically changed First and Second Year training in the MD program at UBC. As part of this program redesign, I was on the front line for one of the most contentious aspects of the medical curriculum—airtime. The redesign transformed courses from lecture-based instruction to tutorials, which forced a reconceptualization and realignment of instructional materials across the curriculum. While every medical discipline clamored for the same amount of student contact time that they had in the lecture-based program, this was not possible with PBL tutorials. Added to this mix was the inclusion of course materials not covered previously—including medical anthropology. I found myself in the midst of established medical specialties vying for students' attention.

This tension was not simply one of professional territoriality, but a reflection of faculty members' legitimate concerns that students develop the necessary competencies in the areas tested by the Medical Council of Canada Qualifying (MCCQ) examinations at the end of students' Fourth Year. I found that the new course content was judged by its ability to cultivate students' professional approach to patients' and communities' health issues, to their medical competence, and to students' preparation for their qualifying exams (Good 1995). The relative strengths of courses were monitored by annual statistical reports about fourth Year students' performances on portions of the MCCQ Examinations and anonymized rankings against other medical schools. UBC saw a significant increase in its students' scores on relevant components following the introduction of DPAS.

During students' first 2 years of medical school, instruction in the medical sciences took place in two sets of courses, Principles of Biology, during the first term of Year One, and the Principles of Medicine courses during the second term of Year One and both terms of Year Two. The Principles of Medicine courses were composed of short blocks of varying lengths devoted to different anatomical organ systems and their related specialties. Students normally worked in the same eight student tutorial groups during their first 2 years, led by the same faculty tutors in the "Prin" courses Principles of Biology and Principles of Medicine.

The new program included three "Longitudinal Courses"—Clinical Skills, Family Practice, and Doctor, Patient and Society that met every week for two terms during the students' first two years. Clinical Skills began with Communication Skills, followed by instruction in clinical procedures. Students' Family Practice Continuum, which began in the early weeks of their first term, took students out of the classroom, and into the clinics of community Family Practice doctors. Students observed their preceptors and took on some basic clinical functions that corresponded with their level of training.

The two DPAS courses were developed to address some of the curricular issues related to the program's social accountability. The DPAS courses for Year One and Year Two revised and integrated the content of several shorter courses from the previous curriculum including Health Care Ethics, Addiction Medicine, Intercollegial Responsibility, Sexual Medicine, Health Care and Epidemiology, Emergency Medicine, and Domestic Violence, and some aspects of introductory courses in Family Practice and Pediatrics. The explicit rationale and guiding principles for the DPAS courses as determined by the Strategic Planning Committee and outlined in the DPAS tutor and student manuals were:

- To respond to the changing needs, expectations and requirements of society and develop physicians and dentists who are competent and sensitive to the ethnic, cultural, and gender diversity of the community;
- To provide learning opportunities (including early access to clinical experience, career counselling, and mentorship) which are student centered, self-directed, responsive to feedback and foster lifelong learning;
- To develop and encourage a spirit of enquiry and collegiality among faculty and maintain academic and clinical excellence; and
- To participate in healthcare management with government, health economists, and administrators responding to national, provincial, and regional distributing issues. (Faculty of Medicine and Faculty of Dentistry 1996: 1)

DPAS classes for Years One and Two followed similar formats, with students meeting once a week for three hours either in tutorial groups, or occasionally in a lecture session followed by a tutorial. The joint lecture session was an opportunity for speakers to introduce concepts that the students may have had little exposure to, or to assure that issues were framed consistently across all 20 or more of the tutorial groups. Each week students received a case study prior to the tutorial that typically concerned a patient or a patient's family, which highlighted particular social issues. Unlike the pure approach to PBL, where students are totally responsible for finding relevant literature, we discovered that they needed to learn where to search for appropriate material in the social sciences and how to assess it. In preparation for each week's tutorial, we provided students with a brief overview of the issues for the week and some related readings, usually from medical anthropology or sociology, community health or epidemiology journals. Students were also expected to find additional journal articles, news articles and other relevant sources that extended beyond the readings.

Thematic material was organized in topical Blocks of several weeks. Though there were some modifications to the material covered as the curriculum evolved, in Year One students received 5–8 weeks devoted primarily to social issues related to health and health care. The material drew on medical anthropology, sociology, and epidemiology to address the social determinants of health, the organization of health systems, families and health seeking, chronic care and disability, cross-cultural care, and Indigenous health. The First Year course also included Blocks on biomedical ethics, the epidemiology of outbreaks, and Evidence Based Medicine. The Second Year course covered community health, occupational health, addictions, domestic violence, death and dying, the impact of medical technologies, and complementary and alternative medicine. Importantly, both courses involved students in activities beyond the classroom.

Evaluating Non-traditional Coursework

A major difference between DPAS and the other courses was evaluation. Evaluation in the Principles of Medicine was dominated by multiple-choice examinations that were familiar to students from their science courses as undergraduates. In DPAS, evaluations were qualitative and intentionally more formative—oriented to the nature of encounters that students might have clinically. Alternatively, they engaged students in projects designed to develop their understanding of their patients and the communities in which they lived.

Evaluating students by their performance on projects required a considerable shift in orientation for both students and faculty. Students, who as undergraduates were concerned with the impact of each test score on their grades and admissibility to medical school, initially found themselves adrift in a program where grades were considerably less significant and marking was less finely quantified. Some faculty were uncertain that students had acquired the requisite information. Our intention was to wean high achieving students from academic measures of individual success to value more global indicators of effective collaboration and professional accomplishment.

Among the new forms of assessment were two major projects, one in each year. In Year One, the "At Home Interview" gave students an intense awareness of patients' experiences. We matched pairs of students with people who had genetic conditions or chronic illnesses (or their parents) for semi-structured interviews that students conducted in the families' homes. The goals were for students to elicit an illness narrative to understand how the condition affected the experiences of the individual and their family, their relationships with their community, and their interaction with medical, social, and educational services (Kleinman 1988; Garro and Mattingly 2000).

During Second Year, groups conducted a "Situation Analysis"—a public health needs assessment. Initially, this began as an investigation of British Columbia's regional health authorities. Students applied concepts from course material on community health, occupational health and health systems in their investigation of the regions' local demographics, vital statistics, and access to transportation and communication, and health and social services (Schmets et al. 2016). Based on their analyses, they designed potential interventions to meet the needs they identified. Students found this project so engaging that we redesigned the Situation Analysis to enable students to pick a specific community for their study.

In both First and Second Year, DPAS and the Clinical Skills courses also assessed students' learning through Objective Structured Clinical Encounters (OSCEs). These scenario-based role-playing activities employed trained actors as patients to simulate the kinds of interactions that students may encounter in clinical practice (Harden 1988; Harden and Gleeson 1979; Turner and Dankoski 2008). We evaluated students on the appropriateness of their interactions with patients on a variety of topics including motivational interviewing for addictions and obtaining information about domestic violence.

Policy, Healthcare, and Medical Education

UBC's Faculty of Medicine policies reflected provincial health priorities and shaped the hidden curriculum through resource allocation for faculty tutors and student admissions. This social milieu formed the learning environment of the students. The PBL model of tutorial teaching created an intensive learning environment that depended upon close interaction between tutors and students. Students and tutors, as a rule, remained in the same tutorial groups for both Principles of Medicine and DPAS for First and Second Year. DPAS had a policy of keeping tutorial groups and tutors together with the explicit intent of developing "learning families," which enabled students to develop sufficient rapport to discuss sensitive topics. Tutors had the option of advancing with their students from First Year to Second Year.

Faculty

Faculty tutors lead the approximately 20 tutorial groups of First and Second Year Doctor, Patient and Society Courses (DPAS). These instructors were drawn from a wide range of disciplines, a variety of medical specialties (from epidemiology to surgery), and diverse backgrounds. Each tutorial group's tutor was an academic or clinical faculty member appointed to the Faculty of Medicine. Approximately 50% of the tutors were practicing clinical physicians, with either appointments as regular university faculty, or community physicians who were hired as clinical faculty. Additional tutors hired by the Faculty from other health disciplines including dentists, nurses, and social workers. We were also able to appoint many of my advanced anthropology, sociology, and interdisciplinary PhD students as faculty tutors. They contributed their research expertise on topics including immigrants' experiences with health care, palliative care, aging and dementia, reproductive technologies, hereditary cancers, genetic testing, alternative and complementary medicine, and drug addiction.

The diversity of the tutor's professional backgrounds and the limited number of tutors with experience in the social sciences meant that it was also necessary to brief tutors in regular meetings prior to the beginning of each topical Block. Many faculty from the medical sciences were eager to participate because they had personal interests in social medicine, while others became more engaged as they recognized new aspects of social issues they had encountered in practice. Many tutors only taught for only one term per year, sharing their teaching and tutorial group with a partner through both First and Second Year.

In addition to the regular tutors, the DPAS block on medical ethics, which was led by a lawyer and a medical ethicist trained in philosophy, included trained ethics tutors who joined the regular tutorials. This interdisciplinary mix was an intentional strategy to expose students to a variety of professional perspectives in anticipation of the multidisciplinary teams that they would encounter during their clerkships and residencies (Hodges and Kuper 2015). However, the degree of interdisciplinary raised some concerns among the physicians who believed that students' professional socialization by physicians was diluted by non-physician tutors.

Students

In the first years that I was involved in the program, each class was composed of 120 medical students, who were taught along with 24 dental students. In 2003, the number of medical students was increased to 200 with the expansion to two additional sites, including the Island Medical Program at the University of Victoria and the Northern Medical program at the University of Northern British Columbia in Prince George. Further expansion of the program to the Southern Medical Program at UBC's Okanagan campus in Kelowna increased the incoming class including all sites to 288 students (University of British Columbia 2018). The increased number of medical students made it impossible to include the dental students in the same courses.

The students who formed each of the medical school classes were primarily from British Columbia, with a smaller component from the rest of Canada. Consequently, the students, like the province were ethnically and culturally diverse, reflecting the population of the province where in 2016 immigrants composed 28.3% of the population, 22.9% were second generation, and visible minorities made up 30.3%. of the population (Canada 2016). Visible minorities however included not only recent immigrants, but also some students who are members of Chinese and South Asian communities that dated from the 1850s as well as more recent immigrants from a variety of countries including China, India, Pakistan, Vietnam, Thailand, Indonesia, and Sri Lanka. The medical school classes were evenly distributed by gender. International students, who lack permanent resident status in Canada, were intentionally excluded from admission as part of the understanding with the provincial government, which would only fund students who were guaranteed to be able to be licensed in Canada when they completed their training.

Though Indigenous people represent about 6% of B.C.'s population, in the early years of the new curriculum the numbers of Indigenous students was small, with only one or two students in each year. In 2002, there were 2 Indigenous students (1.6% in a class of 128 students). In 2001 The Aboriginal, (now Indigenous) Student Initiative was launched by the Faculty to increase the number of Indigenous students by helping them to overcome structural and attitudinal barriers. They received mentoring during their high school and university careers in preparation for the MCATs and admission. This program is in keeping with the goal of developing health care providers for communities in the province. A separate admission stream also enabled Indigenous students to gain admission through a process that considers students' connection to their Indigenous community. As a result of this initiative, the number of Indigenous students grew to 8 students or 4% of the expanded class of 200 students in 2005, and 42 students in 2018.

Our medical students were primarily, but not exclusively natural science majors. Many First Year medical students faced a challenging transition from the precision of academic scientific experiments to the variability of patients and their responses in medical science. Similarly, both the students and many of the faculty tutors discovered that reading material in the social sciences required different strategies than the more predictably structured articles in science and medical journals. After I discovered that one student had highlighted an anthropology article in multiple colors and was concerned about memorizing all of the information, we included a section in the course manual and in tutorials on strategies for reading in the social sciences. Recent changes to admission criteria have placed less emphasis on courses in the natural sciences and increased expectations that students would have some social science background, coupled with the addition of social science material to the MCAT, has resulted in students with strong science backgrounds and familiarity with the social sciences.

Anthropology in the Medical Curriculum

The DPAS courses were successors to material previously taught by epidemiologists, which included introducing students to the EBM model and familiarizing them with the Cochrane Collaboration, an international network of researchers from over 130 countries whose goal is to put "evidence at the heart of health decision-making all over the world" (Cochrane 2019). The premise behind EBM is that physicians should bring the best evidence from meta-analyses, clinical trials, and other methodologically rigorous studies of treatments to the bedside to inform individual patient care. Unfortunately, these studies depend on clearly defined patient populations that do not reflect the conditions and circumstances of particular patients. Perhaps the most important anthropological contribution was to complement the epidemiological approach of Evidence Based Medicine (EBM) and the public health perspective of material on the social determinants of health by introducing a patient-centred, phenomenological perspective that is more suited to physicians' clinical care of individual patients.

The first classes of First Year began with either a discussion of the social determinants of health to demonstrate the impact of social factors on health, or by introducing Kleinman's comparative model, which provided a framework for conceptualizing the relationships among the general public's sources of care and professional medical care (Kleinman 1978). This also helped orient the students to the place of medicine among other health care professionals.

No topic was as effective in grabbing First Year medical students' attention to the social dimensions of health and medicine as the Whitehall Studies that demonstrate the social determinants of health (Marmot et al. 1978, 1991; Hertzman 2001). These epidemiological studies challenged students' assumptions about health and social hierarchy with data that spoke to them in a familiar statistical idiom. The discussion of social gradients demonstrated to them that social factors were not just part of an external context for health care but integral to the well-being of individuals. This epidemiological evidence opened up further discussions of social inequality and the impact of socioeconomic status, economics, and politics on health.

Students assumed that they had a very good grasp of professional health systems. However, discussions about Kleinman's comparative model (1978) and the variability of professional designations surprised students when they began to consider how people sought various forms of health care and became patients. They were also surprised and bewildered when they examined the other health professions to discover that in British Columbia, Traditional Chinese Medicine is a provincially recognized health profession with a self-governing college under the Health Professions Act (British Columbia 2008). In tutorial groups, students developed their understanding of the role of these and other health professions and complementary and alternative medicine to learn about practises that their future patients may employ. Students also went out into the community and interviewed practitioners of Traditional Chinese Medicine, Ayurvedic medicine, and other CAM practitioners in their clinics. Some students went so far as participant observation and underwent treatments.

One aspect of the MD program that pre-dated DPAS was a detailed examination of Canadian health care systems. As mentioned before, health care is primarily a provincial responsibility, with the federal government setting national standards; the system is more intricate when examined in more detail. For example, the federal government retains responsibility for many Indigenous communities, comparable to the US Public Health Service. In addition, each province maintains a special health insurance program for injured workers funded by contributions by employers. Discussion of these systems became part of our discussion of the continuity of care for patients in the province (Miller et al. 2009) and the impact of geographical distribution of health care services on patients, communities and the health care providers who serve them (McKellin 1995). It also raised comparisons between Canadian health care systems and those of other countries.

After the initial discussions about the social determinants of health, health systems, and health seeking behavior, we shifted gears to discuss families. Initially, our goal was to coordinate the concurrent content of the Principles of Biology and Principles of Medicine courses, such as the week when Prin focussed on medical genetics and DPAS examined kinship and family relationships. In their Genetics block, students learned about a priori Mendelian risk based on family histories. In the corresponding DPAS tutorials, students elicited each other's genealogies and discussed family dynamics. This was a surprisingly useful springboard to discuss families and family relationships. It provided students with an opportunity to practice a clinical skill and learn more about each other. The ethnic diversity of the class led to stimulating decisions that moved from medically interesting reports to more personal social observations about each other's families. One student whose family was from Sri Lanka gave an intricate explanation of Dravidian kinship terminology and social relationships that transformed this routine clinical and anthropological practice into an exploration of complex cultural assumptions about social relations.

While we attempted to synchronize some topics like medical genetics in Principles of Biology with DPAS, this proved challenging as the courses evolved. In one instance, the geneticist responsible for a week on common hereditary blood disorders changed the case from a Greek family with thalassemia to a Vietnamese family after a new paper was published (Yong et al. 1999). While the change more closely approximated the characteristics of Vancouver's population and its medical needs, it required a rapid revision of my material about immigrant families and their settlement issues. After several years, we abandoned attempts to coordinate the two courses on a week-by-week basis, but continued to consult across courses to find content synergies.

Patient Experience: Phenomenological Accounts

Students were anxious to learn about patients. The At Home Interview that students conducted in First Year provided students with a window into the everyday experiences of patients with genetic or chronic conditions and their family members and the impact that these conditions had on their family dynamics, friendships, social relationships in their communities, and their interactions with medical, social, and educational services. By conducting these 30–60 min interviews (with occasional follow-up sessions) in participants' homes, the interviewees became the hosts who could set the tenor of the interaction, which was considerably different from clinic-based interchanges (Sankar 1986, 1988). As they elicited these illness narratives (Kleinman 1988; Mattingly 1994; Garro 1994), students learned about the phenomenology of everyday life—the social, psychological, and moral challenges faced by these families. By interviewing them at home, students were also able to observe the physical accommodations that many made to their apartments and houses. In addition, the interviews helped the students to understand how social and cultural assumptions about their conditions shaped individuals' decisions about accessing medical, social, and educational services (Garro 1995; McKellin 1995; Miller et al. 2009). Students were often surprised to learn that patients and families' experiences were often more profoundly affected by the barriers they encountered and the support they received in the community than by their interactions with health professionals in clinics. After the interviews were complete, students wrote brief reports and made oral presentations to their tutorial groups. The interviews helped students to understand how their interviewees made sense of their experiences and they were able to see them without the distortion of the clinical gaze. On exit surveys at the end of their 4-year program, students identified the At Home Interview as one of their most important educational activities because it helped them to see patients as people. These patient-oriented interviews about the social aspects of these chronic conditions was also of particular interest to a national accreditation review committee.

The Social Milieu of Health Care

During Second Year, the curriculum emphasized the social contexts that generated health issues—occupational health and community health, and examined some of the more complex relationships between social and health services. The Situation Analysis contributed to students' understanding of the social foundations of health by applying their knowledge of epidemiology, health seeking behaviour, and family dynamics to an analysis of a specific provincial health authorities' demographics, health statistics, patterns of transportation and communication and access to health, educational, and social services. Due to students' keen interest in these projects, we also gave students the freedom to identify more specific communities for their projects. Typically, these community health initiative projects required some basic ethnography. One project resulted in a new health counselling service in one of Vancouver's neighbourhoods with hard to reach residents that received funding from Vancouver's local health authority. Also in Second Year, lectures and panel discussions tackled challenging topics including death and dying and their social contexts (Gordon and Paci 1997; Akabayashi et al. 1999), the impact of medical technology (Koenig 1988), addictions, and domestic violence. These topics highlighted the contrast between population health and phenomenological approaches. For example, while planning the curriculum on abuse, we faced two alternatives—should we focus on the most common form of domestic abuse—the abuse of women by men, or look at the underlying issues of power and the full range of forms of abuse that students might encounter in practice. Rather than opting to investigate the most epidemiologically prevalent type of violence, we chose to explore the full range of forms of social abuse. Consequently, we were able to have discussions about elder abuse, abuse in same sex relationships, and financial abuse that would have been ignored with the narrower, epidemiological approach.

Anthropologists are assumed to have a special niche in medical education—dealing with cultural diversity. This is usually understood to mean ethno-cultural diversity. In ethno-culturally diverse Vancouver, multiculturalism is not just government policy; it is a fact of everyday life. Students who are members of many different cultural groups brought their own experiences and those of their family members into the discussions. Concern about cultural differences has emerged in the US under the guise of cultural competence, the demonstration of awareness of cultural sensitivity, but it rarely asks how culture is relevant in medicine and in clinical encounters. The phenomenological approach that students were introduced to in their home interviews enabled them to appreciate patients' social contexts and the different perspectives that they bring to clinical interactions. As Kleinman and others have noted, culture is experienced in clinical interactions as the values and assumptions that are relevant to a particular clinical encounter, not the sum total of cultural attributes and assumptions that may be extraneous to the clinical interaction. (Kleinman 1988; Kleinman and Benson 2006; Ming-Cheng and Stacey 2008). This perspective makes it unnecessary to learn about every local ethnic culture. Rather than seeing culture as the vague, distant penumbra of values hanging over interactions between doctors and their patients, students developed strategies to identify assumptions and social factors that were relevant to the patient for their care.

An anthropological perspective also played a role in the Biomedical Ethics coverage in DPAS, which was led by a clinical ethicist trained in philosophy and a lawyer. Ethics complemented the anthropological attention to patients' experiences and the issues of cultural diversity. Clinical ethical problems were posed not only from hypothetical cases to raise specific discussions, but were also derived from issues that students encountered in the news, during their family practice placements, and in their interviews. Differences among students and within their families highlighted the diversity of ethical and cultural values that students were likely to address in practice.

The Canada Health Act's requirement of equitable care across the country also brought to the fore a dimension of medical ethics that is often overlooked—the obligation to treat all patients equitably. The maxim of equality is particularly significant in Canada's publicly funded health care system. In discussions, students struggled with the disparities that arose when priority was given to some conditions over others, inequities that result from family and social dynamics of care, the costs of providing equitable health care to more remote communities, and issues of global health (Bloch et al. 2002).

While medicine has often been characterized as the culture of no culture (Taylor 2003), where the ethno-cultural experience of patients is contrasted with the presumed objectivity and lack of cultural biases of medicine, my physician-educator colleagues were poignantly aware of the culture of their profession and their role in reproducing and modifying its assumptions and practices. An awareness of professional culture pervades admissions, the review of students' term-by-term progress, and their preparation for licensing. Moreover, though there is a strong cultural tendency built into the educational system that advantages class and social background, there is little in the admissions process (other than in the Indigenous Admissions Selection Sub-committee) or the curriculum that considers socioeconomic status. Discussions about socioeconomic inequities during admissions by the Admissions Selection Sub-committee are constrained by the limited kinds and amounts of information collected about students during the admissions process. This reflects the general hesitancy of administrators in Canadian universities to collect socioeconomic data about individual students because there are relatively few means-tested programs.

Professional culture, often a part of the hidden curriculum, is explicitly discussed, modeled and cultivated in many ways, from the explicit statement of expectations of students, the discussions of professional activities between students and their tutors, and the explicit training in clinical and social interaction that molds students' use of language and discourse (Good 1994). Students' professionalism was also monitored by course directors during student assessments at the end of each term. Competence, conscientiousness, respect for patients, fellow students, and instructors, and their ability to work in teams were explicit surrogate markers for students' professional potential and successful socialization. A recent revision of the curriculum framework makes specific reference to medicine's professional culture—both to create a culture of safety for patients and a supportive culture for professional peers (Frank et al. 2015).

In DPAS, with tutors from diverse backgrounds, students received broad interprofessional and interdisciplinary exposure, but we were also careful to guarantee that all students spent time with physician-tutors during their 2 years in DPAS. This provided them with the informal learning from physician-mentors that non-physician could not provide. The tutorials and other interactions between students and tutors cultivated a culture of professionalism that reflected both the aspirational goals and the limitations students would face in practice.

Despite these curricular strategies to develop patient-oriented physicians in Years One and Two, we have found that the processes that contributed to the development of professional identities through the demonstration of clinical competencies during clerkships in Years Three and Four, undercut the attitude cultivated towards patients in DPAS. A sociolinguistic study by one of my physician-graduate students found that during medical students' clerkships in a Clinical Teaching Unit (CTU) the interactions among medical students, residents, and attendings with patients created patients as objects—the "patient-as-disease-category", the "patient-as-educational-commodity" and the "patient-as-marginalized-actor." (Schrewe et al. 2017). Further research on the process of developing competencies and demonstrating professionalization in these clinical settings is needed to minimize the unintended effects on patients, and to create a more patient-centred and socially responsible health care.

Final Reflections

My involvement in the medical curriculum would not have been possible without the conviction of many of my physician colleagues that the interpersonal, social and cultural aspects of medicine were important in training new physicians. They also recognized the need to include someone with expertise in the social sciences, rather than assuming that their own training and experience was sufficient. Perhaps this openness to social issues was due in part because many of my colleagues came from medical disciplines—medical genetics and pediatrics, that are concerned with families, not individual patients. I was challenged to become an ethnographer of a medical school to find synergies with the topics addressed by clinical disciplines and medical specialties to create an anthropologically informed approach to medicine and medical practice.

Since I left teaching in the MD program, I have continued working with physicians, some of whom became graduate students after their initial medical training and others who were tutors in the program. Many of my physician-graduate students have incorporated medical anthropological theories and ethnographic methods into their graduate and subsequent research. In addition to the sociolinguistic research on medical education and the social organization of clinical teaching units (Schrewe et al. 2016, 2017), other physician-graduate students have also incorporated ethnographic and phenomenological approaches. Illness stories and Therapeutic Emplotment, developed by Mattingly (1994, 1998) were employed to reassess the treatment of children with Fetal Alcohol Syndrome Disorder who had sleep problems and adapt their care to their home circumstances (Ipsiroglu et al. 2012, 2013). Phenomenological analysis was also employed to understand the experiences of patients in palliative care (Kuhl 1999, 2006), people with diabetes in Trinidad (Parmasad 2019; Wilson and Parasad 2014), and the issues of patient safety among emergency department staff (Hunte 2010).

Teaching in the MD program also introduced me to new colleagues and new collaborations due to a growing appreciation for ethnographic research where epidemiological approaches are inadequate. Finding the appropriate treatment for a specific patient is still just well informed experimentation. Genetic testing has demonstrated the etiological heterogeneity of many clinically defined diseases such as Duchene Muscular Dystrophy and cancers. Genetic research has also made it possible to develop personalized treatments targeted to the genetic and proteomic characteristics of these genetically defined conditions. Consequently, there is a need for more individually focused methodologies in the growing movement to personalized medicine (Collins and Varmus 2015; Leplege et al. 2007). One approach that I am developing with a former DPAS colleague, other physicians, and a graduate student is a strategy that employs Therapeutic Emplotment to identify the Personally Meaningful Outcome goals of individuals receiving treatments (Jaggumantri et al. 2015, 2016). In combination with more conventional n = 1 clinical trial strategies, this approach will reduce the dependence on surrogate outcome markers and overly broad quality of life scales.

Collaborations with former tutors has also led to work developing programs for hereditary cancer (Horsman et al. 2007), studies of the continuity of care for children with chronic conditions, using illness narratives and Social Network Theory (Miller et al. 2009; Dewan 2017), studies of communication issues in a pediatric intensive care unit (Collet et al. 2014), and involvement in drafting curriculum guidelines for the Medical Genetics portion of UBC's newest curriculum.

While I wish that I could claim that the DPAS program that we developed still continues to operate as we designed it, the staffing demands of the medical school expansion and a new national strategy that focuses on explicit competencies (Frank et al. 2015) have resulted in the approval of a new curriculum in 2017. However, the collaborative, patient-oriented approach that we took in DPAS has continued in different forms that still reflect the importance of medicine's social responsibility to patients, families, and communities and some of the innovations that I introduced. The interviewing skills that initially brought me into medical education are specifically identified as a competency in the new CanMeds framework which cites the need to elicit and synthesize relevant information that incorporates the perspectives of patients and their families and the ability to " Use patient-centred interviewing skills to effectively gather relevant biomedical and psychosocial information" (Frank et al. 2015: 17).

Community engagement and the social responsibility of medicine to meet the needs of the community has also developed both at UBC and nationally. The community advisory group composed of representatives of patient organizations who helped us recruit interviewees for DPAS, was first expanded to serve the whole Faculty of Medicine, and more recently it has contributed to the development of UBC' Partners in Care, which matches students in the health professions with chronic care patients, and UBC's Health's Patient & Community Partnership for Education. Their goals are to promote inter-professional patient-centered, community-based, team-oriented, and evidence-based health strategies, which were summarized in the Vancouver Statement on patient involvement in health and social care education (Towle et al. 2016).

Also, the student directed community projects that began in Second Year DPAS provided the seed for the new FLEX (Flexible and Enhanced Learning) program that enables students in Years 1, 2, and 4 to engage in research under the supervision of a faculty member. While some projects are very clinical in orientation, many retain the community and patient focus of the original activities. In recent years, I have been involved in two patient-oriented FLEX projects. The first emerged from my collaborative research with the Pediatric Intensive Care Unit (PICU) at the British Columbia Children's Hospital (Collet et al. 2014). Students developed new resources for parents with children in the PICU, updated existing materials, and integrated them into the hospital's website. The second, recently completed student project, was conducted in Nepal in conjunction with a local NGO. In this project students investigated the informational and public health needs of health care providers and members of a community composed of members of an ethnic minority with a high incidence of genetic hemoglobinopathies.

Nationally, new funding streams for Canadian health research also reflect this desire to address the needs of patients and their communities. The Canada Institutes for Health Research program, Strategy for Patient-Oriented Research prioritizes "a continuum of research that engages patients as partners, focuses on patient-identified priorities and improves patient outcomes" by funding provincial centers and national collaborative networks (Canadian Institutes of Health Research 2014: 5).

Both the formal and the "not-so-hidden" curricula that I helped to introduce were intentionally designed to address the social responsibilities of the medical profession and more particularly those of the medical school and its graduates. This mandate enabled me to include anthropological content because my colleagues were socially engaged physician-educators. They also recognized, and continue to value the clinical relevance of anthropology for medical students and physicians who see their patients not only as individuals, but also as members of families and communities. This collaboration also required me to set aside the conventional anthropological stereotypes of privileged physicians, to appreciate their positions, and their understanding of their roles within the healthcare system, and the future roles of our medical students.

Acknowledgements I would like to thank my colleagues who served in various capacities in the DPAS courses during their development and implementation including Doctor, Patient, and Society (DPAS) Course Directors Dr. Barbara McGillivray (Medical Genetics), Dr. Christine Loock (Developmental and Social Pediatrics), Dr. Michael Whitfield (Neonatology); Associate Director Dr. Gary Poole (Health Care and Epidemiology), and additional committee members: Dr. Rosalind Harrison (Dentistry), Dr. Jane Garland (Psychiatry), Dr. William Webber (Anatomy), Dr. Allister Browne, (Philosophy) and the Associate Dean for Undergraduate Medical Education, Dr. Angela Towle. Dr. Towle has also developed patient-oriented activities, Partners in Care, and the Health's Patient & Community Partnership for medical students since leaving the Dean's Office.

References

Adam, S., S. Wiggins, K. Lawson, B. McKellin, and M. Hayden. 1995. Predictive testing for Huntington disease (HD): Differences in uptake and characteristics of linked marker and direct test cohorts. *American Journal of Human Genetics* 57 (4): 1698–1698.

Akabayashi, Akira, Michael Fettters, and Todd Elwyn. 1999. Family consent, communication, and advance directives for cancer disclosure: A Japanese case and discussion. *Journal of Medical Ethics* 25: 296–301.

Albanese, M.A., and S. Mitchell. 1993. Problem-based learning: A review of literature on its outcomes and implementation issues. *Academic Medicine* 68 (1): 52–81. https://doi.org/10.1097/00001888-199301000-00012.

Bates, Joanna, Chris Lovato, and Terri Buller-Taylor. 2008. "Mind the gap": Seven key issues in aligning medical education and healthcare policy. *Healthcare Policy* 4 (2): 46–58.

Benjamin, C.M., S. Adam, S. Wiggins, J.L. Theilmann, T.T. Copely, M. Bloch, F. Squitieri, W. McKellin, et al. 1994. Proceed with care: Direct predictive testing for Huntington disease. *American Journal of Human Genetics* 55: 606–617.

Bloch, Gary, Daniel Roth, and W. McKellin. 2002. *Linking ethics and equity in global health. Paper presented at the Canadian Conference on International Health.* Ontario: Ottawa.

British Columbia. 2008. Health Professions Act. R.S.B.C. 1996, c. 183.

Canada. 1985. Canada Health Act. Revised Statutes of Canada 1985, c.C-6R.S.C., 1985, c. C-6.

Canada, Statistics Canada. 2016. *The 2016 census program.* http://www12.statcan.gc.ca/census-recensement/index-eng.cfm?GC=59&RELEASE_TOPIC_ID=7#keystats. Accessed 03 July 2018.

Canadian Institutes of Health Research. 2014. *Strategy for patient-oriented research: Putting patients first.* http://www.cihr-irsc.gc.ca/e/48413.html.

Cochrane. 2019. *Our mission.* https://www.cochrane.org/about-us. Accessed 10 Jan 2019.

Collet, Jean-Paul, Peter Skippen, Mir Mosavianpour, Alexander Pitfield, Bubli Chakraborty, Garth Hunte, Ronald Lindstrom, Niranjan Kissoon, and William McKellin. 2014. Engaging pediatric intensive care unit (PICU) clinical staff to lead practice improvement: The PICU participatory action research project (PICU-PAR). *Implementation Science* 9 (1): 6. https://doi.org/10.1186/1748-5908-9-6.

Collins, Francis S., and Harold Varmus. 2015. A new initiative on precision medicine. *New England Journal of Medicine* 372 (9): 793–795. https://doi.org/10.1056/NEJMp1500523.

Copley, T.T., S. Wiggins, S. Dufrasne, M. Bloch, S. Danam, W. McKellin, M.R. Hayden, and Canadian Collaborative Study for Predictive Testing. 1995. Are we all of one mind?: Clinicians and patients' opinions regarding the development of a service protocol for predictive testing for Huntington disease. *American Journal of Human Genetics* 58 (1): 59–69.

Cox, Susan M., and William McKellin. 1999. 'There's this thing in our family': Predictive testing and the construction of risk for Huntington disease. *Sociology of Health & Illness* 21 (5): 622–646.

Dewan, Tammie Joanne. 2017. *Characterizing the experience of accessing medical care for children with rare and undiagnosed complex conditions.* MS Thesis, Experimental Medicine, University of British Columbia, Vancouver.

Faculty of Medicine and Faculty of Dentistry, University of British Columbia. 1996. *Doctor, patient, and society tutor manual.* Vancouver: Faculty of Medicine and Faculty of Dentistry, University of British Columbia.

Frank, J.R., L. Snell, and J. Sherbino. 2015. *CanMEDS 2015 physician competency framework.* Ottawa: Royal College of Physicians and Surgeons of Canada.

Garro, Linda C. 1994. Narrative representations of chronic illness experience: Cultural models of illness, mind, and body in stories concerning the temporomandibular joint (TMJ). *Social Science and Medicine* 38 (6): 775–788.

Garro, L. 1995. Individual or societal responsibility? Explanations of diabetes in an Anishinaabe (Ojibway) community. *Social Science and Medicine* 40 (1): 37–46.

Garro, Linda C., and Cheryl Mattingly. 2000. Narrative as construct and construction. In *Narrative and the cultural construction of illness and healing*, ed. Cheryl Mattingly and Linda C. Garro, 1–49. Berkeley: University of California Press.

Good, Byron. 1994. *Medicine, rationality, and experience: An anthropological perspective.* Lewis Henry Morgan lectures; 1990. Cambridge: Cambridge University Press.

Good, Mary-Jo DelVecchio. 1995. *American medicine, the quest for competence*. Berkeley: University of California Press.

Good, Byron, and Mary-Jo DelVecchio Good. 1993. "Learning medicine": The construction of medical knowledge at the Harvard Medical School. In *Knowledge, power, and practice: The anthropolgy of medicine and everday life*, ed. Shirley Lindenbaum and Margaret M. Lock, 81–107. Berkeley: University of California Press.

Gordon, Deborah R., and Eugenio Paci. 1997. Disclosure practices and cultural narratives: Understanding concealment and silence around cancer in Tuscany, Italy. *Social Science and Medicine* 44 (10): 1433–1452.

Guyatt, Gordon, John Cairns, David Churchill, Deborah Cook, Brian Haynes, Jack Hirsh, Jan Irvine, Mark Levine, et al. 1992. Evidence-based medicine: A new approach to teaching the practice of medicine. *JAMA* 268 (17): 2420–2425. https://doi.org/10.1001/jama.1992.03490170092032.

Hafferty, F.W. 1998. Beyond curriculum reform: Confronting medicine's hidden curriculum. *Academic Medicine* 73 (4): 403–407. https://doi.org/10.1097/00001888-199804000-00013.

Harden, R.M. 1988. What is an OSCE? *Medical Teacher* 10 (1): 19–22.

Harden, Ronald M., and F.A. Gleeson. 1979. Assessment of clinical competence using an objective structured clinical examination (OSCE). *Medical Education* 13 (1): 39–54.

Hertzman, Clyde. 2001. Health and human society: Wealthier nations are not always healthier, and efforts to improve health can be swamped by the effects of inequality and conflict. *American Scientist* 89 (6): 538–545. https://doi.org/10.2307/27857565.

Hodges, Brian David, and Ayelet Kuper. 2015. Education reform and the hidden curriculum: The Canadian journey. In *The hidden curriculum in health professional education*, ed. Frederic W. Hafferty, Joseph F. O'Donnell, M.D. DeWitt, and C.Jr. Baldwin, 41–50. Hanover: Dartmouth College Press.

Horsman, Doug, Brenda J. Wilson, Denise Avard, Wendy S. Meschino, Charmaine Kim Sing, Marie Plante, Andrea Eisen, Heather E. Howley, and Jacques Simard. 2007. Clinical management recommendations for surveillance and risk-reduction strategies for hereditary breast and ovarian cancer among individuals carrying a deleterious BRCA1 or BRCA2 mutation. *Journal of Obstetrics and Gynaecology Canada* 29 (1): 45–60. https://doi.org/10.1016/S1701-2163(16)32349-0.

Hunte, Garth Stephen. 2010. *Creating safety in an emergency department*. PhD dissertation, Health Care and Epidemiology, University of British Columbia, Vancouver.

Ipsiroglu, Osman S., William McKellin, and Eric Vatikiotis-Bateson. 2012. In*dividualized medicine: From narratives to videos. The concept of therapeutic emplotment*. Presented at Grand Rounds, British Columbia Children's Hospital, January 13, 2012.

Ipsiroglu, Osman S., William H. McKellin, Norma Carey, and Christine Loock. 2013. "They silently live in terror..." why sleep problems and night-time related quality-of-life are missed in children with a fetal alcohol spectrum disorder. *Social Science & Medicine* 79: 76–83. https://doi.org/10.1016/j.socscimed.2012.10.027.

Jaggumantri, Sravan, William McKellin, Sylvia Stockler, Clara van Karnebeek, and Jean Paul Collet. 2015. Personalized evaluation model for making informed decisions in treatments for individuals with intellectual disability. *International Journal of Developmental Neuroscience* 47, Part A: 66. doi:https://doi.org/10.1016/j.ijdevneu.2015.04.182.

Jaggumantri, Sravan, William McKellin, and Jean Paul Collet. 2016. Evaluating treatment effect in rare diseases: Are we measuring the right outcomes? A qualitative study to evaluate clinical endpoints with patient preferences. Paper presented at the International Congress on Personalized Health Care, Montreal, June 2016.

Kleinman, Arthur. 1978. Concepts and a model for the comparison of medical systems as cultural systems. *Social Science & Medicine. Part B: Medical Anthropology* 12 (0): 85–93. https://doi.org/10.1016/0160-7987(78)90014-5.

———. 1988. *The illness narrative*. New York: Basic Books.

Kleinman, Arthur, and Peter Benson. 2006. Anthropology in the clinic: The problem of cultural competency and how to fix it. *PLoS Medicine* 3 (10): e294.

Koenig, Barbara. 1988. The technological imperative. In *Biomedicine examined*, ed. Margaret M. Lock and Deborah R. Gordon. Dordrecht: Kluwer Academic Publishers.

Kuhl, David. 1999. *Exploring spiritual and psychological issues at the end of life*. PhD Dissertation: Interdisciplinary Studies, University of British Columbia, Vancouver.

Kuhl, David. 2006. *Facing death, embracing life: Understanding what dying people want*. Toronto: Doubleday.

Leplege, Alain, Fabrice Gzil, Michele Cammelli, Celine Lefeve, Bernard Pachoud, and Isabelle Ville. 2007. Person-centredness: Conceptual and historical perspectives. *Disability & Rehabilitation* 29 (20–21): 1555–1565. https://doi.org/10.1080/09638280701618661.

Marmot, M.G., G. Rose, M. Shipley, and P.J. Hamilton. 1978. Employment grade and coronary heart disease in British civil servants. *Journal of Epidemiology and Community Health* 32 (4): 244–249.

Marmot, M.G., S. Stansfeld, C. Patel, F. North, J. Head, I. White, E. Brunner, A. Feeney, M.G. Marmot, and G. Davey Smith. 1991. Health inequalities among British civil servants: The whitehall ii study. *The Lancet* 337 (8754): 1387–1393. https://doi.org/10.1016/0140-6736(91)93068-K.

Martinez, Iveris. 2015. Integrating anthropology in medical education: Opportunities, challenges, and lessons. *Practicing Anthropology* 37 (1): 35–39. https://doi.org/10.17730/praa.37.1.tu6753574487nx84.

Mattingly, Cheryl. 1994. The concept of therapeutic 'emplotment'. *Social Science & Medicine* 38 (6): 811–822. https://doi.org/10.1016/0277-9536(94)90153-8.

———. 1998. *Healing dramas and clinical plots: The narrative structure of experience*. New York: Cambridge University Press.

———. 2000. Emergent narratives. In *Narrative and the cultural construction of illness and healing*, ed. Cheryl Mattingly and Linda C. Garro, 181–211. Berkeley: University of California Press.

McKellin, William H. 1995. Hearing impaired families: The social ecology of hearing loss. *Social Science and Medicine* 40 (11): 1468–1480.

———. 2001. Clinical ethics and family morality. *The American Journal of Bioethics* 1 (3): 31–32. https://doi.org/10.1162/152651601750417928.

Miller, Anton, Christopher Condin, William McKellin, Nicola Shaw, Anne Klassen, and Sam Sheps. 2009. Continuity of care for children with complex chronic health conditions: Parents' perspectives. *BMC Health Services Research* 9 (1): 242. https://doi.org/10.1186/1472-6963-9-242.

Ming-Cheng, M.L., and Clare L. Stacey. 2008. Beyond cultural competency: Bourdieu, patients and clinical encounters. *Sociology of Health & Illness* 30 (5): 741–755. https://doi.org/10.1111/j.1467-9566.2008.01091.x.

Neufeld, Victor R., Thomas S. Inui, Richard J. Pickering, Beverly C. Walters, and Jeffrey M. Turnbull. 1991. Curriculum design in response to societal needs and expectations: Educating future physicians for Ontario. *Academic Medicine* 66 (Supplement): S86–S87. https://doi.org/10.1097/00001888-199109001-00034.

Neufeld, V.R., R.F. Maudsley, R.J. Pickering, B.C. Walters, J.M. Turnbull, R.A. Spasoff, D.J. Hollomby, and K.J. LaVigne. 1993. Demand-side medical education: Educating future physicians for Ontario. *Canadian Medical Association Journal* 148 (9): 1471–1477.

Parmasad, Vishala. 2019. *Sick with sugar: The sociocultural dimensions of managing diabetes in a semi-urban indian trinidadian community*. PhD Dissertation: Anthropology, University of British Columbia, Vancouver.

Romanow, R. 2002. *Building on values: The future of health care in Canada-final report*. Commission on the future of health care in Canada. Canada. Privy Council Office. http://publications.gc.ca/collections/Collection/CP32-85-2002E.pdf.

Sackett, David L. 1991. *Clinical epidemiology: A basic science for clinical medicine*. 2nd ed. Boston: Little Brown.

Sackett, David L., William M.C. Rosenberg, J.A. Muir Gray, R. Brian Haynes, and W. Scott Richardson. 1996. Evidence based medicine: What it is and what it isn't: It's about integrating individual clinical expertise and the best external evidence. *British Medical Journal* 312 (7023): 71–72.

Sankar, Andrea. 1986. Out of the clinic into the home: Control and patient-physician communication. *Social Science & Medicine* 22 (9): 973–982.

———. 1988. Patients, physicians and context: Medical care in the home. In *Biomedicine re-examined*, ed. Margaret Lock and Deborah Gordon, 155–178. Amsterdam: Kluwer.

Schmets, Gerard, Dheepa Rajan, and Sowmya Kadandale. 2016. *Strategizing national health in the 21st century: A handbook*. World Health Organization. http://apps.who.int/iris/bitstream/10665/250221/41/9789241549745-eng.pdf?ua=1.

Schrewe, Brett, Daniel Pratt, and William H. McKellin. 2016. Adapting the forms of yesterday to the functions of today and the needs of tomorrow: A genealogical case study of clinical teaching units in Canada. *Advances in Health Sciences Education* 21 (2): 475–499. https://doi.org/10.1007/s10459-015-9608-y.

Schrewe, Brett, Joanna Bates, Dan Pratt, Claudia W. Ruitenberg, and William H. McKellin. 2017. The big d(eal): Professional identity through discursive constructions of 'patient'. *Medical Education* 51 (6): 656–668. https://doi.org/10.1111/medu.13299.

Servant-Miklos, Virginie F.C. 2018. Fifty years on: A retrospective on the world's first problem-based learning programme at mcmaster university medical school. *Health Professions Education*. https://doi.org/10.1016/j.hpe.2018.04.002.

Shah, Chandrakant P. 2003. *Public health and preventive medicine in Canada*. 5th ed., vol. Book, Whole. Toronto: Elsevier Saunders.

Snadden, David, and Joanna Bates. 2005. Expanding undergraduate medical education in British Columbia: A distributed campus model. *Canadian Medical Association Journal* 173 (6): 589–590. https://doi.org/10.1503/cmaj.050439.

Spaulding, William Bray, and Janet Cochran. 1991. *Revitalizing medical education: Mcmaster medical school, the early years 1965-1974*. Hamilton, Ontario: BC Decker.

Taylor, Janelle S. 2003. Confronting culture in medicine's culture of no culture. *Academic Medicine* 78 (6): 555–559.

Towle, Angela, Christine Farrell, Martha E. Gaines, William Godolphin, Gabrielle John, Cathy Kline, Beth Lown, Penny Morris, Jools Symons, and Jill Thistlethwaite. 2016. The patients voice in health and social care professional education: The Vancouver statement. *International Journal of Health Governance* 21 (1): 18–25. https://doi.org/10.1108/IJHG-01-2016-0003.

Turner, John L., and Mary E. Dankoski. 2008. Objective structured clinical exams: A critical review. *Family Medicine* 40 (8): 574–578.

University of British Columbia, Faculty of Medicine. 2018. *Admission statistics*. http://mdprogram.med.ubc.ca/files/2017/10/FINAL-MED-2021-Admissions-Statistics-website.pdf. Accessed 02 July 2018.

Wiedman, Dennis, and Iveris L. Martinez. 2017. Organizational culture theme theory and analysis of strategic planning for a new medical school. *Human Organization* 76 (3): 264–274.

Wilson, Marisa, and Vishala Parmasad. 2014. Political economies of sugar: Views from a former sugarcane industry. In *Dietary sugars and health*, ed. Luc Tappy, Lê Kim-Anne, and Michael I. Goran, 13–26. Boca Raton: CRC Press.

Yong, Karina N., Louis D. Wadsworth, Sylvie Langlois, Siu Li Yong, and R. Douglas Wilson. 1999. Thalassemia carrier screening and prenatal diagnosis among the British Columbia (Canada) population of Chinese descent. *Clinical Genetics* 55 (1): 20–25. https://doi.org/10.1034/j.1399-0004.1999.550104.x.

William H. McKellin, PhD is a medical, social, and linguistic anthropologist in the Department of Anthropology, University of British Columbia (UBC). He has had extensive involvement in medical education at the undergraduate (MD) and graduate levels, and in medical education administration. He was a curriculum consultant (1994–2005), and Associate Course Director (2001–2005) for the Doctor, Patient and Society Courses in the MD program at the University of British Columbia. He was also a content consultant in a collaboration between UBC and the University of Cape Town's Child Health Unit to develop an MPhil program in Maternal and Child Health. He served has a member of the UBC Faculty of Medicine's MD program Admissions Sub-Selection Committee, and the Indigenous MD Admissions Sub-Committee. In 2002 he received an award for Excellence in Medical Education from the British Columbia Children's and Women's Hospitals. His current research focuses on the experiences of families whose children have rare diseases and neurological developmental conditions. He is a founder of the Rare Disease Foundation.

Chapter 9
Medical Anthropology Teaching at the National Autonomous University of Mexico Medical School: A Reflexive Analysis of Programmatic Development, Challenges, and Future Directions

Alfredo Paulo Maya and Rosalynn A. Vega

Introduction

This chapter explores anthropological instruction within medical education at the National Autonomous University of Mexico (UNAM), focusing on the curriculum's strengths, limitations, and potential directions for future growth. Since graduate programs (ranging from focused certificates to the PhD) and tenured faculty in medical anthropology are housed in the medical school (not a college of liberal arts, as in most U.S. institutions), the curriculum offered to medical students reflects a uniquely anthropological approach to patient care and population health.

This chapter will explore how many of the ethical commitments that shape medical education in the U.S. are also paramount in Mexico, but often use terminology and concepts that are tailored to the Mexican social context. More specifically, in Mexico, intersecting axes of inequality (including indigeneity, gender, poverty, and limited infrastructure in rural regions) all play a role as social determinants of health. Since cultural (not racial) difference is often the rhetoric used when describing indigenous others, Mexican medical education emphasizes "pluriculturality" and "intercultural health" where the U.S. system might argue for "diversity." At the same time, the chapter reveals an ongoing struggle to resist potential tendencies within biomedicine towards reducing medical anthropology to an atheoretical, qualitative method that exoticizes indigeneity.

A. P. Maya (✉)
Faculty of Medicine, Department of History and Philosophy of Medicine, National Autonomous University of Mexico, Mexico City, Mexico
e-mail: alfpaulo@comunidad.unam.mx

R. A. Vega
Department of Anthropology, University of Texas Rio Grande Valley, Edinburg, Texas, USA
e-mail: rosalynn.vega@gmail.com

I. L. Martinez, D. W. Wiedman (eds.), *Anthropology in Medical Education*,
https://doi.org/10.1007/978-3-030-62277-0_9

In essence, the chapter is a reflexive analysis of the program's strengths and shortcomings. At UNAM, patient-centered strategies have championed equitable engagement with ethnomedicine and increased humanism through not only awareness, but an active embrace, of the patient's cosmovision. The chapter thus provides medical educators with recommendations for integrating anthropology, and greater competency regarding patient-physician communication in a variety of sociocultural contexts, into their pre-med and medical school curriculums.

Background: The History of Anthropology Instruction Within UNAM Medical School

In Mexico, the medical degree (referred to as the Bachelor of Surgery) is earned through an undergraduate course of study. Thus, directly after completing high school, students enter into 4 years of medical school. When compared to the United States, Mexico's higher education is more professionally oriented. That is, while the United States' higher education system focuses on a liberal education (for example, through general education requirements at most colleges), bachelor's degrees in Mexico are most often geared towards developing one area of practical expertise, thus resembling graduate- and professional-level education in the United States. Thus, anthropology has been included within the medical school curriculum because of the practical expertise it is thought to provide for medical students.

The development of medical anthropology as a discipline in Mexico is characterized by discontinuity. Historically, physical anthropologists, ethnohistorians, and, to a lesser extent, cultural anthropologists were responsible for the study of medical and therapeutic knowledge of indigenous peoples. However, while the emphasis of physical anthropology on biological evolution and the physiological adaptation of human beings favored dialogue between physical anthropologists and health professionals, the discipline's theoretical corpus is limited with regard to the relationship between culture and the socio-cultural factors of health. It was not until the mid-1980s that medical anthropology consolidated itself as a disciplinary field and began to define the health care process as an object of study.

In the UNAM Medical School, elective subjects related to anthropology have been offered since the mid-1960s. These elective courses basically addressed issues relating to physical anthropology and ethnohistorical measurements of pre-Hispanic cultures. It was not until 1985 that the course "History and Philosophy of Medicine" was included as a required course in the "Sole Plan" curriculum at the medical school. The course was classified as a Socio-medical Science and included 80 h of classroom instruction. The subjects included in this extensive course included the history of medicine, medical ethics, and medical anthropology.

With respect to Medical Anthropology in particular, cultural diversity and the presence of indigenous peoples in contemporary Mexico were key topics. As such, a primary focus was explaining the persistence of traditional medicines, which although they were not recognized legally, were practiced daily across Mexico. The faculty explored diverse aspects of this focus, including the coexistence and/or resistance between alternative medicines and biomedicine; invisible medicine; and the relationship between traditional medicine and the socio-cultural identity of indigenous peoples.

While students were taught to recognize the political economic context within which medical pluralism unfolds, during this period, the predominance of a culturalist approach that primarily emphasized the importance of the indigenous "worldviews" was notorious. Examples, rooted in the pre-Hispanic past, include notions of the world around space (four cardinal points and a center) to notions of time (revolving around the agricultural cycle of corn), and notions about the person (composed of animistic entities).

At present, some of these notions continue to define how indigenous people understand and experience their being-in-the world. A pervasive prejudice in the field of medicine is that the indigenous "worldview" is what is hindering contemporary populations from fully accepting "scientific biomedicine." Given this background, anthropology instruction in medical education tries to demonstrate that although the traditional indigenous medicine differs from "medical scientific knowledge", it is a knowledge system that includes precise knowledge of the human body, therapeutic resources, healing practices, and the etiology of disease. Furthermore, traditional indigenous medicine encompasses both general practitioners and specialists. This approach argues for the equal valuation of traditional indigenous medicine and biomedicine as medical models.

From 1970 to 1985, Dr. Fernando Martínez Cortés, from the Biopsychosocial Medicine Unit of the General Hospital of Mexico, proposed the curricular integration of biological, psychological, historical, social and cultural aspects of health. The Medical School at UNAM has heeded his proposal by including a focus on patients' suffering and personal experiences of the medical clinic in the curriculum. This proposal led to an expanded focus on the ideas and experiences of patients regarding the disease. Under the influence of Dr. Luis Vargas, biocultural processes were also included in the curriculum in 1985. This inclusion highlighted the biocultural aspects of pregnancy, childbirth, puerperium, feeding, old age, and death.

The greatest criticism of anthropological teaching in medical education at UNAM during the following epoch is its omission of clinical anthropology approaches proposed by Arthur Kleinman (1988) and Byron Good (1994). Although students studied notions such as suffering, medical practice, and the health process, this new emphasis was not undergirded by a solid theoretical framework. This theoretical dearth has since been rectified in the intervening years. The work of Kleinman and Good, along with a strong biocultural focus, continue to be featured prominently within the medical school curriculum to this day.

As the Department of History and Philosophy of Medicine hired anthropologists, who specialized in the field of medical anthropology, the medical school curriculum gradually adopted the theoretical approach developed by Dr. Eduardo Menendez (1983). Menendez' theoretical orientation is anchored in Gramscian Marxism. He therefore suggests that the characteristics of illness and death, such as differential morbidity and mortality, highlight how the capitalist system produces social inequality. Furthermore, Menendez argues that the "biomedical model", apart from fulfilling curative and preventive functions, also exercises functions of control, normalization, and legitimation. He argues that through biomedicine, the dominant classes exercise and reproduce problematic relations of hegemony/subalternity.

Menendez' approach unfolds in opposition to those who criticize the resistance of indigenous peoples to biomedicine. Instead, he notes how indigenous people have used biomedicine on the one hand, while indigenous medicine and culture has been appropriated by non-indigenous people on the other hand. Thus, rather than researching issues related to indigenous medicines and the indigenous "worldview," Menendez is concerned with what he defines as the health/disease/care continuum. In contrast to biomedicine, in which a patient's history begins with illness and is hopefully later resolved by treatment and a cure, Menendez' approach begins with the patient in full health before contracting disease and seeking care. Using Menendez' approach, one must account for the articulation between economic, political, and ideological-cultural dimensions affecting the patient's health/disease/care process. The Menendez school of medical anthropological thought continues to be the most influential in the present day.

Teaching Concepts Tailored to the Mexican Social Context

To begin describing how anthropological instruction in medical education unfolds within the context of contemporary Mexico, we must first focus on how humanism, holism, and social justice (often represented in U.S. medical education through emphasis on diversity, social determinants of health, and patient-centered care) has been tailored to the Mexican social context. Specific differences between the concepts used in the United States and those developed in Mexico are described in further detail, below.

Diversity vs. Pluriculturality/Interculturality

While U.S. medical education may incorporate a focus on "diversity," medical education at UNAM emphasizes "pluriculturality." This is not to say that one Word has simply replaced another. Instead, important differences between the U.S. social context and that of Mexico undergird tendencies towards these different conceptual frameworks for understanding differences within the nations' populations. Within the United States, "diversity" primarily refers to inclusion across racial differences, while simultaneously referencing a history of multiple movements for civil rights, women's liberation, and LGBTQ rights.

Pluriculturalism refers to a specifically Mexican sociocultural phenomenon: ethnic diversity and the demographic importance and presence of the indigenous population in the "Mexican nation." For example, in the 2000 census, a total of 6044, 547 speakers of indigenous language older than 5 years were registered, but when adding 1,233,455 children under 5, whose head of household was HLI and 1,103,312 of inhabitants who were considered indigenous, result in an estimated indigenous population of 8,331,314.

However, while Mexico is a multiethnic and pluricultural country, in which the indigenous population has an important weight in the demographic structure, indigenous interests have not been adequately represented in the design and implementation of public policies. The lack of respect for the rights of this sector of the population has historically caused indigenous organizations and communities to seek and demand citizenship-based resources through ongoing political conflict and, at times, they have even resorted to violent acts against government offices at the federal and state levels. Meanwhile, national and international human rights organizations have placed constant pressure on the Mexican State to comply with the constitutional commitments to the rights of all citizens.

For example, on January 1, 1994 in the State of Chiapas, the Zapatista Army of National Liberation (EZLN) took up arms, which prompted representatives of the Mexican State to negotiate with indigenous organizations and the EZLN, resulting in the polemical "Indigenous Reform." In 2001, the Mexican government passed the reformation of Article 2 of the Political Constitution of the United Mexican States, in which the "multicultural composition" of the Mexican nation, with origins rooted among the indigenous peoples, is highlighted. Its impact implied reforming various government offices and federal norms, such as the General Health Law. In particular, Article 6 instructs the National Health System to "promote the knowledge and development of indigenous traditional medicine and its practice in suitable conditions." In response to this article, the Mexican government developed The Office of Traditional Medicine and Intercultural Development.

Furthermore, the National Commission of Human Rights has forcefully expressed the need to respect and fulfill international commitments made in the "Agenda on Traditional Medicine 2014-2023" by the Mexican State to the World Health Organization's Sustainable Development Goals of 2030. The primary thrust of these commitments is that the indigenous population must be able to access public health services in conditions of equality and without discrimination.

This social context is reflected in the medical curriculum at the National Autonomous University of Mexico. Specific research focuses, "chair" positions, and office spaces have been established to address unequal access to citizenship and political conflicts among indigenous communities. The medical curriculum at UNAM has incorporated anthropological instruction in order to teach students to embrace cultural differences by taking a "pluricultural" approach that understands Mexico, and thus, their patients, composed of many rich cultures. That is, in an attempt to uncover health-related aspects of indigenous cultures across Mexico, including familiarization with traditional ethnomedicines, the medical curriculum has gradually integrated anthropological content.

In 1975, UNAM implemented a pilot program known as "A-36", which incorporated anthropological instruction and offered optional subjects dealing with traditional indigenous medicine. In 1985, as part of the "Single Plan of Studies", the subject "History and Philosophy of Medicine" was designed and promoted, in which both indigenous traditional medicine and the socio-cultural aspects of medicine were addressed.

More recently, in the 2010 competency-based study plan, students are required to demonstrate competency in medical anthropology and interculturality. Interculturality in Mexico aims to reduce the effects of xenophobia by incorporating indigenous cultural elements into government-provisioned services, including in the area of health care. This competency includes making culturally sensitive adaptations when providing health care to indigenous peoples and conducting a sociocultural analysis of the health-care-disease process.

"Interculturality" is explicitly mentioned as a priority in the second article of the Mexican constitution. The article states, "The nation has a pluricultural composition originally sustained by indigenous peoples who are the descendants of those who inhabited the present-day territory of our country at the initiation of colonization and who preserve their own social, economic, cultural, and political institutions.... Awareness of their indigenous identity should be a fundamental criteria for determining who undertakes the ruling over indigenous peoples" (my translation). The article goes on to state that, in an effort to ameliorate the *rezagos* (backwardness)[1] in indigenous communities, authorities are obligated to assure effective access to health services that make the most of traditional medicine, as well as support the nutrition of *indígenas* through food programs, especially for the child population (Article 2, Section B III). Furthermore, authorities are obligated to foster the incorporation of indigenous women into development through support for productive projects, the protection of women's health, and granting incentives to boost women's education and participation in decision-making related to community life (Article 2, Section B V).

Social Determinants of Health

The Bachelor of Surgery degree requirements have been designed to provide the medical student with first-hand knowledge of health problems facing the diverse populations that make up the Mexican nation. All students who are in the terminal stage of the Medical Surgery Career Study Plan have the obligation to provide their medical services for 1 year free of charge, in a community of the Mexican republic. This year-long social service requirement was first instituted in 1936, and has been carried out uninterruptedly to date. Although students' social service requirement has undergone important transformations, its main objective is to apply previous

[1]The inclusionary intent of interculturality can often conceal discriminatory undertones embedded in its discourse. We will discuss the limitations of interculturality as a concept in the section on "Successes and Limitations."

years' classroom-based learning experiences about health-disease problems to community-based circumstances, especially in populations of the country where the presence of health professionals are lacking or insufficient.

In practice, the communities that are lacking in the presence of health professionals are impoverished, indigenous communities. Health professionals do not choose to develop their careers, reside, and make out their lives in these zones due to the utter dearth of resources. These communities often have no infrastructure, which means there is no running water or electricity. As a result, accessing potable water, or even bathing water, is a challenge. Likewise, there are no communication services—no telephone lines, no internet, no cell phone reception, and no television, etc. The same factors that discourage medical professionals also discourage teachers from making out their careers in these zones, so even when students from all over the region hike through the rural terrain to elementary school (sometimes carrying their own chair on their back), the presence of a teacher at the school house is inconsistent.

If health professionals were to choose to work in these communities long-term, they would be choosing regions where there is no private sector and where the public sector is under-funded or mismanaged, leading to a lack of equipment and medications for treating patients. Furthermore, they would be exposing themselves and their families to multiple health threats, and their children would not have access to a proper education.

During their required year of social service, students become all-too-well acquainted with the harsh realities of these impoverished, indigenous zones. Over the course of the year, many students, the sole health care personnel at rural outposts, receive patients undergoing medical emergencies. They struggle to resolve these emergencies without even the most standard equipment, and often have to decide whether or not to risk transporting the case on treacherous rural roads to the nearest emergency-equipped hospital. Unfortunately, it is not uncommon for these experiences to end in fatalities.

This year-long experience provides medical students with an up-close view of dire effects of structural violence (Farmer 2003). That is, their social service is designed as a sustained experiential learning experience so that they may not only witness, but also contend, with how social determinants of health—specifically, gender inequality, poverty, political disempowerment, isolation in rural environments, lack of education, and racial discrimination—determine health outcomes, including who lives and who dies.

The year-long social service requirement has not solved the insufficient health care problem in rural, impoverished, and indigenous zones. Ethnographic research in Mexico (Vega 2018) has described the frustration of indigenous villagers with the cyclical presence of medical school students at rural outposts, in the absence of permanent medical staff who are fully-trained. However, the social service requirement nonetheless forms an integral part within the medical curriculum. Specifically, it provides students with an intimate and tragic perspective of the social determinants of health.

Humanistic, Patient-Centered Care

The School of Medicine of the National Autonomous University of Mexico has identified its mission to be "a public institution that trains highly qualified, ethical, critical and humanistic professionals, capable of investigating and disseminating knowledge for the solution of health problems and other areas for the benefit of the human being and the nation. In its vision, the school points to "being at the forefront to exercise leadership in education, research and dissemination in health and other scientific areas for the benefit of the human being and the nation."

Since the beginning of the 1980s, the theoretical interventions of Dr. Martínez Cortés (2003) have strongly shaped humanistic, patient-centered approaches at UNAM medical school. Martínez Cortés signaled how biomedicine fragmented individuals, separating their biological etiology from their identity as a person. That is, biomedicine often fails to treat the patient in a holistic fashion, paying careful attention to psychological and cultural factors, the patient's life experiences, and the patient's place in the social order. As a result of Martínez Cortés' proposals, the UNAM curriculum strives to teach medical students to recognize how biological symptoms are phenomenologically experienced by individual patients. Humanism in Mexico is aligned with holism—humanistic medicine deals with health problems as belonging to a person who is one indivisible whole. The future doctor is taught to heal the person while providing relief or ongoing management of the disease, thus paying attention to how the disease affects the person on psychological, cultural, and social levels (Campos-Navarro et al. 2016).

How Anthropological Concepts Unfold in Contemporary Mexican Medical Education

The Medical Degree: The 2010 Competency-Based Curriculum

In 2010, the School of Medicine implemented a new competency-based curriculum for the Bachelor of Surgery Degree. As a result, the entire curriculum was restructured. Competencies were designed as part of a holistic pedagogical strategy that is expected to generate "knowledge, skills, attitudes, and values" in future medical professionals. Particular emphasis is placed on the development of "communication, critical and reflective judgment, ethics and attitude", as well as constant improvement of capabilities. Through "problem solving and the process of searching for evidence" the student is expected to develop "integrated skills." Thus, the competency-based approach requires both individual and group activities that allow students to apply skills as they are learning. This approach affirms that self-learning is a key formative process throughout the medical curriculum.

The 2010 Competency-Based Curriculum is designed to develop the following eight competencies:

1. Critical thinking, clinical judgment, decision making and information management.
2. Self-regulated and permanent learning.
3. Effective communication.
4. Knowledge and application of the biomedical, sociomedical and clinical sciences in the practice of medicine.
5. Clinical skills of diagnosis, prognosis, treatment and rehabilitation.
6. Professionalism, ethical aspects and legal responsibilities.
7. Population health and health system: health promotion and disease prevention.
8. Development and personal growth.

The Department of History and Philosophy of Medicine was placed within the field of Socio-medical and Humanistic Medicine. Meanwhile, the required "History and Philosophy of Medicine" course was radically restructured and divided into three compulsory subjects, taught across the eighth and ninth semesters: medical ethics and professionalism; history of medicine; and medical anthropology and interculturality. The subject of "medical anthropology and interculturality" is expected to contribute to the following competences, in order of importance: professionalism, ethical aspects, and legal responsibilities (Competency 6); effective communication (Competency 3); critical thinking, clinical judgment, decision making, and information management (Competency 1), and development and personal growth (Competency 8).

With respect to the medical anthropology content delivered in the 2010 curriculum, it has remained basically the same as the previous "Single Plan." However, the 2010 curriculum allots fewer classroom hours to the delivery of "medical anthropology and interculturality" as a subject, thus significantly impacting how the content is delivered. The anthropology faculty within UNAM Medical School have agreed on an operative plan that prioritizes certain topics and subtopics.

At the outset, medical anthropology faculty explain the theories and methods of anthropology. Specifically, students learn about the distinct fields of anthropology, and focus on medical anthropology as a subfield of social anthropology. The course teaches students about qualitative research methods and techniques. Importantly, the course focuses on diversity and interculturality. Students are taught to consider the impacts of culture, so that when they are exploring a health problem, they are expected to recognize different ways in which culture is expressed, as well as its relationship with the health disease process. Similarly, students are instructed on how belief systems, such as the indigenous "worldview," shapes everyday practice. Here, the class defines the distinctions between enculturation, acculturation, pluriculturality, multiculturalism, interculturality, and transculturality. In doing so, the subject material throws into question the binary nature of the normal and the pathological. More specifically, students are taught to consider health and illness as biocultural processes.

Furthermore, when researching a problem, the medical student is expected to identify the role of culture in the life cycle processes of every human being. The subject material explores notions of the human body and what it means to be a person; the meaning of sexuality and the construction of gender; pregnancy, childbirth, and puerperium as a life stage; the processes of taking in food; and end of life issues such as senescence and death. Returning to the theme of interculturality—an important underlying theme throughout the subject material—students are taught to uncover the intercultural contexts within which biocultural processes unfold.

The subject material then focuses on medical pluralism, with the objective of helping students identify relations of hegemony and subalternity that are established within the trajectory of patient care. Specifically, faculty describe different medical models, and identify the biomedical model as one of multiple models in operation, albeit the hegemonic medical model. The relationship between hegemony/subalternity, harking back to Menendez (1983) provides the theoretical anchor for this portion of the subject material. Students explore structural characteristics that shape the trajectory and therapeutic itinerary of the patient. In essence, students learn that, contrary to assumptions about the bilateral "flow" of culture, interculturality is often transactional, and is therefore, laden with all of the socioeconomic inequality that structures society.

The subject material also focuses on the doctor-patient relationship. Students are taught to evaluate the main aspects of the patient physician relationship, which includes: respect for personal space; the potential for different worldviews between patient and provider; how disparate roles and perceived "status" may influence the interaction; the importance of the patient's illness experience and individual suffering; and the pragmatics of resisting medicalization through intercultural communication.

Subsequently, students are taught to face a reality: in the health/disease/care process, patients dealing with chronic illness usually turn to different therapies and resources in medically pluralistic ways. Topics include self-care and self-medication; alternative and complementary medicines; care in the home setting, and the patient's embodied knowledge.

The subject material also explores traditional Mexican medicine. The objective is that when dealing with a particular patient's health problem, the medical student is familiar with and can recognize the traditional medicine techniques, resources, and practitioners that the patient may be turning to in medically pluralistic ways. Faculty discuss culture-bound syndromes, along with the material and symbolic resources used to treat them.

Finally, the subject material explores applied medical anthropology, with the goal of analyzing the characteristics of medical practice in intercultural contexts. In this final section, the role of cultural competency and interculturality in the provision of health care is discussed. To "flesh out" this concept, faculty provide examples of medical practice in intercultural contexts.

Graduate Degrees in Medical Anthropology

UNAM Medical School houses The Medical and Dental Health Sciences Graduate Program. Seven academic entities of the National Autonomous University of Mexico and eight entities of the Health Sector also participate in the program. The graduate program is organized into seven disciplinary fields, each with their own theoretical focus. As a whole, this program specifically emphasizes social determinants of the health-disease process since students in this program study the correlation between epidemiological trends and structural inequalities. The objective of this social epidemiological approach is to expose the fundamental social causes of public health events, including discrimination, stigma, and poverty.

The Medical and Dental Health Sciences Graduate Program opened the field of Anthropology in Health in 2011. Within this field of study, interculturality in health is indicated as a research and action strategy. While this is not a specific objective of the Anthropology in Health graduate program, current graduate students are gravitating towards issues relating to maternal health. In fact, almost 50% of the enrollment of PhD students are conducting research that addresses obstetric violence and control over the sexuality of low-income women. In most cases, these students conceptualize health professionals as agents that reproduce patriarchal logics.

Certificate-Granting Workshops

The Ministry of Medical Education of the Faculty of Medicine has sponsored certificate-granting workshops in which the importance of "dialogical communication" is addressed (Hamui et al. 2018). These workshops are offered to medical professionals in hopes that what they learn will be applied and implemented in their daily practice of medicine.

The workshop introduces current anthropological and ethnographic perspectives, thus making a case for ethnography as an epistemological and methodological tool for studying social phenomena in the field of health. The workshop incorporates global health perspectives when it examines macro-social factors shaping health. At the meso-social level, it uncovers how institutional logics within the clinic prefigure care. The workshop also examines the micro-social factors that influence individual care trajectories.

The workshop also delves into communication and social interactions among the doctor, the patient, and health care institutions. Specifically, the workshop teaches providers to be self-reflexive of how they have been taught to cycle through the phases of the medical consultation, taking a primarily biological approach. The workshop furthermore analyzes different pedagogical techniques used across the socio-medical sciences—these range from competency-based medical school education models and social studies-oriented educational models.

The workshop then refocuses providers so that they can better understand the patient's social, cultural, and embodied experiences of suffering, and how their individual life story frames those experiences. In this module, workshop attendees also focus on the effects of the institution within which patient-doctor communication unfolds—specifically, the workshop analyzes the administrative logic that regulates the clinical setting (including bureaucratic and structural factors that heavily predetermine the tenor of patient-doctor interactions, such as the spatial orientation of people and objects within the clinic, and the time allotted for each medical consultation). Importantly, the workshop also examines illness narratives (Kleinman 1988) and familiarizes students with the theoretical-methodological articulations that allow anthropologists to uncover sociocultural meanings concealed within individuals' narrated experiences of suffering from disease and other forms of malaise.

Successes and Limitations

The incorporation of anthropology content into UNAM Medical School course offerings and degree requirements has both produced successes and revealed limitations. To begin with, while anthropological perspectives have been incorporated into the medical school curriculum for decades—beginning with elective subjects relating to medical anthropology in the mid-1960s and culminating in "History and Philosophy of Medicine," a required socio-medical science course introduced into the curriculum in 1985—the 2010 Plan marks the first time that medical anthropology has been taught as a stand-alone requirement. While this would be considered a "success," the medical anthropology requirement lasts only 20 h (8 theoretical hours and 12 practical hours), distributed over eight sessions. This very limited duration signals that curriculum planners consider medical anthropology to be relatively less vital to medical education than other subjects.

The limited course hours devoted to medical anthropology is also noted by students. Between 2015 and 2016, anthropology faculty at UNAM Medical School administered a survey to evaluate the contents of the "Medical Anthropology and Interculturality" subject material. Analysis of the survey revealed that medical students expressed heightened interest in subjects related to traditional or indigenous medicine and felt that the time devoted to the subject was insufficient.[2]

Not only are anthropology faculty challenged by limited course hours, anthropology faculty have faced curricular restrictions regarding what topics within medical anthropology they are allowed to include. Given the competency-based

[2]The evaluation presented important methodological difficulties, since only the survey experienced 20% loss to follow-up among the students. Furthermore, the survey results are potentially biased: the survey was administered by the same teacher who taught the subject, thus throwing into question the validity of the results.

program's emphasis on "integrated skills," faculty have encountered the challenge of structuring their coursework around problem-solving practices that complement the medical training process. Another challenge that anthropology faculty face is how to adapt the content of "Medical Anthropology and Interculturality" so that it is relevant to the eight specific competencies targeted in the 2010 Plan. Thus, much of the coursework addresses Competency 5 by attempting to improve patient-doctor communication. The majority of the anthropology faculty at UNAM Medical School agree that "Medical Anthropology and Interculturality" contributes to Competency 1 (Critical thinking, clinical judgment, decision making and information management); however, it does so in a way that may not be what the authors of the 2010 Plan had intended, since their objective was to train students to make clinical decisions using evidence-based criteria. Anthropology faculty hope that exposure to the course content contributes to Competency 8 (Development and personal growth); however, the actual impact on individual students can be difficult to measure.

While on one hand, using "applied" anthropology to improve the quality of patient-doctor interactions in clinic based settings can be considered a "success," on the other hand, faculty are unable to teach according to their true interests in anthropology. Instead, students are offered a very limited view of medical anthropology, and are largely unaware of many of the innovative theoretical frameworks being produced in the field. The narrow focus on developing clinic-based skills is of concern to the anthropology faculty, since they believe that medical anthropology must question the social conditions of the disease, particularly economic and political factors. Given the very short duration and limited topics addressed in the course, to what degree has the inclusion of "Medical Anthropology and Interculturality" disrupted the mechanisms that reproduce health professionals as actors operating according to the logics of the hegemonic biomedical model?

The heavy focus of the course on the concept of "interculturality"—signaled by the inclusion of this concept in the title of the and expounded upon multiple times throughout its teaching—reveals the predominantly cultural-symbolic approach of the course. "Interculturality" is a concept that informs policy in Mexico. Following the recommendations of the World Health Organization, in relation to the biomedical health programs implemented in the indigenous communities, the Mexican configuration of medical and anthropological education has been designed with the intention of solving health problems in a nation characterized by "multiculturalism." In theory, this approach aims to resist assumptions that the "indigenous worldviews" are opposed to the logic of biomedical knowledge. That is, the intention of the course design is to prepare medical professionals to develop cultural competencies and make cultural adaptations in clinic settings in order to ensure health care access for the indigenous population (to what degree this is accomplished will be discussed further, below).

While students express heightened interest in traditional or indigenous medicine, excessive emphasis on "culture" can lead to another limitation: students may be less attuned to issues relating to social inequality. Similarly, while the terminology of pluriculturality underscores the demographic importance of indigenous people in Mexico, it is not without critique. In Mexico, a history of colonialism and subsequent racial admixture (mestizaje) between Spanish and indigenous groups has led to a focus on "culture" as the primary factor distinguishing social groups, even when indigenous groups continue to suffer racial discrimination and structural inequality (Vega 2017, 2018; and Paulo Maya). In this way, "culture" collapses onto phenotypic, linguistic, socioeconomic, and rural vs. urban differences, often using the terminology of different "cosmovisions" across the Mexican population.

In 2016, a follow-up with five of the students surveyed was conducted while they were completing their social service requirement in health centers located in Mixtec indigenous communities of Oaxaca. The students were visited by anthropology faculty in February and June, with the intention of recording narratives regarding their experiences during completion of their social service. Through in-depth interviews, it was found that students held romanticized notions of indigeneity and indigenous health. While the students described these communities as isolated from modern development, in actuality, emigration has linked these rural localities with urban centers in Mexico and the United States. Students' notions about "the indigenous worldview" contrast with the clinical prevalence of chronic degenerative diseases, contagious diseases, and injuries caused by violence—all linked to grinding poverty and structural inequality.

We argue that the culturalist approach, in emphasizing the importance of "indigenous worldviews" and highlighting the continuity of the "pre-Hispanic" to contemporary Mexico, inadvertently exoticizes indigenous culture. Our framing signals the inadequate attention of "interculturality" to gender, racial discrimination, and political economic factors. Furthermore, our perspective on intersectional racialization processes (Vega 2018) questions the reification of cultures upon which "interculturality" is premised. Specifically, in respect to health, focusing on culturalist logic and belief systems that undergird "traditional indigenous medicine" has, in practice, resulted in the erasure of critical perspectives on determinants of health and the political economic conditions of the health/disease/care process. That is, highlighting the cultural symbolic aspects of "traditional medicines" has lapsed into the exoticization of health problems faced by indigenous population; thus disabling the potential of the "interculturality" concept to productively facilitate medical pluralism in a way that is responsive to the economic and political conditions of the health/disease/care process and the sociocultural context of the clinic.

Just as troubling, this limitation means that, in the Faculty of Medicine of the UNAM, the discipline of medical anthropology is primarily associated with the study of indigenous peoples. Instead of viewing indigenous people as a sector of the population that faces urgent poverty-related health problems, medical anthropology has been too readily considered a discipline that preserves exotic knowledge of traditional indigenous medicines rooted in a pre-Hispanic past.

This culturalist approach, in the absence of critical perspectives on political economic determinants of health, has paved the way for the misapplication of the "interculturality" concept in clinical settings. Vega (2018) has noted how interculturality has been deployed by Mexican Secretary of Health in ways that juxtapose allopathic medical services with "traditional indigenous" services, instead of actually integrating them. She observes the consistent privileging of allopathic medicine over "traditional indigenous" services offered in disjointed, decontextualized forms. For example, patrons of "traditional indigenous" services are often charged a fee, while allopathic services in government hospitals are always free of charge (resulting in further commodification of "indigeneity" and an upsurge of "traditional medicine" tourism among nonindigenous people while indigenous individuals seek remedies elsewhere). Vega argues that "interculturality" has done little to challenge hegemonic biomedicine, leaving relationships of domination/subordination intact.

In a subversive turn, Maya opines that while the purported goal of "interculturality" is not met, its actual aims are adroitly accomplished. During a September 10, 2014 seminar at the Center for Superior Research and Studies in Social Anthropology (CIESAS), Mexico City, he argued that "intercultural" programs are exculpation strategies whose true purpose (placating human rights groups by developing programs for which *"indios"* are purported beneficiaries) is routinely and satisfactorily met—thus the continuity of "interculturality" as a political goal over time.

We suggest that inequity in how disciplines are valued is what actually undergirds the misapplication of the "interculturality" concept. More specifically, the biomedical sciences have tended to reduce the sociomedical sciences, including medical anthropology, to a series of qualitative research techniques. The interest of biomedical colleagues, including those who design curricular requirements, have focused on the ethnographic method without incorporating the theoretical arguments of medical anthropology. The result has been the reduction of medical anthropology's transformative potential in clinic-based settings.

Future Directions

While there are numerous strengths with regards to anthropology instruction at the UNAM medical school, the limitations outlined in the prior section require improvement in the future. To that end, this section outlines the future directions of the anthropology program at UNAM. Since 2014, UNAM Medical school has turned to collaborations between the Ministry of Medical Education, the Department of Family Medicine, and the Department of History, and Philosophy of Medicine in order to strengthen competency-based content relating to the health humanities.

Firstly, the anthropology program plans to expand its research focus. With regards to the subject material delivered to students of medicine, there is an undue emphasis on "interculturality." With regards to graduate studies in Anthropology of Health, there are similar limitations with respect to political and economic theorizations on determinants of health. Furthermore, the graduate program currently has a disproportionate emphasis on research topics related to reproductive health. Both groups of students would benefit from further analysis of the intersectional conditions (Crenshaw 2014) that affect the well-being and health status of all social groups across Mexico—not only indigenous peoples.

With the support of the Ministry of Medical Education at the Faculty of Medicine, and with the participation of graduate students, two new research areas have been introduced: "physician-patient communication" and "narratives of suffering." These new research areas will facilitate greater emphasis on how the habitus of health professionals is reproduced; frameworks that shape interpersonal interactions in hospital contexts; potential for conflict among the differing agendas held by the doctor, the patient and the institution; and the patient's subjective experiences of suffering from malaise and/or illness.

To that end, a doctor-patient communication seminar has been introduced. The seminar resulted in a research project, "Teaching Patient Medical Communication," funded by the Support Program for Innovation and Improvement of Teaching (PAPIME) at UNAM. One of the primary achievements of this research project was the design of an innovative teaching strategy for health professionals, and the publication of the book, *Dialogical Communication as Essential Medical Competence*.

Furthermore, two collaborations with researchers at other academic institutions are shaping anthropology instruction at UNAM Medical School in important ways. For example, UNAM Medical School has created an agreement with the University of Lausanne in Switzerland to create a research area focused on the sociocultural context of the clinic. This research area will address processes of neglect and structural violence (specifically, corruption within hospital settings); moralities, citizenship, and medical professionalism.

The UNAM-UNIL agreement laid the foundation for a workshop-seminar, "Clinical Anthropology and Public Health, Interdisciplinary and Interprofessional Perspectives, offered by Dr. Mario Rossi, Professor of Medical and Health Anthropology at THEMA Laboratory (Théorie Sociale, Etiquete Critique, Médiations, Action Publiqué) of the University of Lausanne, Switzerland (Rossi 2018). Finally, with the support of Dr. Rosalynn Vega at the University of Texas Rio Grande Valley (Department of Sociology and Anthropology), the anthropology faculty at UNAM Medical School, plans to develop a research area focused on syndemics (Singer and Clair 2003). This research area would uncover synergistic mechanisms behind multiple, overlapping chronic diseases unfolding in different social and economic contexts. Specific interests include the sociocultural epidemiology of leukemia, nutritional deficiencies, and neurological disorders in children.

Recommendations for Integrating Anthropology into Medical School Curriculums

In the concluding section of this chapter, we provide medical educators with recommendations for integrating anthropology, and greater competency regarding patient-physician communication in a variety of sociocultural contexts, into their pre-med and medical school curriculums.

First and foremost, we recommend that the medical anthropology instruction be incorporated within the biomedical academic structure in such a way that facilitates articulation with Health Sector institutions while ensuring that this does not inadvertently subordinate the theoretical-methodological approaches of anthropology to biomedical logic. That is, anthropology should be incorporated into medical school curriculums in a way that combines biomedical expertise regarding disease etiology with theoretically grounded anthropology perspectives. Too often, anthropology is taught in medical schools in ways that reduce the discipline to a qualitative research technique, thus eliminating possibilities for theoretically robust analysis of clinical experiences. Subsequently, anthropological methods can be dismissed as subjective, anecdotal, and not statistically valid. We argue that medical school curriculums should incorporate anthropological theory and qualitative research methods in a way that validates its importance for improving patient care. This assertion is supported by the World Health Organization's definition of health: "the state of complete physical, mental and social well-being, and not only the absence of diseases or illnesses." In the process, we insist that biomedicine not be demonized. Specifically, we resist uncritical assumptions that cast health providers as co-reproducers of structural violence and biopolitical control. What we suggest is not subordinating biomedical approaches to anthropological perspectives, but rather, a truly integrative combination of both.

Secondly, we suggest that medical schools resist totalizing culturalist approaches. By attributing all social differences with "culture," these approaches can nullify important concepts such as medical pluralism, racialization, citizenship, the biopolitical body, and social determinants of health. In Mexico, these cultural approaches have focused on the "worldview" of indigenous people, thus emphasizing the importance of "intercultural health" strategies that adapt biomedical treatments to incorporate symbolic aspects of indigenous culture (Campos-Navarro 1997, 1999, 2010; Paulo Maya and Cruz Sanchez 2018). In the United States, cultural approaches have often been dubbed "cultural competency" in medical school curriculums. In both countries, these totalizing perspectives eliminate a critical analysis of different forms of inequality by likening difference to the patient's "culture."

Third, we suggest that medical school curriculums incorporate anthropology in ways that explore patient-doctor communication. This exploration should include how both the individual behaviors of patients and health professionals shape interactions between the two. Furthermore, medical students should be made aware of institutional factors—for example, schedules determining how long the patient has to consult the physician, and the consultation room layout which influences how the patient and physician are physically oriented vis a vis each other. This administrative logic, which usually prioritizes efficiency and cost-effectiveness over the patient's experience, should also be analyzed (Cruz et al. 2018).

Finally, we suggest greater interdisciplinarity by using medical anthropology theory to analyze epidemiological data, for example, through the concept of syndemics (how coexisting epidemics, nested in specific sociocultural contexts, interact in ways that produce an excess burden of disease). This type of interdisciplinarity within medical school curriculums would also require a deep engagement with bioethical and human rights arguments. This final suggestion would transform anthropology instruction within medical schools so that the discipline is not only positioned to analyze existing disease, but rather, to seek and promote humanistic, patient-centered health and wellbeing (Baer et al. 2006).

References

Baer, Hans A., Merrill Singer, Debbi Long, and Pamela Erickson. 2006. Rebranding our field?: Toward an articulation of health. *Current Anthropology* 57 (4): 494–510.

Campos-Navarro, Roberto. 1997. La satisfacción del enfermo hospitalizado: empleo de hamacas en un hospital rural del sureste de México [The satisfaction of a hospitalized patient: The role of hammocks in a rural hospital in southeast Mexico]. *Revista Médica del Instituto Mexicano del Seguro Social* 35 (4): 265–272.

———. 1999. La enseñanza de la medicina popular tradicional en la Facultad de Medicina de la Universidad Nacional Autónoma de México. [The teaching of popular traditional medicine at the medical school of the National Autonomous University of Mexico]. *Kallawaya* 6: 7–18.

———. 2010. La enseñanza de la antropología médica y la salud intercultural en México: del indigenismo culturalista del siglo xx a la interculturalidad (Salud del siglo XXI.) [The teaching of medical anthropology and the intercultural health in Mexico: From the culturalist indigenism of the xx century to the interculturality (Health in 21st century)]. *Revista Peruana de Medicina Experimental y Salud Pública* 27 (1): 114–122.

Campos-Navarro, Roberto, Alfredo Paulo Maya, and Adriana Ruiz Llanos. 2016. Capítulo 15: Profesionalismo y humanismo e interculturalidad en medicina [Chapter 15: Professionalism and humanism and interculturality in medicine]. In *Educación médica y profesionalismo?* ed. C. Leobardo, Ruiz Perez, and Liz Hamui, 227–242. Mexico City: Editorial Mc. Graw Hill.

Crenshaw, Kimberlé Williams. 2014. The structural and political dimensions of intersectional oppression. In *Intersectionality: A foundations and frontiers reader*, ed. Patrick R. Granzka. Boulder, CO: Westview Press.

Cruz Sánchez, Martha, Jessica Margarita González Rojas, Alfredo Paulo Maya, and Pedro Dorantes. 2018. Capítulo 3: El ejercicio de la profesión médica y la comunicación médico-paciente en contextos situacionales [Chapter 3: The practice of the medical profession and the doctor-patient communication in situational contexts]. In *La comunicación dialógica como competencia médica esencial*, 58–100. Mexico City: El Manual Moderno.

Farmer, Paul. 2003. *Pathologies of power: Health, human rights, and the new war on the poor.* Berkeley, CA: University of California Press.

Good, Byron J. 1994. *Medicine, rationality, and experience: An anthropological perspective.* Cambridge, UK: Cambridge University Press.

Hamui, Liz, Alfredo Paulo Maya, and Isaías Hernández Torres. 2018. *La comunicación dialógica como competencia médica esencial.* Mexico City: El Manual Moderno.

Kleinman, Arthur. 1988. *The illness narratives: Suffering, healing and the human condition.* New York: Basic Books.

Martínez Cortés, Fernando. 2003. *Ciencia y humanismo al servicio del enfermo [Science and humanism at the service of the ill].* 2nd ed. Mexico City: El Manual Moderno.

Menéndez, Eduardo. 1983. Modelo hegemónico, modelo alternativo subordinado, modelo de autoatención: Caracteres estructurales [Hegemonic model, alternative subordinate model, self-care model: Structural characters]. In *Hacia una práctica médica alternativa: Hegemonía y autoatención (gestión) en salud*, ed. Eduardo Menéndez. Mexico City: Ediciones de la Casa Chata N° 86.

Paulo Maya, Alfredo, and Martha Cruz Sánchez. 2018. De eso que se ha llamado interculturalidad en salud: un enfoque reflexivo [That has been called health interculturality: A approach focus]. *Revista de la Universidad Industrial de Santander, Salud* 50 (4): 366–384.

Rossi, Ilario. 2018. Capítulo 2. La clínica como espacio social ¿Época de cambios o cambio de época? [Chapter 2: The clinic like a social space. Time to change or changing times?]. In *La comunicación dialógica como competencia médica esencial*, ed. Liz Hamui, Alfredo Paulo Maya, and Isaías Hernández Torres, 38–53. Mexico City: El Manual Moderno.

Singer, Merrill, and Scott Clair. 2003. Syndemics and public health: Reconceptualizing disease in bio-social context. *Medical Anthropology Quarterly* 17 (4): 423–441.

Vega, Rosalynn. (2017). Racial I(nter)dentification: The racialization of maternal health through oportunidades in Government clinics. *Salud Colectiva, 13*(3), 489–505. https://doi.org/10.18294/sc.2017.1114.

———. 2018. *No alternative: Childbirth, citizenship and indigenous culture in Mexico*. Austin, TX: University of Texas Press.

Alfredo Paulo Maya, PhD is Professor of the Faculty of Medicine of the National Autonomous University of Mexico. He has been faculty in the Department of History and Philosophy of Medicine since 1992 and Senior Coordinator of the Medical Anthropology Diploma since 2005. He also serves as Tutor for the disciplinary field Anthropology in Health Program and the Master and Doctorate in Dental and Health Medical Sciences since 2011. His recent books include *La comunicación dialógica como competencia médica esencial* (2018) y *Narrativas del padecer: aproximaciones teórico-metodológicas* (2019) both by the Faculty of Medicine of the National Autonomous University of Mexico. His research has focused on global discourses and their impacts on national health policies, as well as critical approach to interculturality in health and sociocultural context of the clinic. He has experience in the field of planning, and execution of health promotion programs in indigenous communities in Chile, Venezuela, Peru, and Mexico.

Rosalynn A. Vega, PhD is Assistant Professor of Medical Anthropology and Global Health at the University of Texas Rio Grande Valley (2016–present). Prior to her current appointment, she was a research scientist at Centro for Research and Advanced Studies in Social Anthropology-Mexico City (2014–2015) and Adjunct Faculty at National Autonomous University of Mexico Medical School (2013–2014). Her ethnographic monograph, *No Alternative: Childbirth, Citizenship, and Indigenous Culture in Mexico*, was published by the University of Texas Press in 2018. She has published numerous articles, including "Commodifying Indigeneity: How the Humanization of Birth Reinforces racialized inequality in Mexico," which appeared in *Medical Anthropology Quarterly* in 2017. Her research has been supported by NSF STEM ADVANCE, the Ford Foundation, UC MEXUS, the UC Global Health Institute, the UC Human Rights Center, and the Jacob K. Javits Foundation. Furthermore, she has been awarded the Complementary and Alternative Medicine/Integrative Medicine Paper Prize from the Society for Medical Anthropology. With the goal of reaching international audiences, she has published in bilingual English-Spanish formats, and her English-language publications have been translated into Spanish and Portuguese. Her research has been presented and published across the Americas, Europe, and Asia.

Part III
Ethics and Humanities

Chapter 10
Translation Without Medicalization: Ethnographic Notes on the Planning and Development of a Health Humanities Program in California

Sharon Rushing and Juliet McMullin

Introduction

> In my dream I sat at a conference table, arguing with a group of frustrated physicians who were earnestly urging me to see their point: "If it looks like a duck, walks like a duck, and quacks like a duck, it's a duck!" one shouted. Equally frustrated, I shouted back: "What do you mean by 'a duck'?" (Hunt 1994).

For the most recent generation of mid-career medical anthropologists who have ventured into the halls of medical education, there is a sense that important work has already been done however, there is still much to do. Arthur Kleinman's "The Illness Narratives" (1988) has provided a framework for discerning the relationship of individual suffering and one's social context. A generation of medical students have read Kleinman's illness narratives, followed by Anne Fadiman's "The Spirit Catches You and You Fall Down" (1997) just a decade later. Their works highlight the importance of eliciting patients' stories of disease to understand the impact of a patient's social context (beliefs, care access, culture, resources, environment, etc.,) on health and treatment approaches. In the last two decades, frameworks of structural competency import the necessity for medical curricula to address growing health inequities and focus on social, economic, and political factors (structural determinants) that result in illness (LaVeist and Isaac 2012; Holmes and Pointe 2011; Metzl and Hansen 2014). The work around structural competency has encouraged our sense of what more can be done to intentionally integrate knowledge of structural inequities into clinical encounters. Changes in the Medical College Admission Test (MCAT) and American Association of Medical Colleges (AAMC) competencies require physicians and physicians-in-training to understand the impact of social and

S. Rushing · J. McMullin (✉)
Department of Anthropology, University of California, Riverside, CA, USA
e-mail: srush001@ucr.edu; julietm@ucr.edu

I. L. Martinez, D. W. Wiedman (eds.), *Anthropology in Medical Education*,
https://doi.org/10.1007/978-3-030-62277-0_10

cultural contexts in their work. Anthropology has increasingly become part of the electives, and at times a requirement in medical training. Within this history, the 2000s saw an increase in Medical and Health Humanities programs in medical schools, emphasizing interdisciplinary goals and reminding institutions, again, that medicine is a practice of humans interacting, not just medicine as the science of humans. Each iteration forwards the integration of humanistic epistemologies into medical education, reiterating the tension between categorization and context, competency and instrumental knowledge, and reductionism/scientism. In this chapter, we describe both the observations and roles of anthropologists in the planning process of building an interdisciplinary health humanities program where multiple paradigms and pedagogy are translated to create integrated content. We attend to the tension between previous accomplishments and the nuances of institutional change that demand continuous repetition of anthropological ways of thinking and performing medicine. Notably, there are institutional and programmatic expectations that regularly require discussion and support. Continual and attentive regard of anthropological ways of knowing in medical education emphasizes context, communication, and emancipatory forms of knowledge that may otherwise be foreclosed in the institutionalization of medical education. This sense of revisiting and redefining ways of knowing is also a moment for anthropologists to better understand their contributions to sustain equitably translated (and integrated) content in Medical and Health Humanities Programs that are on the rise.

It is a rare opportunity to be on site and a participant in building a new medical school. It is also a unique moment to conduct an ethnography in the first public medical school west of the Mississippi in over 40 years. Administrators, researchers, physicians, and communities who were involved in developing the University of California, Riverside's School of Medicine (UCR SOM), wanted the school to be something different (Olds and Barton 2015). They wanted to address the long-standing physician shortages and structural health inequities in the surrounding Inland Valley communities. Hence, the school of medicine's mission seeks to increase the number of physicians who would stay and practice in the county and to train those physicians to be attuned to local community health experiences and health inequities. As anthropologists, it was a prime opportunity to parse out the recurring debates over knowledge and practices that support cultural competency as required by the AAMC, the instrumentalism of humanistic knowledge, and what Kumagai (2014) calls the emancipatory knowledge that supports social justice in medicine. Our chapter is organized as both ethnography and reflection on the role of anthropologists, specifically the two authors', experiences and observations of building an interdisciplinary health humanities program in the new medical school. Juliet McMullin (JM) is a faculty member who was on-site and participating at the start of the conversations for the medical school in the early 2000s, was the lead or co-lead for much of the development and implementation of the health humanities program, and ultimately moved her faculty appointment to the School of Medicine in 2014. Sharon Rushing (SR) is a PhD candidate with a background in public health and healthcare. She joined the anthropology PhD program at UCR in 2012 and became part of the health humanities effort in 2013, the moment when the campus was hiring new faculty for the School of Medicine. SR's ethnographic fieldwork is centered on how medical schools incorporate humanities into their curriculum. The combination of anthropologists who were interested in a holistic and social justice form of medical education and practice and the school's mission facilitated the examination of processes that can create time and space to address recurring debates on the integration of social context in medical education. This was, indeed, a rare moment for anthropologists to be involved in medical education

The conversation to build a full medical school began in the mid-2000s. While JM watched the inclusion of many social sciences in the development of the effort, she wondered how the voices of the humanities faculty were included. How might the school attain greater inclusion in this foundational conversation? To address this concern, an interdisciplinary team of UCR faculty (anthropologists, gender and sexuality studies, history, English, theater, and medicine), led by JM and Chikako Takeshita (a faculty member in gender and sexuality studies), came together to engage the campus and medical school. The faculty created opportunities to engage through a regular dialogue with administrations and intra- and extramural funding (the universal language in a university). The interdisciplinary group decided to develop health humanities programming in the new medical school. Medical humanities are multi-disciplinary fields of the humanities, arts, and some social sciences dedicated to the provisions of humanistic education in medicine. Historically tied to Renaissance humanism, the role of medical humanities in medical education has had a long standing conversation centered on the concerns of medical reductionism and scientism in medical education and practice (Bouwsma 1990; Carson 2007; Anderson 2011; Podolsky and Greene 2014; Jones and Tansey 2015). More aptly defined as a movement, its continued and recursive discourse has responded to the changes in and over time to an increasingly specialized and technologically-driven medical culture seen as depersonalized care through "mechanistic" medicine (Fox 1985; Callahan 1999; Tierney 2004; Arbuckle 2012; Cole et al. 2015). Drawing on multiple epistemological frames, the medical humanities advocates for the understanding of the complexities of modern lives and illness experiences in the clinical encounter (Carson 2007; Crawford et al. 2010; Metzl 2012; Boudreau and Fuks 2015). More recently, there has been a turn toward the Health Humanities, a more inclusive movement that considers health and healing outside of clinic and hospital walls. The broader scope of the health humanities encompasses caretakers and the host of allied health professionals that deliver patient care services and support care. Notably, this inclusion is an ideal collaborator for anthropologists (Jones et al. 2014; Crawford et al. 2015; Atkinson et al. 2015). Throughout the remainder of the paper, we will refer to our programming as health humanities. Like medical anthropology, health humanities seek to effect change in reductive medical education approaches. Approaches that may impede a physicians' ability to provide contextualized patient-centered care inclusive of the social, economic and political realities of disease and illness. The health humanities forwards paradigms and pedagogies of co-constructed humanistic learning where humanities philosophies and biological training benefit both patient and doctor. Current national and international discourse in the health humanities retains the movement's recurrent themes of the ethical-vocational obligations of integrating humanities content into medical curricula (Dror 2011; Shapiro 2012; Jones et al. 2014; Bleakley 2015; Westerhaus et al. 2015). It continues to call out hegemonic ideologies in biomedicine that preclude value-supported inclusion of the humanities in medical education. The health humanities push back against an economic and political climate, where medicine and health care seem fundamentally in opposition to core components of the humanities (Rorty 2007; Bullon et al. 2011; Good 2011a, b).

This last decade has brought greater accountability for including social or structural determinants on health and health care delivery in medical education. Health humanities scholars and biomedical educators alike argue for medical curricula that focuses attention on social, economic, and political factors that result in symptoms (Gravlee 2009; LaVeist and Isaac 2012; Metzl 2012; Metzl and Hansen 2014) and influence patient adherence and prognosis. Humanities scholars, such as Bleakly (2015) call for democratizing medicine, in which medical education and practice shift away from an authority-led hierarchy toward patient-centered, socially equitable care. Care practices that are fostered through the health humanities is a core discipline of medical education. Within academic institutions, debates center on how best to implement and evaluate humanities, as well as content in medical education. Discussions center on the differences in medical curricula quantitative frames and the interpretative qualitative frames of the humanities as well as contributing disciplines, desirable content, differing pedagogic approaches, and assessing learning outcomes (Schwartz et al. 2009; Wear 2009; Coria et al. 2013; Shankar 2014; Valsangkar et al. 2014; Bleakley et al. 2015; Cole et al. 2015; Tsevat et al. 2015). Coupled with these debates are concerns of humanities content drifting into the competency-based skill sets that lend themselves to the realm of biomedical clinical governance (Foucault 1975, 1977; Petersen et al. 2008) or medicalization (Clarke and Shim 2011; Dror 2011).

The increasing creation of health humanities courses and programs in medical schools has revived the emphasis of illness meanings and structural inequities in medical education, creating new opportunities for the current generation of anthropologists. More than conveying anthropological theories and methods into medical education and practice, ethnographic understanding of how efforts to transform medical education itself are necessary for sustainable contributions to the human experience of treating and living with illness. Drawing on our larger ethnographic research of a multidisciplinary effort to build a health humanities program, we highlight *processual aspects* of bringing together multiple humanities pedagogies and paradigms with those of medical education. Today's emphasis on interdisciplinary work coupled with the history of how anthropology has been used to reinforce cultural stereotyping rather than provoke an imagination of how to do things differently provided us with a unique opportunity.

Context and Structure

Using ethnographic methodologies SR documented, observed, participated in, and at times contributed to the building of the health humanities program at UCR. Anthropological theories of critical medical anthropology, political economy of health and structural determinants of health framed the ethnographic inquiry. The ethnography sought to explore how multiple fields of study, some with foundationally different approaches to knowledge generation and application, co-construct new paradigms in medical curricula and institute a health humanities program. A primary strength in selecting an ethnography to study the development of a medical humanities program is its inherently inclusive (democratizing) approach. As such, ethnographic methodologies allowed us to capture perspectives and voices of the multiple stakeholders in which developing and implementing a health humanities program could affect. In-depth exploration and documentation of the process of bringing multiple institutions, academic departments and faculty together with varying standpoints opened space for reflective understanding. It made visible how individuals (faculty) and institutions comprehend their role and culture in relation to transforming medical education, as well as conceptualize the medical humanities as a core part of medical education. To this extent, using an ethnographic approach allowed for interpretation of multiple perspectives in the processual development of the health humanities program. It helped to highlight the applied role, strengths and challenges of sustainable anthropological contributions in transforming medical education.

Through ethnographic methods of engaging the process of program development (the convening of multiple disciplines and schools, working across university institutions, and co-construction and implementation of program content), we asked: what mechanism opened space for, supported, independent faculty to convene; how are disciplinary boundaries and paradigms reconstituted to co-construct new frames; and whose knowledges are validated in program development? Observing how the multiple disciplines worked together offered insight into the ways in which the humanities and biomedicine translated their knowledge frames and practice paradigms. As well as, how the various humanities translated their disciplines' knowledge among themselves to engage and adapt their approaches to medical education. In doing so we examined institutional aspects of development across multiple administrative levels and systems, academic calendars, faculty permissions and institutional justifications for humanities content in medical curriculum. We documented the academic process of content development and pedagogical formulations and adaptations. Finally, once content was created, we observed how courses were implemented and received within medical education. Through our reflective and ethnographic experiences, we found that there is great potential for change, as there always has been, but that change towards humanities and social justice requires continual support (administrative, financial, and theoretical) from individuals and institutions.

UCR SOM is located in a medically underserved region, with a notable physician shortage, and poor population health indicators (Conduent Healthy Communities

Institute 2017; Riverside County Department of Public Health 2013). Referred to as the Inland Valleys, the region is economically and ethnically diverse. Riverside County's vast and fertile lands have been home to multiple Native American tribes, to the Spanish missions and Mexican land grants, European colonies and citrus farming, China towns of Chinese rail laborers, and has played a role in African-American civil rights. It is home to working undocumented immigrant populations and the second largest number of federally recognized tribes in the United States (U.S. Census Bureau 2017). In addition to the importance of UCR's location in addressing population health needs, UCR was uniquely positioned to host a medical school. For the past 30 years, UCR has implemented the UCR/University of California, Los Angeles (UCLA) Thomas Haider Biomedical Sciences program. Through the Haider program, medical students would complete the first 2 years of training at UCR, then transfer to UCLA's David Geffen School of Medicine for the third and fourth years. Because of the Haider program UCR already had both medical sciences and clinical faculty on campus to transition the program into the medical school. Distinctive to UCR's SOM is its establishment as a community-based medical model, in which there is no primary teaching hospital, but rather medical students train in the local community health systems. This model positions the SOM to meet its social mission to serve the medically underserved and train physicians who will stay in the local Inland Valley and southern California regions. With its social mission that emphasizes a physician workforce committed to wellness and health for the underserved regions of Riverside and the Inland Valley communities (Olds and Barton 2015), UCR SOM is a unique opportunity to improve doctor-patient encounters through humanities epistemological frames. In keeping with its social mission, its goal is to train doctors to address population needs for family, general internal, primary care pediatrics, obstetrics/gynecology and psychiatric medicine. UCR SOM's admission application includes a focus on medical students interested in health inequities and social justice. It retains 24 seats for UCR undergraduates, promoting inclusion of local students. Within its original curriculum development, the first 2 years are designated pass-fail in order to reduce competition among students and increase cooperative and effective learning. Unlike other medical schools, UCR's SOM students begin clinical work in their first year and its 4-year curriculum includes required courses designed to help students understand and address health disparities and population health. Finally, UCR SOM students are offered a loan forgiveness program for those who commit to practicing in the Inland Valley region for 5 years. In 2013, UCR SOM enrolled its inaugural cohort of 40 medical students, which graduated in 2017. All students matched for their residencies, 25% of its students will complete residencies in Riverside County, and 63% in Southern California.

The Health Humanities Work Group

It is worth noting that our ethnography of the development of the health humanities program began in 2012 with participant-observation of the UCR Health Humanities Work Group, 1 year prior to the SOM admitting medical students. The Health Humanities Work Group (the work group) is a core group of multi-disciplinary faculty that actively built UCR's health humanities program. Documenting its genesis, we describe how it was formed, and how it collaboratively produced and sustained itself over 3 years to create a recognized interdisciplinary health humanities program at UCR. We argue that without the development of the space for this collaborative effort, anthropological perspectives and faculty would not have been able to participate in the educational mission of the school of medicine.

Initial inter-campus discussion for humanities pedagogy in medical education at UCR was initiated between anthropology faculty and biomedical sciences faculty several years prior to enrollment of medical students. JM had engaged biomedical faculty directing the Thomas Haider Program in conversations regarding anthropological collaboration with the then existing program. Faculty in the biomedical program were interested in a more focused conversation on health inequalities for their students. This effort led to invited lectures by medical anthropologists during the first 2 years of the existing Thomas Haider Program. While these conversations were sporadic, interest in nurturing community-centered medical students led to continued conversations.

A Medical Narratives Colloquium, initiated and led by JM and Chikako Takeshita, was established in 2011 through an Andrew W. Mellon Foundation grant with UCR's Center for Ideas and Society. This Medical Narratives group housed in the College of Humanities and Social Science (CHASS) brought together interdisciplinary scholars for theoretical and research-based discussions, workshops and debates centered on the intersections of humanities and medicine. Faculty participation in the work group varied, at times including faculty representing anthropology, art history, creative writing, history, psychology, science and technology, School of Medicine, theater, and women's studies. A smaller contingent of six CHASS and SOM faculty from this interdisciplinary group would make up a core work group dedicated to regular meetings, dialogue, education, material, and content development. Aspects of their work can be found at https://mednarratives.com/. The primary aim was to strengthen interdisciplinary conversations around that role of narrative in medical practice and education. Our conceptualization of narrative ranged from the central work of Arthur Kleinman (illness narratives) to Rita Charon (narrative medicine) and Michel Foucault (power/knowledge and discourse). The work group sought to foreground the interpretive-dialogical engagement—the dynamics of the clinical encounter and medicine more broadly that address the knowledge perspectives, power relations and collaborations between patient and provider. In other words, the dialogue that takes place between patient and provider that is weighted with plural worldviews, ontologies, and epistemologies. Additionally, the work group sought to address institutionalized aspects of medical education that create conflict with medical students' personal and ethical values and ability to build a productive patient-provider relationship.

With the opportunity to meet regularly and consider our interdisciplinary perspectives, JM, Tiffany Lopez (Professor of Theater, Film, and Digital Production) and Paul Lyons (Professor and Senior Associate Dean for Medical Education) developed a proposal for the National Endowment for the Humanities (NEH), Humanities Initiatives program in 2014 and was awarded 3-years of funding for "Narratives in Tandem: Creating New Medical and Health Humanities Programming". The NEH award represented how scholars from across campus could collaborate toward a common goal, facilitating conversations between humanities and medical faculty. Collaborations addressed among the interdisciplinary group included the cultural, economic, historical, and philosophical complexities of medical encounters of health and illness; as well as delivery of quality care. Over the 3-year period, the core working group designed and received institutional approval for a PhD Designated Emphasis (DE) in medical and health humanities. Because the processes for the PhD DE is on a different timeline and approval process for medical students, a second DE for medical students was developed. The Medical and Health Humanities DE for medical students, developed by JM and supported by Dr. Lyons, includes over ten courses. The DE courses link seven humanities disciplinary knowledge paradigms with expected medical student research (practice improvement projects), clinical (Longitudinal Ambulatory Care Experience (LACE), and course work (Clinical Reasoning). Some of the more traditional humanities courses in the DE include *Introduction to Medical and Health Humanities, Narrative Pathways*, *Literature and Disabilities,* and *Indigenous Literature*. While the group had hoped to have greater integration with the broader medical school curriculum, to date, mechanisms to be integral partners in curriculum building have not been achieved. Prior to the official implementation of the DE, the core work group designed and implemented two mandatory courses, Clinical Reasoning and Medical Humanities and Narratives plus one selective course, graphic medicine with an artist-in-residence. In 2017 the DE for medical students was opened and 6.5% of the 4-year medical student body self-enrolled during its first block. This number is extraordinary. Reports from colleagues in other medical schools who have initiated a DE or certificate program in medical humanities report less than 1% of the students enroll in these elective programs.

While the intra- and extramural funding that we received put our group on the map and much had been achieved, it was not clear that humanities, outside of our group, would ever play a significant role in medical education unless we translated our goals, making them legible to the institution. This meant that our goals had to take on more utilitarian forms—they needed to address institutional academic goals of "increasing empathy" in medical students or fit into the goals of a select group of students who were motivated toward social justice. On the "practical" institutional level, funding is eligible to institutions. If a medical and health humanities focus can bring insufficient indirects, then ways can be found to accommodate its presence. Importantly, our group included individuals, Associate Deans, and senior level faculty in the School of Medicine who also supported our efforts.

Making Space and Stitching Pieces Together

Convening Faculty

Over the course of 3 years of bi-monthly meetings and quarterly seminars with outside speakers, three persistent practices in the planning and implementing of our program were observed and documented. These recurring practices included a highly dialogical engagement, iterative progression, and participating faculty's educational investment. Ideally each practice would have informed the translation of multiple paradigms and pedagogy in program content. In reality, interdisciplinary work in a medical school is challenging. Disciplinary investments, individual personalities, and institutional expectations are ready to thwart attempts to include anything new into medical education, particularly courses that are not taught by Medical Doctors (MDs).

Dialogical Engagement, Iterative Processes, and Education Investment

In our effort to make space for broader experiences in medical education, dialogical engagement among the work group was observed to be most critical and frequent in the initial stages of development. This engagement required anthropological skills of determining individual and disciplinary (i.e., cultural) expectations and how to stitch those desires alongside the goals of creating transformative spaces that also met the expectations of the AAMC. Over the course of 2 years, discussions involved understanding the varying disciplinary ideologies of knowledge paradigms and pedagogical approaches. Dialogical engagement and framing occurred in the form of meetings, emails, and hallway conversations. Meetings could draw upwards of 20 faculty representing the various humanities disciplines and medical school faculty. However, faculty participation attrition was one of the first challenges faced in advancing toward a program. In fact, no one in our group had been trained in Medical or Health Humanities. We all had research that focused on health, illness, and health inequalities, but those interests were bound by our respective disciplines. In addition, faculty participating in the initiatives and development process had several duties within their own departments. For some scholars, disciplinary boundaries are difficult to cross. There are a host of reasons that these divides occur, for some stages of career may hang in the balance. How is someone to obtain tenure or subsequent promotions if their work does not obviously and significantly contribute to their field? For example, as an anthropologist, JM was often questioned about how her work promoted the goals of the field and that if she did not become more focused her research would suffer. While on one hand, anthropological contributions to addressing health inequalities and how to collaborate and understand diverse communities were highly valued, to transform those research endeavors into the needs of a professional school, like medicine, raises questions about how to situate the resulting knowledge within disciplinary fields.

How to stitch together the needs of the institution, discipline, and contribute to medical education is an ongoing and challenging question. It is challenging because of the mechanisms required to make space for remembering that medicine is about humans, not only science. In our case, an instrumental asset to meeting shifting educational goals for the work group was funding. External funding afforded opportunities to invite medical humanities scholars from multiple universities to take part in half-day workshops with the work group. More importantly, it demonstrated that what we were doing had value to scholars and professionals outside of our small group. Bringing experts to our campus made space for our group to show our dialogical engagement, both as actors and creators in this multi-voiced effort. Our guest scholars provided insight, direction, guidance and recommendations on program development and implementation. The repetitive process of hearing other voices then returning to the table for dialogue on how to stitch together those aspects of the various disciplines' frames and methods drafted a targeted, inclusive, and integrated program. Thus, external funding made space for transformations in medical education. It also meant that one discipline could not dominate the effort. And yet, it was challenging because aspects of the humanities, arts, and social sciences that are not as complicated to integrate into medical education, are the first to be taken up in the curriculum. A secondary problem with external funding is that projects that focus on health inequalities and community engaged research are easier to fund in Schools of Medicine than humanities and medical education projects. As the anthropologist in the SOM, JM found that there was a greater push to secure external funding for research on health inequity rather than in humanistic arts focused endeavors. While this could have been an additional opportunity to include medical students in multiple forms of health equity and humanistic research, there was insufficient infrastructure at the beginning to actually make that happen.

JM was the primary organizer of the regular meetings with the interdisciplinary faculty. Some meetings were dynamic, and others were contemplative. Even though we are academics used to debating and considering different ideas, we found that it is often difficult to hear differing perspectives and definitions of common place terms and jargon. For example, as the work group engaged theoretical premises of knowledge production and ways of knowing, it required reception to multiple explications of the ways in which the body is known, from art to history and medicine. Understandings of the production and meaning of the phenomena of "disease," "illness," and "patient-lived experience" had to not only be understood in the context of the mechanics of anatomy, but also from a social context. Dialogue around the dominant narratives of both medicine and the humanities (and medicine versus the humanities) necessitated reflection and telling truths in order to push past divides to work toward inclusive change—such as medicine's medical hegemony and ambiguity and, even, what constitutes a narrative and its meaning. In another example, comprehension of the nature of the clinical encounter required care in consideration of the multiple views of the encounter: interpretive and patient-centered, co-constructed narrative, regulatory and time-driven, as well as its financial and paper life. Despite the effort to be inclusive, understanding, and to make space, each of these conversations was a power struggle. Questions about clinical encounters are not just about the patient and the physician, they are also about diversity. Who should teach the course? Whose voices will be heard? Will minority voices be included, or will we continue to have non-BIPOC teaching diverse humanistic perspectives on medicine? Anthropology and the humanities more broadly have their own problems with inclusion. Staying with the trouble of making space and fostering dialogic engagement is that we are human, some people do not want to hear other perspectives, or are easily offended when a different path is offered. Others do not understand why different voices should be included. To say that our group did not argue, and that people were not dismayed would be a lie. Our desire to make bigger changes, however, allowed us to stitch together the pieces. It is unclear to JM that this was actually the better approach, but it is what we did.

On our lighter days of conversation, the work group often assumed that the best approach for our program in the medical school was to "highlight the unique opportunity to embed humanities into the curriculum. Not as an elective." Prompted by an outside speaker, an intensive debate ensued around this question. What use was it to have angry students in a humanities lecture who did not want to be there and whose only goal was to disrupt the class because "what they were learning had nothing to do with medicine." On the other hand, what use was it to have students who self-select into the class as they were likely those students who were already seeking better ways to humanistically practice medicine? At other times, convening multiple paradigms and pedagogy could beg the question, *Does disciplinary jargon make us illegible to each other?* What is most important about this iterative process of dialogical engagement is that it gave the group a center, a space to work from and toward integration with medical education. These iterative conversations allowed for moments of attentive care to draw out and move toward informed understandings among the group. Questions about jargon, and the time necessary to transform thinking from utilitarian to emancipatory highlighted the divergent knowledge frames and approaches among humanities disciplines at the table. But they were also questions that through iterative dialogue brought forth the shared ideologies between humanities and biomedicine—of medicine as a social discipline.

Within the context of these conversations, the work group recognized not only the need to educate each other about their disciplines' paradigms and pedagogy, but also their perspectives on their own disciplinary contributions to medical education. Planning time for "education sessions" among the work group presented a challenge to program development due to the varying faculty schedules and responsibilities. The education sessions however were deemed an essential asset in being able to academically and ideologically create an inclusive and co-constructed medical and health humanities program. Individual members of the work group prepared written descriptions of knowledge frames and methods from their perspective disciplines as it related to medicine. Additionally, each recommended articles, texts, and works that exemplified their discipline. One dynamic conversation focused on narrative in theater and in the clinic. Faculty participants recognized that when they spoke about narrative for the arts versus narrative as a way to co-construct a treatment itinerary for patients and physicians, what each wanted to include as significant in the narrative was at odds. In addition to learning the multiple disciplinary frames, the work group sought to explore what constituted the "medical and health humanities" and what were the key debates and calls within the health humanities both nationally and locally. This debate, at times, reductively centered on not wanting "health humanities" because it sounded like a physical education class, something to not be taken seriously. Parsing out these debates and preferences required research by work group members on defining medical and health humanities, identifying existing programs, approaches, and outcomes on medical education. A primary goal of the work group in building the health humanities program was a program that would support the vision that "Humanities is medicine.", a phrase coined by Paul Lyons.

Despite the commitment of the work group, sustaining engagement required commitment from individuals in the group to organize and host meetings to further previous discourse through meeting agendas and goals. In this regard, one of the assets in building the UCR SOM health humanities program was an advocate of the cause; someone driven to keep the momentum of the development on track and visible. Within the work group JM, with the enduring collaboration of Tiffany Lopez and Paul Lyons, continuously moved the dialogical, educational, and translational process along. Their collaboration ensured that we would convene regular meetings, secure locations for meetings, coordinate faculty availability, investigate funding opportunities, and manage program and content development. Collaboration with a key person in the SOM, and then JM's move to the SOM, was critical as it built a bridge, ensuring that the work that the faculty outside of the SOM was engaging in would ultimately be included in medical education.

Working Across Schools/Disciplines

Although the work group had refined and merged paradigmatic approaches for program goals and content, cultural differences between the humanities and medicine did present challenges. The work group encountered professional and institutional norm differences between the schools. As anthropologists leading the effort to broaden medical education on our campus, it was critical that we understood how medical schools functioned. One of the first challenges faced as the work group began to institutionally formalize the health humanities program was the requirement to justify the need for humanities content in the medical curriculum for SOM administrators. Like the majority of medical schools, UCR's SOM medical curriculum is identified as "impacted" and/or often under pressure to include more material. Because the work group included senior medical faculty, they were able to guide us in the challenges we would encounter in bringing and justifying the program in the professional structures of a medical institution.

For the humanities faculty in the work group it was observed that understanding, engaging and working within the culture of medical education presented a critical learning component for developing and implementing humanities program content. As stated by a medical faculty work group member, "Humanities needs to be exposed and aware of medical culture." While Western biomedicine's culture of hierarchical structure and erudite reverence are more well-known and evident in working across institutions, the work group's experience here focuses on didactic norms and expectations. For example, as program content began to take shape, dialogue emerged around the fundamental differences in arriving at or achieving intended objectives in learning. In translating medical and health humanities content the work group identified that, "in medicine the correlative of being better means they get narrower in what they take in for a diagnosis," and that medicine, "is an information field but. . . .Students don't know what to do with information outside of biomedical science." Consequently, as identified by the work group's medical faculty, medical students "are not being trained on relationships of providing care" that draw on more interpretive frames found in the humanities.

These examples of learning premises presented the work group with the challenge of developing content that was inclusive of biomedical and humanities approaches. As such, it was noted that the work group sought to address an integrative approach asking *How do we create content that engages the medical tool of differential diagnosis without foreclosing valuable and essential humanities knowledge?* Developing content that was co-constructed or representative and inclusive of the disciplinary composition of the work group was predicated on the work groups continuous dialogical engagement. An engagement that required a translation process where the multiple disciplinary paradigms were visited and revisited, imagined and created, and re-imagined and re-created into co-constructed content. It required disciplinary boundaries to be deconstructed in ways that did more than lend disciplinary theories and methodologies to medical training for consideration. Co-constructed translation meant content that was built into medical training in a manner in which its application was made visible as a vital variable. A primary asset the work group held in addressing and developing such content was the diverse and inclusive disciplinary composition of the faculty within the group itself. The work group was well equipped to respond, drawing on its dialogical, iterative and educational approaches in building the program's foundation. Hence, the design of the health humanities program was both embedded within existing UCR SOM medical training courses and also focused on clinical practice. Noted was the work group's approach of providing justification by showing how the program lent itself to meeting aspects of the SOM's mission, training values, and strategic plan:

- *Inclusion—Embracing diversity in the broadest sense and appreciating all points of view.* (mission)
- *Developing innovative research and healthcare delivery programs ... and become a model to be emulated throughout the state and nation.* (mission statement)
- *Education Objective #4 Augment undergraduate and graduate medical education programs with new opportunities in inter-professional education, community service and outreach.* (strategic plan)

- Innovative training that *emphasizes patient continuity, progressive learning, public health, social determinants of health, and practice improvement research.* (strategic plan)

Could this work have been done by anyone other than an anthropologist? Probably. But anthropology is positioned in a unique space that is ideally suited for dialogical engagement. In fact, other Medical and Health Humanities programming that are emerging across the US are often started by anthropologists. If we are to make space for a diversity of voices and alternative ways of encountering medicine or encountering humans, then anthropologists must be key players. We must find a way to be outside of our disciplinary boundaries and critiques of medicine, so that we can make space for actually educating and doing medicine differently.

The Liminal Road Between Towers: Anthropology and Medicine—An Ethnographer's Experience

A critical component in the methodological process of an ethnography is the reflective process of the ethnographer. Reflexivity allows for understanding of how one's encounters, experiences, and comprehension may be influenced during the ethnographic process and more importantly, determining where, how, or if those experiences may inform data collection and analysis. The reflective process at this moment adds the perspective of a generation of anthropological training in medical education. While much of the program building was done by JM and colleagues farther along in their academic careers, the view from the beginning of a career is critical in understanding the impact of interdisciplinary and professional education on anthropological training and disciplinary assumptions. In this section, SR shares her experiences as an ethnographer working between and among two divergent fields: Anthropology and Medicine.

Selecting to be a participant-observer within the work group provided a unique opportunity to observe the multi-voice perspectives of the various disciplines engaged in program development. It also helped to establish familiarity and trust among the participating faculty as a researcher with genuine interest in the debates, processes and nuances of co-constructing change in medical education. Unquestionably, committed and regular participant-observation created a relationship that fostered introduction and access to a network of additional and alternative voices in the development of the health humanities program. It is not novel within ethnographic work to struggle to gain an audience with those considered to hold the power within a given culture. And while my work with and within the work group afforded opportunities to engage those with power among the two fields (humanities and medicine), responses to ethnographic inquiries were expressly different and reflective of the differing cultures. Responses from faculty within CHASS for interviews or meetings with a graduate researcher tended to be received as an exchange typifying their academic roles in serving students. Although often busy or overextended, CHASS faculty interactions conveyed a more equitable position deference. CHASS faculty were overall more accessible in contacting them without colleague introductions or recommendations for contact, and more likely to respond to requests to meet without introductions. While this is not the case of CHASS faculty disciplines wide, my time and work overall was demonstrated as relevant via acts of engendered moments for sharing their positions and perspectives in translating their paradigms in medical training. CHASS faculty interactions most often exhibited recognition of the value of such studies even when it was not related to their own work or positions. This is not to say that SOM faculty were better or worse, but rather to convey a fundamental difference experienced between the cultures and cultural expectations of medical training and humanities education. Those SOM faculty explicitly interested and supportive of the role of humanities in medicine provided time and moments to share their perspectives, often deferring to the knowledge of the humanities scholars and my own as an anthropologist researching and working with medicine. Access to and response from faculty and administration in the SOM were greatly facilitated by participation in the work group. Because the work group had several medical school faculty, including two departmental deans from the school of medicine, introductions to medical administration and faculty were made on my behalf. This is not to say however, that requests for interviews were always accepted. In some cases, those medical faculty who declined interviews cited their unfamiliarity with my area of study. Interestingly, those who cited lack of knowledge on the topic had been selected for their role, in some way, in fostering more humanistic learning. Although this may have presented a challenge to my study goals, I sought it as an opportunity to explore the "semantics" of humanities in medical education. How were those existing, sporadic courses within the medical curriculum which drew from humanities frames understood within the curriculum? How do medical institutions, administration and faculty conceptualize the humanities? What are the mechanisms that make such courses acceptable within the medical culture, while direct intentional development of humanities courses in medical education can generate such resistance? Inquires that lead to examining whose voice is heard and whose knowledge is validated.

A principle tenet of anthropological ethnographies is the immersing of oneself in the subject culture while maintaining object reflexivity. As an anthropologist studying within the SOM, I encountered as much, and at times, more challenges from within my own field. Having entered the ethnography with a working background in healthcare as an anthropologist and training in public health, I was repeatedly told to change the language I used to more "anthropological" terms. In part, I understood this criticism as the tension between academia and the medicalization and misappropriation of "culture in medicine" and perhaps stemming from decades of cultural competency approaches in healthcare, that could cause more harm than good. However, given that anthropologists conducting ethnographies in cultures with languages and terminology other than their own are expected to learn and speak the language and/or jargon, being repeatedly called out in the use of terminology/language that was used in the structures of medicine was both frustrating and discouraging. Was using the language of my study site making me less of an anthropologist? Does its use hinder or facilitate comprehension and translation of paradigmatic approaches?

As an applied medical anthropologist with a focus on health disparities and inequities studying in a research institution, the very process of merging my health training with academic anthropological theory seemed to parallel the observation of the work group in developing the health humanities program. In one tower, I am too clinical in my application to theory and approach, while in the other too theoretical for discernible value-driven application. For me, this tension spoke to the heart of the matter: finding the line of perceptible and appreciable translation among divergent paradigms and pedagogy. To be clear, I hold paramount the significance of anthropological theory and methodological approaches in my research. They are the scope through which I explore the power dynamics at play in health inequities and structural determinants. My experience, however, left me often pondering why I would have to relinquish the very premises of what brought me to medical education as an anthropologist in order to be considered anthropologically trained.

Most anthropologists having worked or working in medicine and healthcare are likely to have experienced the medical regard of anthropology as "complementary" or "value-added." In other words, nice to know but not of practical value in "real medical" training. In this ethnography, anthropology and humanities were not broadly recognized for their real and practical applications in medical training. There were however a number of SOM faculty, to include those of significant position that not only recognized its applications, but also who were advocates of integrating humanities into medical training. This experience could be biased however by the number of faculty who sought employment at the medical school due to its mission. The medical regard of anthropology among medical students somewhat mimicked that of the faculty. The student body of the medical school has shown a considerable interest (by comparative percent enrollments) in medical humanities courses and social justice, an observation potentially biased by the school's mission and application/acceptance process. What I did observe with enrolled medical students was students either tended to be aware and interested in the role of humanities in their medical training or dismissive of its use in their training schedule. The latter often seemed to be reinforced by standard medical institution expectations and culture. When conducting participant-observation among the medical students, I experienced encounters when students behaved, approached, and spoke to me differently when they learned I was not medical faculty. An experience also shared by some humanities faculty during interviews. In the competitive culture of medical training, it is not uncommon for the medical students to be keenly focused and attentive to those persons, activities, and interactions that serve their current and future standing.

Observing medicine as an institution, beginning to embrace the concepts of social determinants and structural competency in health and health outcomes, is both promising and intriguing. The relationship of social determinants and political economy of health on health care outcomes is not new to anthropologist or humanities scholars. Hence, it is promising to see medical training (and the medical students on their own initiative) seek knowledge frames and pedagogy to address structural impacts in provisions of patient care—a noted turn from its delegation by medicine to social work. For certain, the language and definitions of social determinants can be found in biomedical associations such as the American Medical Association, Institute of Medicine, and others; and glimpsed in medical literature. At present, as observed at the UCR SOM, structural determinants are moving toward application in training and practice supported by key faculty and medical student special interest groups. This embrace mirrors tensions around the validation of knowledge, application and knowledge-power itself, yet, also affords anthropologists a space and moment for humanistic pedagogy in medical education. This turn, too, offers a moment and space for ethnographic observation of the course of the institution of medicine's integration of social/structural determinants in medical training. How will they be forwarded and tied to competencies? How might integration avoid drift into medicalizing or distilling of structural determinants into quick reference for differential diagnoses.

None of these shared experiences are necessarily new or groundbreaking. They are however being shared for those anthropologists entering or considering work as an anthropologist in medicine. Like the study of all cultures, there are learning curves and hard lessons, but unlike a bounded study discernible translation between paradigmatically different fields requires persistent reflection. Ultimately, as an anthropologist working in medicine and health care, the renewed attention to the fundamental role of humanities knowledge and approaches in medical training is both exciting and encouraging. And perhaps a pathway to sustainable translation.

Table 10.1 provides a list of strengths, challenges, and outcomes identified in our ethnographic and reflective work on the building of a health humanities program. We found that co-constructing content that forwards humanistic knowledge in medical education, requires continuous dialogical engagement and attentiveness to systems and practices that foreclose alternative paradigms in medical education. The revisiting and redefining ways of knowing in medical practices is a moment for anthropologists to better understand their contributions to sustaining perceptible and equitable content in medical education.

Conclusion

The co-constructed translation of multiple disciplines' knowledge paradigms and pedagogies in building UCR's health humanities program was observed ethnographically as a central premise to bringing the program to fruition. In our study, the act of effectively translating disciplinary frames for collaboration was contingent upon the enacted dialogical, educational, and iterative processes. Processes that required balancing the integration of humanities and medical knowledges between unintelligible translation and reductive medicalization. Anthropologists working in medical education and practice are and have been keenly aware of the dangers or unintended consequences of the translation of their knowledge frames into utilitarian

Table 10.1 Strengths, challenges, and outcomes in building a health humanities program

Strengths
• 3-year National Endowment for the Humanities funding
• Advocate or champion to sustain momentum
• Supported by the UCR SOM Dean of Education and Dean of Clinical Affairs
• Education investment of faculty work group members
• External health humanities scholar workshops for the work group
• New medical school with social mission to address health inequities
• Commitment to dialogical engagement
• Commitment to reiterative processes of program development
• Program content objectives aligned with UCR SOM mission and strategic plan
Challenges
• Interested and participating faculty schedules
• Disciplinary boundaries and institutional expectation of faculty members
• Disciplinary jargon
• Deconstructing ways of knowing among multiple disciplines
• Culture differences between medicine and humanities
• Funding
• Differing academic calendars
• Funding faculty working across disciplines—time designations
• Developing content that would avoid utilitarian forms, medicalization
• Medical student resistance to new course content
• Acceptance by medical students of humanities scholars teaching in SOM
Outcomes
• Health Humanities Designated Emphasis for UCR's medical students
• 6.5% self-enrollment of medical students in Health Humanities DE
• Health Humanities Designated Emphasis for UCR's PhD students
• Humanities content linked to medical education research, clinical and course work
• Required longitudinal course for medical students
• Interdisciplinary faculty teaching courses in SOM

skill sets and competencies for medical training purposes; or medicalization (Browner 1999; Clarke and Shim 2011; Dror 2011). Humanities knowledge paradigms translated without working knowledge of their intersection with medical knowledge and practice can fail to contribute to humanistic and equitable quality care.

Like medicine, anthropology (and the humanities) is a calling. A vocation that is a politicizing, ethnicizing, and ideological critique (Dror 2011) of the world and societies in which we all live. For those anthropologists drawing from critical theory, such as critical medical anthropologists, working in biomedicine requires recognition of space and moments in which their translation of critical contributions exposes them to criticism from the medical institution. And certainly not to be overlooked, draws out professional frustrations of working as an anthropologist in biomedicine. Critical medical anthropology and critical medical humanities is often understood, and unfortunately at times poorly translated by anthropologists and medical humanities scholars as portraying medicine as Machiavellian or viewed as determined in its agenda to define medicine as a conscious oppressor of patient agency, and specifically of the underserved. These critiques are well documented in literature and discourse on the anthropological role in medical education and practice, citing the perception of anthropological knowledge and approach as a harsh and critical voice, one that is counterproductive to advocating for humanities in medicine (Peterson 2008; Shapiro et al. 2009; Jones et al. 2014; Atkinson et al. 2015).

However, from the anthropologist's paradigmatic perspective it is their obligation to respond to the positions of social structures and most specifically the effects those structures have on the people they serve. Yet, retaining discipline ideology within medical culture, like translation, requires critical reflexivity from anthropologists. It is equally important to call out the responsibility that critical medical anthropologists and critical medical humanities must take in responding to biomedicine's critiques and resistance to inclusions of humanities knowledge frames. As a collaborator in a medical humanities program or as an anthropologist working in medicine, Goffey (2015) suggests that critical insights that build upon the insistence of the acceptance of biomedical knowledge as social constructs can themselves produce hierarchies.

In sustaining anthropological work in biomedicine, anthropologists might benefit from viewing themselves as what Viney et al. (2015) call a *critical collaborator*: a complex role "based on the notions of entanglement, rather than servility or antagonism" (Viney et al. 2015) where enacting critical theories, welded reflexively, are our core strength. For those anthropologists in biomedicine the turn may become how we then respond to collaborations with biomedicine "while retaining the uniqueness of our anthropological perspective" (Browner 1999). Our commitment to the vocation of anthropology that forwards collaborations with biomedicine which engage a politicizing, ethicizing, and ideological critique (Dror 2011) co-constructs change.

In the last round of increased anthropological presence in medical education, Nancy Scheper-Hughes (1990) warned us that we needed to cut loose our "moorings from conventional biomedical premises and epistemologies." That becoming part of a system premised on funding and hegemonic models of bodies and knowledge would undermine the goals of anthropology. She reminded us that, "Ours must be an anthropology of affliction and not simply an anthropology of medicine." Our reiterations of medicine as a practice of human interaction in medical education is a struggle, a constant institutional reminding of what is at stake when we only teach future physicians about the workings of the body. They are also reiterations to ourselves—a constant reminder that we do not live in a world of anthropologically-minded people, but rather we have to find a way to translate, transform, and continually reiterate that there is ambiguity in medicine, there are other ways to understand context and suffering. To think like an anthropologist, whether it is under the guise of medical and health humanities, global health, medical anthropology, or any other current name, is to create opportunities for alternatives, and to change systems of power that have for too long lead to sustained health inequalities.

References

Anderson, Warren. 2011. Outside looking in: Observations on medical education since the flexner report. *Medical Education* 45: 29–35.
Arbuckle, Gerald. 2012. *Humanizing healthcare reforms*. London: Jessica Kingsley Publishers.
Atkinson, Sarah, Bethan Evans, Angela Woods, and Robin Kearns. 2015. The 'Medical' and 'Health' in a critical medical humanities. *Journal of Medical Humanities* 36: 71–81.
Bleakley, Alan. 2015. *Medical humanities and medical education: How the medical humanities can shape better doctors*. New York: Routledge.
Boudreau, J., and Abraham Fuks. 2015. The humanities in medical education: Ways of knowing, doing and being. *Journal of Medical Humanities* 36: 321–336.
Bouwsma, William J. 1990. *A usable past: Essays in european cultural history*. Berkeley, CA: University of California Press.
Browner, Carole. 1999. On the medicalization of medical anthropology. *Medical Anthropology Quarterly* 13: 135–140.
Bullon, Antonio, Mary-Jo DelVecchio Good, and Elizabeth Carpenter-Song. 2011. The paper life of minority and low-income patient care. In *Shattering culture: American medicine responds to cultural diversity*, ed. Mary-Jo DelVecchio Good, Sarah S. Willen, Seth Donal Hannah, Ken Vickery, and Lawrence Taeseng Park, 200–216. New York: Russell Sage Foundation.
Callahan, Daniel. 1999. The hastings center and the early years of bioethics. *Kennedy Institute of Ethics Journal* 9: 53–71.
Carson, Ronald. 2007. Engaged humanities: Moral work in the precincts of medicine. *Perspectives in Biology and Medicine* 50: 321–333.
Clarke, Adele, and Janet Shim. 2011. Medicalization and biomedicalization revisited: Technoscience and transformations of health, illness and american medicine. In *Handbook of the sociology of health, illness, and healing*, ed. Bernice A. Pescosolido, Jack K. Martin, Jane D. McLeod, and Anne Rogers, 173–199. New York: Springer New York.
Cole, Thomas R., Nathan S. Carlin, and Ronald A. Carson. 2015. *Medical humanities: An introduction*. New York: Cambridge University Press.
Conduent Healthy Communities Institute. 2017. *The 2017 socioneeds index, strategic health alliance pursuing equity*. www.shaperivco.org/Socioneeds. Accessed 20 Jan 2018.
Coria, Alexandra, T. Greg McKelvey, Paul Charlton, Michael H. Woodworth, and Timothy Lahey. 2013. The design of a medical school social justice curriculum. *Academic Medicine* 88: 1442–1449.
Crawford, Paul, Brian Brown, Charley Baker, Victoria Tischler, and Brian Abrams. 2015. *Health humanities*. New York: Palgrave Macmillan.
Crawford, Paul, Brian Brown, Victoria Tischler, and Charley Baker. 2010. Health humanities: The future of medical humanities? *Mental Health Review Journal* 15: 4–10.
Dror, Otniel. 2011. De-medicalizing the medical humanities. *The European Legacy* 16: 317–326.
Fadiman, Anne. 1997. *The Spirit catches you and you fall down: A hmong child, her american doctors, and the collision of two cultures*. New York: Farrar, Straus, and Giroux.
Foucault, Michel. 1975. *The birth of the clinic*. Trans. A.M. Sheridan Smith. New York: Vintage Books.
———. 1977. *Discipline and punish: The birth of the prison*. New York: Vintage Books.
Fox, Daniel. 1985. Who we are: The political origins of the medical humanities. *Theoretical Medicine* 6: 327–341.
Goffey, Andrew. 2015. Homo immunologicus: On the limits of critique. *Medical Humanities* 41: 8–13.
Good, Mary-Jo DelVecchio. 2011a. Shattering culture: An introduction. In *Shattering culture: American medicine responds to cultural diversity*, ed. Mary-Jo DelVecchio Good, Sarah S. Willen, Seth Donal Hannah, Ken Vickery, and Lawrence Taeseng Park, 1–30. New York: Russell Sage Foundation.

———. 2011b. The inner life of medicine: A commentary on anthropologies of clinical training in the twenty-first century. *Culture, Medicine, and Psychiatry* 35: 321–327.

Gravlee, Clarence. 2009. How race becomes biology: Embodiment of social inequality. *American Journal of Physical Anthropology* 139: 47–57.

Holmes, Seth M. and Maya Pointe. (2011). En-case-ing the patient: disciplining uncertainty in medical student patient presentations. Culture, Medicine, and Psychiatry, 35(2), 163–182.

Hunt, Linda (1994). An Anthropologist in the Land of Clinical Research: Quagmires of Collaborative Inquiry. Paper presented at the 93rd Annual Meeting of the American Anthropological Association, Atlanta, GA.

Jones, E., and E. Tansey, eds. 2015. *The development of narrative practices in medicine c. 1960-c. 2000*. London: Queen Mary, University of London.

Jones, Therese, Delese Wear, and Lester Friedman. 2014. *Health humanities reader*. New Brunswick: Rutgers University Press.

Kleinman, Arthur. 1988. *The illness narratives: Suffering, healing, and the human condition*. New York: Basic Books.

Kumagai, Arno. 2014. From competencies to human interests: Ways of knowing and understanding in medical education. *Academic Medicine* 89: 978–983.

LaVeist, Thomas, and Lydia Isaac. 2012. *Race, ethnicity, and health: A public health reader*. New Jersey: Wiley.

Metzl, Jonathan. 2012. Structural competency. *American Quarterly* 64: 213–218.

Metzl, Jonathan, and Helena Hansen. 2014. Structural competency: Theorizing a new medical engagement with stigma and inequality. *Social Science & Medicine* 103: 126–133.

Olds, G., and Kathryn Barton. 2015. Building medical schools around social missions: The case of the university of california, riverside. *Health Systems & Reform* 1: 200–206.

Petersen, Alan, Alan Bleakley, Rainer Brömer, and Rob Marshal. 2008. The medical humanities today: Humane health care or tool of governance? *Journal of Medical Humanities* 29: 1–4.

Podolsky, Scott, and Jeremy Greene. 2014. Are the medical humanities for sale? Lessons from a historical debate. *Journal of Medical Humanities* 37: 355–370.

Riverside County Department of Public Health. 2013. https://www.rivcoph.org/Portals/0/pdf/2013_Community_Health_Profile.pdf. Accessed 20 Jan 2018. Community health profile.

Rorty, Richard. 2007. *Philosophy as cultural politics: Vol. 4. Philosophical papers*. New York: Cambridge University Press.

Scheper-Hughes, Nancy. 1990. Three propositions for a critically applied medical anthropology. *Social Science & Medicine* 30: 189–197.

Schwartz, Andrea, Jeremy Abramson, Israel Wojnowich, Robert Accordino Edward Rona, and Mary Rifkin. 2009. Evaluating the impact of the humanities in medical education. *Mount Sinai Journal of Medicine* 76: 372–380.

Shankar, P. 2014. Medical humanities: Developing into a mainstream discipline. *Journal of Educational Evaluation for Health Professions* 11: 32.

Shapiro, Johanna. 2012. Whither (whether) medical humanities? The future of humanities and arts in medical education. *Journal for Learning Through the Arts* 8.

Shapiro, Johanna, Jack Coulehan, Delese Wear, and Martha Montello. 2009. Medical humanities and their discontents: Definitions, critiques, and implications. *Academic Medicine* 84: 192–198.

Tierney, Thomas. 2004. Foucault on the case: The pastoral and juridical foundation of medical power. *Journal of Medical Humanities 25*: 271–290.

Tsevat, Rebecca, Anoushka Sinha, Kevin Gutierrez, and Sayantani DasGupta. 2015. Bringing home the health humanities: Narrative humility, structural competency, and engaged pedagogy. *Academic Medicine* (11): 1462–1465.

U.S. Census Bureau. 2017. *QuickFacts: Riverside county, California*. https://www.census.gov/quickfacts/map/IPE120213/06065. Accessed 20 Jan 2018.

Valsangkar, Bina, Candice Chen, Hannah Wohltjen, and Fitzhugh Mullan. 2014. Do medical school mission statements align with the nation's health care needs? *Academic Medicine* 89: 892–895.

Viney, William, Felicity Callard, and Angela Woods. 2015. Critical medical humanities: Embracing entanglement, taking risks. *Medical Humanities* 41: 2–7.
Wear, Delese. 2009. The medical humanities: Toward a renewed praxis. *Journal of Medical Humanities* 30: 209–220.
Westerhaus, Michael, Amy Finnegan, Mona Haidar, Arthur Kleinman, Joia Mukherjee, and Paul Farmer. 2015. The necessity of social medicine in medical education. *Academic Medicine* 90: 565–568.

Sharon Rushing, MPH, MA is a medical anthropology PhD candidate at the University of California, Riverside. She has a background in health inequities, structural determinants of health, and patient-provider communication. She has worked as an anthropologist and public health professional in southern California health maintenance organizations and federally qualified health centers and taught in both global health and anthropology. Her doctoral research focuses on the integration of the humanities in medical education to forward the inclusion of social and structural contexts of health and health care.

Juliet McMullin, PhD is Professor and Chair of the Department of Anthropology at University of California, Riverside and is currently the co-Director for the Center for Health Disparities Research. She specializes in Cultural and Medical Anthropology, as well as Health Humanities. Professor McMullin's research interests include the political economy of health and the role of narrative in medical encounters, particularly in cancer narratives. She is the author of *The Healthy Ancestor: Embodied Inequality and the Revitalization of Native Hawaiian Health*, co-editor of the School of Advanced Research volume *Confronting Cancer: Metaphors, Advocacy, and Anthropology*, and author of numerous articles. Professor McMullin has an enduring interest in the production of health knowledge and inequalities, and a passion for translating that interest to her work with local communities and students. She currently has two parallel projects. The first examines the growing field of graphic medicine, and is creating a graphic storytelling intervention for cancer patient supportive care. Her second project is a community engaged project that examines the concept of historical trauma and its role in the delivery of healthcare with Native Americans. As a community-engaged scholar, her goal is to facilitate sharing knowledge and resources while being critical of the ways in which these collaborations can co-produce the inequalities they seek to alleviate.

Chapter 11
Wearing a Cloak and Many Hats: Expectations of Anthropologists in an Academic Health Science Center in Texas

Arlene L. Macdonald and Jerome W. Crowder

Humanities, Anthropology and Medical Education

As anthropologists our tenure at an academic health science university has been an uphill struggle. In saying this, we do not differ substantially from the many reports that have emphasized the difficulties of being a non-clinician in clinical education (Chrisman and Maretzki 1982: 1–34), the marginalization that comes from offering epistemic challenges to scientific 'certainties' (Anderson 2008), the divided loyalties anthropologists feel between the patients they seek to understand and the clinicians they seek to support (Kleinman 1982), the challenge of moving anthropological research practices and views into the world of medicine (Albert et al. 2015), or the uncertainties of professional recognition and advancement in academic health science environments (Scheper-Hughes 1990, 196–197). There are, of course, positive collaborations and growing recognition for the role anthropologists play in medical education. Strong and flourishing programs such as McGill's Department of Social Studies of Medicine in the Faculty of Medicine and the joint UCSF/UCB Medical Anthropology program that offers an MD/PhD in UCSF's Medical Sciences Training Program are clear evidence of the acknowledged contribution medical anthropology makes to medicine. This recognition is further illustrated by the National

Arlene Macdonald and Jerome W. Crowder made equal contributions to this chapter.

A. L. Macdonald
Institute for the Medical Humanities, University of Texas Medical Branch, Galveston, TX, USA
e-mail: almacdon@utmb.edu

J. W. Crowder (✉)
Department of Behavioral and Social Sciences, University of Houston, College of Medicine, Houston, TX, USA
e-mail: jcrowder@central.uh.edu

I. L. Martinez, D. W. Wiedman (eds.), *Anthropology in Medical Education*,
https://doi.org/10.1007/978-3-030-62277-0_11

Institutes of Health (NIH) supported Medical Scientist Training Program (MSTP) that includes Medical Anthropology as a funded option for students seeking both the MD and PhD degrees. We are hopeful for the opportunities of medical anthropologists in two newly created medical schools in Texas: the University of Houston College of Medicine (opening August 2020) with a mission to close the primary care gap by "engaging, collaborating, and empowering patient populations and community partners to improve their health and healthcare" (https://www.uh.edu/medicine/about/) and the University of Texas Rio Grande Valley School of Medicine whose mission is shaped by their location in a region historically burdened by health disparities. But our uphill struggle has been both as anthropologists at the oldest medical school in Texas—a stand-alone academic health science university without the buttress of a school of liberal arts—and as anthropologists in a traditionally-oriented medical humanities program. It is this dual emplacement that this paper wishes to explore.

We are faculty members in an interdisciplinary medical humanities institute at an academic health sciences university. We are dually charged with bringing the insights of "medical humanities" into the medical school curriculum and furthering the scholarship of the medical humanities by training graduate students in this field. Both charges have held challenges, challenges specific to the "epistemic habitus" (Albert et al. 2015, 18) of faculties of medicine and challenges specific to the tensile relationship between the Western humanist tradition (that animates many medical humanities programs and most certainly our own) and the discipline of anthropology. Medical humanities may offer a viable entrée for anthropologists seeking to work in medical education. However, as the chapter elaborates, the 'humanist self' that animates many medical humanities endeavors is increasingly under siege from several disciplinary vantage points, including anthropology—which has had its own evolving and ambivalent relationship with the humanist self. This chapter seeks to do three things: 1) outline the shifting terrain of humanities education in medicine that is the context for the challenges anthropologists in humanities program may face; 2) document the strategies of legitimation that we undertook as anthropologists teaching in these programs; 3) suggest key opportunities for, and obstacles to, making the terrain a little less "uphill" for future anthropologists entering the field of medical humanities.

Despite the long associations between the humanities and medicine—both ancient and modern—the rise of formal humanities programs in medical education is a late twentieth century intervention. Dating the origins of the medical humanities to the decade of the 1970s, Jones et al. (2017) outline how concerns about medicalization, subsequent lobbying for 'patient autonomy', advancing movements for 'patients' rights', and the ethical and human quandaries raised by new biotechnologies set in motion a cry—from intellectuals, activists, and physicians—for 'human values' to be brought to bear on the complex human and ethical issues that animated contemporary medical arenas (c.f. Daniel Fox 1985). Programs and courses drawing on traditional humanities fields (by and large: philosophy, literature, history, religious studies) began to proliferate in medical schools (see Cole et al. 2015).

According to Viney et al. (2015), the foci and the strengths of the medical humanities through the decades of the late twentieth century were:

> Its resistance to positivist biomedical 'reductionism', its sensitivity to narrative-based interventions and their limitations, its designation of the patient–clinician relation as a renewed focus of attention, its interest in concepts of disease and practices of diagnosis, the dynamic role of the arts in health, and the therapeutic importance of comparative histories (p. 2).

These foci have been strategic gains for the medical humanities, Viney et al. (2015) argue. However, they also wish to remind us that these areas of focus have been enabled "by particular—humanist—models of the self, of the ill and suffering body, and of modes of intervention and care" (p. 3) whose normative and individualist tendencies have been restrictive in the light of biomedicine.

A humanist model of the self owes much of its ontology, its normativity, and its cultivation to the persuasive power and pervasive practices of the western humanist tradition. Central to this model of the self is the phenomenological attestation of the centrality of first-person access to one's own experiential life and the enduring individual who experiences (Mattingly 2012, 170). Humanism understands such a self to be 'knowable to itself', commends such knowledge, and consigns any number of moral practices and pedagogies to this end, many of them drawn from Renaissance repertoires (Kutac et al. 2016). It posits both indefatigable freedom and relentless responsibility to engage in the cultivation of self (be it via the *studia humanitatis* of the renaissance era, Kant's imperative of the free use of reason, or existential projects of self-making) and generally sees self-cultivation as an ethical foundation to civic and collective processes. Informed by Enlightenment ideals of coherence, centering, singularity, and authenticity (de Freitas and Paton 2009, 484), humanism fundamentally distinguishes such an experiencing, enduring, reflexive first person 'anthropos' from the 'natural' world it experiences. And while many strands of humanism have appealed to God's relationship to humans to justify our inherent dignity and liberty, Charles Taylor argues that modernist renditions present "a humanism accepting no final goals beyond human flourishing, nor any allegiance to anything else beyond this flourishing" (2007, 18).

This humanist self—so central to the traditional missions and methods of the medical humanities—is under siege from many sides. "A series of profound challenges," writes Nikolas Rose, have been directed towards 'the self' understood as "coherent, bounded, individualized, intentional, the locus of thought, action, and belief, the origin of its own actions, the beneficiary of a unique biography" (1998, 3). In a cogent passage (1998, 3–9), he summarizes the ways biotechnical advances have problematized the uniqueness of human embodiment (and its related demarcations of self from both 'nature' and 'machine') and he illuminates the ways various strands of social theory (feminist philosophy, anthropology, psychoanalytic theory, and poststructuralism among others) have historicized, relativized, and fractured the primacy, unity, and givenness of the self, which is revealed "not as our inner truth but as our last illusion, not as our ultimate comfort but as an element in circuits of power that make some of us selves while denying full selfhood to others and thus performing an act of domination on both sides" (1998, 5).

Anthropology has had its own complicated relationship with the western humanist tradition. The widely held conviction that anthropology was centrally concerned with understanding the 'human endeavor' in all its cultural variety stood largely unchallenged until the 1980s. However, the "cultural critique" leveled by Clifford (1988) and others (Clifford and Marcus 1986; Marcus and Fischer 2014), drew attention to the situatedness of the ethnographer in search of such an "anthropological humanism", troubled the homogenous and static versions of culture that defined the ethnographer's fields, and questioned the hegemony of the humanist tradition that sought to classify all that was 'different' in 'familiar' (aka western) epistemologies and ontologies of the human. This critique has had long lasting and wide ranging impacts on the field of anthropology and its relationship with humanism. In applied anthropology, for instance, Trevor Purcell (1998) writes of a "general dissatisfaction with the process of Westernization, a dissatisfaction linked to a humanist tradition associated with the study and understanding of non-Western peoples" (p. 258). In feminist anthropology, there has been influential calls to subject "secular humanism" (and its attendant visions of gender equality and freedom) to the same scrutiny afforded the gendered desires of Islamic subjects (Abu-Lughod 2002; Mahmood 2001, 2005). Moreover, anthropology has contributed directly to the postmodern fracturing of the humanist self in multiple ways. For instance, anthropology has been fundamental in revealing the cultural specificity of the Western ideal of the self and related values of individualism. A large body of anthropological research has explored cultural variations on 'personhood', arguing for ethnographers and others to recognize the cultural, historical, political and technological conditions that have made possible not only the selves of "other" places, but also the constructions of the Western self (for a helpful review, see Smith 2012). Anthropology has also provided illuminating accounts of the ways medical technologies are fundamentally rupturing the 'naturalness' of the self, its corporeal boundaries, its biological processes, and its social matrices. Strathern's (1992) early work on reproductive technologies and the disruption of kinship, Lock's (2002) revealing work on organ transplant and the remaking of death, and Dumit's (2004) provocative account of the ways PET brain scans recalibrate popular and personal understandings of the self are prime examples of the ways that medical anthropology (in particular) has added to the diminution of the coherent, 'natural', and knowable self that has animated much of the western humanist tradition.

This series of challenges to the western humanist self has galvanized much of the humanities for the past several decades. However, it is only in the last decade and only tentatively, that the medical humanities—a discipline so closely articulated with the western humanist tradition, so strongly committed to cultivating "human values" in medicine, so preoccupied with the individuated self, its experiences of suffering, and its need for meaning—has begun to call for a more sustained engagement with these critiques of the western humanist self, and by extension, the centrality of the western humanist tradition to its endeavors.

The "health humanities" is an emergent initiative whose aim is to recalibrate the 'medical humanities'. Couching their concerns in language of "democratization" and "inclusiveness" (Crawford et al. 2015, 19), various proponents of the 'health humanities' emphasize a wider constituency of healthcare professions and personnel (including informal caregivers and patients themselves) as the partners and beneficiaries of a "health" (rather than a "medical") humanities (Crawford et al. 2015, 1). Moreover, "health" signals a broader purview than does "medicine": a commitment to engaging with a broader and more culturally diverse array of therapeutics than biomedicine (Crawford et al. 2015, 2), a recognition that "medicine is only a minor determinant of health in human populations alongside social and cultural factors" (Jones et al. 2017, 1), and a call to revision an "instrumentalist" humanities designed to enhance medicine to a "critical" humanities that probes the making, meaning, and authority of health knowledges and practices (Bishop 2008). The health humanities' explicit allegiance to "the thoroughgoing development of critique and critical theory" (Crawford et al. 2015, 13) has been influential in multiple ways. A subset of scholars has made the "critical medical humanities" their foremost project (cf Whitehead and Woods 2016; Viney et al. 2015). The project of the 'critical medical humanities' has been characterized as:

> (i) a widening of the sites and scales of 'the medical' beyond the primal scene of the clinical encounter; (ii) greater attention not simply to the context and experience of health and illness, but to their constitution at multiple levels; (iii) closer engagement with critical theory, queer and disability studies, activist politics and other allied fields; (iv) recognition that the arts, humanities and social sciences are best viewed not as in service or in opposition to the clinical and life sciences, but as productively entangled with a 'biomedical culture'; and, following on from this, (v) robust commitment to new forms of interdisciplinary and cross-sector collaboration. (Viney et al. 2015, 2)

The call for more "intensive engagement...with how health, illness, and treatment are constituted in and through tangled webs of human and nonhuman biosocial organisms, political-economic formations, discourses, and affects" closely aligns with the "profound challenges" to the humanist self outlined above. And their urging of "critique"—"explicit attempts to reflect upon the underlying suppositions that ground the knowledges it produces" (Viney et al. 2015, 3)—can be read as an invitation to query the hegemonic force of the western humanist tradition in the project of the medical humanities.

Commitments to "inclusiveness", "interdisciplinarity", "cross-sector collaboration", a "closer engagement with critical theory" and "activist politics" in the new strains of "health humanities" and "critical medical humanities", have broadened the traditional disciplinary scope of the medical humanities. Anthropology, disability studies, science and technology studies, political science, women's studies, queer studies, postcolonial studies and others have become viable (if not always fully understood) partners in the revitalization of the medical humanities. Our own program aimed to partake of these movements when it hired (2010) a political scientist (since departed), two anthropologists (one since departed), and a religious studies scholar firmly centered in critical social theory and anthropological methods. While the "new hires" quickly found common ground in critical and engaged projects and pedagogies, the receiving group of medical humanists became increasingly estranged from what they saw as anthropology's "political" and "activist" nature, its scholarly commitments to understanding health beyond the immediate environs of the Gulf Coast, and its critical appraisal of the humanist 'self' and western humanist tradition that anchored both graduate training and medical humanities teaching in our institution. Anecdotally, when one of us stated at a faculty discussion that she didn't consider herself a 'humanist', the retort from one of the receiving groups was "then we shouldn't have hired you". In short, the progressive health humanities' discourses of "inclusiveness", "democratization", and "entanglement" are enticing—even to traditional medical humanists—but they can mask the real epistemological challenges, ethical orientations, institutional politics, and academic commitments that anthropologists and others informed by critical theory bring. The 'health humanities' and the 'critical medical humanities' may need to grapple more explicitly with their ambivalent relationship to humanism if the entanglements they call for are to be productive.

Recently, Cheryl Mattingly (2012) has written evocatively of the tangles of humanism and poststructuralism in the anthropology of morality. Her arguments may be especially germane to the challenges faced by anthropologists in medical education because 'morality' is a central preoccupation in the training of health professionals (and what it means to be professional), in the lifeworlds of illness, and in the projects of the medical humanities. Specifically, Mattingly wishes to highlight current researches that seek to move anthropology past its fixation on a Durkheimian-inherited reduction of morality to "unreflective norm following" without resorting to western modernity's 'freedom' based moral schemes and thereby abandoning key anthropological insights about "the social force of moral norms and practices within particular historical communities" (p. 162). She finds two viable trajectories emerging in the anthropology of morality, trajectories that seem complementary and entangled, but ultimately, she argues, make "irreconcilable claims" (p. 161).

According to Mattingly, contemporary work in the anthropology of morality varyingly situates itself in the neo-Aristotelian revival of 'first-person' or 'humanist' virtue ethics and/or the poststructural conception of ethics largely inspired by Foucault. What these trajectories share is a sense that moralities are always (to some extent) "unfree"—they are "contextualized…constituted by local and traditional practices" albeit with possibilities (to some extent) for "moral scrutiny, reflection, and choice in the cultivation of a moral self" (p. 162). Where they differ is what intrigues her. First-person/humanist virtue ethics draws from moral and political philosophy (e.g. MacIntyre, Taylor, Nussbaum, Arendt, Ricoeur) that reclaims Aristotle's emphasis on the task of cultivating virtues, a task bounded by one's moral horizons, and predicated on a robust notion of some kind of biographical integrity and narrative arc of a life. Those anthropologists of morality working in the first-person humanist virtue tradition "tend to emphasize the singularities and exigencies of practical judgment and the moral struggles involved in inhabiting one's everyday life" (p. 170). Conversely, poststructural virtue ethics looks to Foucault, and in particular his genealogical reading of the texts of classic Greek and Greco-Roman antiquity (History of Sexuality v 2 and 3). What emerges from his close review of the habits, practices, and curricula of cultivating an ethical self is "the pedagogical nature of becoming a certain sort of ethical subject... the striving toward the occupancy of a 'subject position'...the reproduction of an ethical regime through training in self-care practices within predefined ethical modes of life" (p. 172). Poststructural virtue ethics reject 'the self' as posited in first-person virtue ethics. They emphasize "how easily moral practices of self-cultivation can be no more than (or less than) practices of normalization of a particular regime of truth" (p. 173). Anthropologists of morality working in this tradition "foreground the shared practices, technologies and discourses that form ethical subjectivity" (p. 175).

Rather than merging post-structural and first person accounts of morality, Mattingly recommends that we can benefit from both of these approaches if we ask such questions as "What does a conceptual framework allow us to see and what does it hide?" (p. 179). Her recommendations for anthropology are germane to the revisionary ambitions of the health humanities and the critical medical humanities. "Thorough-going development of critique and critical theory"—particularly where it builds on poststructuralist frameworks—poses both implicit and explicit challenges to the humanist self, the humanist tradition, and first-person virtue ethics that have traditionally animated the medical humanities. As Da Silva (2018) notes: "virtue ethics is the ethical theory most suited to humanism, and humanism offers an educational ideal that perfectly complements virtue ethics. One can plausibly claim that virtue ethics and humanistic education are two faces of the same coin". But as Mattingly makes clear, poststructural understandings of the virtuous projects of the subject are another coin altogether.

Buoyed by a spirit of "inclusiveness" and "democratization", there was no recognition when our department sought to add anthropologists to its roster of medical humanists that they might bring alternate theories of morality, ethics, and the self, and with them a profound ambivalence about the humanist tradition. When those challenges became obvious, there was no mechanism that allowed the group to see what our varied conceptual frameworks revealed and hid. Instead we, as anthropologists, junior scholars, and new hires, felt the need to hide our frameworks.

Wearing a Cloak and Many Hats: Strategies of Legitimation

The divides in our own department between commitments to first-person virtue ethics and poststructuralist inquiries into the subjects of a regime of truth have increased the difficulty of introducing medical students to the key insights that anthropology might offer them. Beyond the perennial challenge of finding adequate time and space in the medical school curriculum, expanding the traditional medical humanities foci (ethical principles, empathetic professionals, and agentic individuals) to encompass anthropological insights (an understanding of the social determinants of disease, the role of social factors in patient health outcomes, the socially constructed nature of health and illness, critical appraisal of health science knowledges, issues of power, conflict, and representation in medical encounters and narratives of illness) met strong resistance from our established humanities colleagues who traditionally directed the various curricula our faculty delivered in the medical school. Our primary teaching commitments include the Humanities, Ethics and Professionalism (HEP) modules, incorporated into the required "Practice of Medicine" (POM) course delivered to both first and second-year medical students. Additionally, our medical humanities faculty deliver a series of electives (2-week intensive minimesters, semester long electives and selectives, honors research supervision) to medical school students.

Most particularly in the required HEP modules, we effectively worked by stealth, "cloaking" anthropological insights in the delivery of more established medical humanities fare. We taught Francis Peabody's customary early twentieth century classic, *The Care of the Patient* (1927), and asked pointed questions about gender and professionalism. We taught the four-box method of ethical decision-making (Jonsen et al. 2015) and expanded the fourth box, "Contextual Features", beyond bioethical recognition. We taught the requisite ethical, legal, and policy concerns about organ transplant in North America, and then refracted those concerns through anthropological insights about "artificial scarcity" (Scheper-Hughes 2001), "invented kinship" (Sharp 2006), "hybridity" (Lock 2002) and global organs markets (Sharp 2007). We used the assigned humanities materials to generate more reflexive positions on difference, simultaneously drawing from anthropological insights to question and decode the very categories of difference (race, gender, sex, religion) rather than emphasizing "empathy" for differences that were often naturalized by traditional ethics approaches.

We found it necessary to 'cloak' our anthropological knowledge and critical theoretical commitments in certain settings and simultaneously find terrain in the health sciences curriculum where we could more freely advance anthropological insights. We found ourselves wearing many hats (including that of the ethnographer to understand our own position within the system itself) as we moved between established and emerging curricula. Such a strategy went a considerable way to securing some sense of anthropology's legitimate place in an academic health sciences university. But cloaks are heavy, and they are cumbersome. And they didn't do much to dissuade our colleagues from their suspicions of anthropological subterfuge: the sense that anthropologists were surreptitiously refiguring the humanist self at the center of long-standing pedagogies, and substituting a critical poststructuralist view of ethics in place of the virtue ethics that was widely held to be vital to the professional development of medical trainees.

Strategies of Legitimation: The Interprofessionalism Hat (Macdonald)

My anthropological engagement in medical education became substantially more rewarding when I changed hats, adding teaching and curriculum development responsibilities in interprofessionalism to my acknowledged role in bringing humanities to medical students. A series of chance encounters with Interprofessional Education (IPE) has evolved into an appreciation for its vision and values, as well as the critical interest in the socio-political forces behind it. Making anthropology matter in the training of health professionals (rather than simply physicians) also seems germane to the ambitions of the health humanities. My forays into IPE are born of equal parts frustration (with the existing disciplinary politics and the heavy weight of cloaks), optimism (for the inclusive vision of IPE and the special role that anthropology might play in this fledgling educational initiative), and a hermeneutic of suspicion (regarding the neoliberal tendencies that IPE discourses may mask). Having already alluded to my frustrations, let me articulate the ways that anthropology might matter to the IPE endeavor. Newly hired into academic medicine in 2011, I found my degree in Religious Studies, my training in the anthropology of religion, my post-structural approaches to health and religion, and my undergraduate liberal arts teaching experience had not prepared me for the translational challenges that faced me. As a tenure-track faculty member teaching Medical Humanities graduate students, I joined other new hires in developing and delivering a concentration in "Social Medicine". Here I contributed courses such as "Ritual Bodies", "Social Rites", and "Religion & the Politics of Health". These drew directly on my academic background in the anthropology of religion, but were a large departure from traditional medical humanities offerings in religion that typically foreground theology, religious ethics, and comparative religions. "Do you even teach about religion?" an interim director of our program queried me at one memorable faculty meeting, highlighting how little medical humanists knew about the anthropological discipline they had so eagerly sought out. In medical school teaching, I "cloaked" my anthropological training, as described above, but this always felt like a rather anemic approach to teaching. Wondering how to make my background in the anthropology of religion relevant, I stumbled upon an interprofessional "Spirituality and Clinical Care" course. The "Spirituality and Care" course had been one of the early interprofessional initiatives at our institution. The course was developed with a John Templeton Spirituality and Medicine award from the National Institute for Healthcare Research in 1999. (For further detail see Sandor et al. 2006).

The course had been championed by faculty across professional schools with special commitments to the subject matter, and had been mandatory for medical students, nursing students, and many of the allied health professions students for several years. I contacted the course directors, was welcomed to their planning meetings, and found this interprofessional group of faculty generally receptive to the anthropological insights I brought. Indeed, negotiations about content and approaches in interprofessional courses, while they are no doubt fraught with very real differences in professional orientations and cultures (Martinez 2015, 37), are at the very least *expected.* No one was surprised that I had a different perspective on the material or the objectives for the course; everyone did. We were all expected to wear different hats and speak from those differing positions in order to provide an interprofessional framework that reflected the diverse learners in the course.

The course was canceled shortly after I had joined it, effectively dismantled by the retirement of key faculty champions in two of the professional schools, a chronic impediment of interprofessional efforts that are insufficiently institutionalized (Nelson et al. 2014). But I was intrigued by the effort to teach and learn interprofessionally, the relative openness to negotiated curricula, and the pervasive aim of inculcating a 'team' of health professionals. My participation in this course also laid bare, as shifting cultural locations often does, my own myopic preoccupation with educating doctors—a preoccupation that has too often been normative in both medical humanities (see above) and medical anthropology (which will be addressed later in the chapter). Recently, my university has taken steps to institutionalize interprofessional competencies in teamwork, communication, ethics/values, roles and responsibilities (IPECEP 2011) across the educational mission. A new vice-president position has been created with direct oversight for interprofessional education. In the latest Southern Association of Colleges and Schools (SACS) accreditation of our institution in 2017, interprofessionalism was selected as the focus of a 5-year Quality Enhancement Plan (QEP). The Office of Interprofessional Education features an ever-increasing array of interprofessional electives and events and a growing roster of Interprofessional Scholars. How effective these measures will be, and how effectively anthropology can be embedded in them, remains to be seen. But there are encouraging signs.

The campus-wide mandatory interprofessional case study, "What's Wrong with Warren?", began as an exercise for nursing, medical, and allied health professions students to better understand their own and others "roles and responsibilities" in the delivery of care, one of the basic interprofessional competencies. Within their own academic silos, first-year students are presented with the case of Warren: a 16 year old boy who presents in the ER with an acute and complex condition, is diagnosed with an infectious condition that necessitates a community health response, and eventually morphs into a long-term convalescent phase. Students identify their specific professional roles and responsibilities in the case, but are then tasked with soliciting "consults" from other professional groups across campus while simultaneously providing "consults" about their own profession. The consultation phase of Warren turns the campus into a positive hubbub of intermingling students trading "Warren dollars" for the interprofessional information they need to activate best care strategies. The event wraps up with a "debrief" session where close to 1000 students recapitulate the knowledge they have acquired about the diverse roles and responsibilities of a healthcare team dealing with a complex case (Rowan et al. 2016) (Fig. 11.1).

Originally, none of the case writers remotely thought of including anthropologists, medical humanists, ethicists, chaplains, bench scientists, or any of the other "non-professional" students on campus in an exchange of information about interprofessional "roles and responsibilities". But those same groups had no difficulty in seeing their relevance to Warren's health—and they wanted in on the action. Interprofessionalism (at least on our campus) has wrestled with defining its mandate: is it about synchronizing and enhancing the professional healthcare delivery team? Or is it a broader vision of the many professions that contribute to the definition,

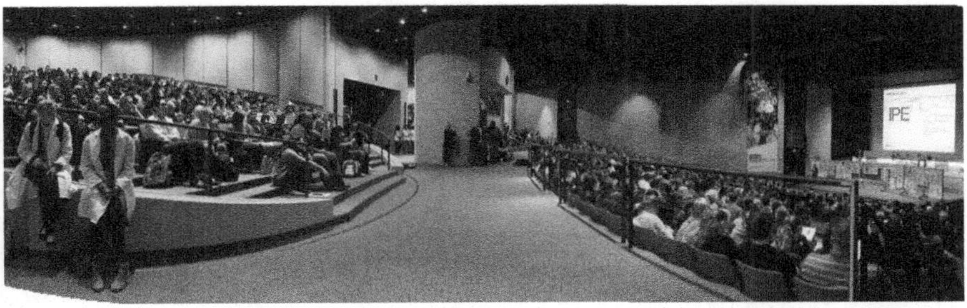

Fig. 11.1 Debrief meeting in Levin Hall, UTMB, "What's Wrong with Warren" event (Photo: J. Crowder 2018)

delivery, and development of 'health' writ large? In the Warren case the latter, broader, vision won out. Biomedical engineering students now discuss their role and responsibility in developing new prosthetic devices for patients like Warren and trade that information with other health students. The Pastoral Care office has a "consultancy" booth. Infectious disease scholars at the Galveston National Lab offer their knowledge of vaccine development and learn something about occupational therapy or pharmacy professions in exchange.

However, the faculty and graduate students of the Institute for Medical Humanities, including the anthropologically minded among us, struggled with how to define an anthropologist's or a humanist's "role and responsibility" in a case scenario such as Warren. Ultimately, we are moving towards cultivating Scheper-Hughes and Lock's (1987) "mindful body" as our own particular 'role and responsibility'. In addition to addressing ethical conflicts that arise in the case, medical humanities graduate students emphasize the phenomenally experienced individual body-self in their consultations with students from other professions and ask anthropologically inspired questions about voice and representation in the portrayal of the fictitious "Warren". In the first year they participated, medical humanities students were quick to recognize that the human being at the center of the case ("Warren") became more and more invisible as the number of professionals involved in his care multiplied. When medical humanities students were approached for "consultation", they raised questions about Warren's experience of his own illness (and the difficulties of accessing such an experience) and they brought structural and social justice concerns into view (Fig. 11.2).

In 2017, we piloted an art workshop, led by Amerisa Waters, PhD from Medical Humanities, that allowed students to explore the "social body" of Warren—a movement into the symbolic and cultural representations of ill, amputated, and youthful bodies, the social stigma they carry, and the social forces that shape them. In 2018, we featured an exhibit of anatomical and pathological specimens related to the Warren case. "Making Warren Matter," co-developed with Paula Summerly, PhD, Research Project Manager from the Old Red Medical Museum, allowed diverse learners to situate their roles and responsibilities in medical, institutional, and social histories—histories that make clear the ambivalent (and

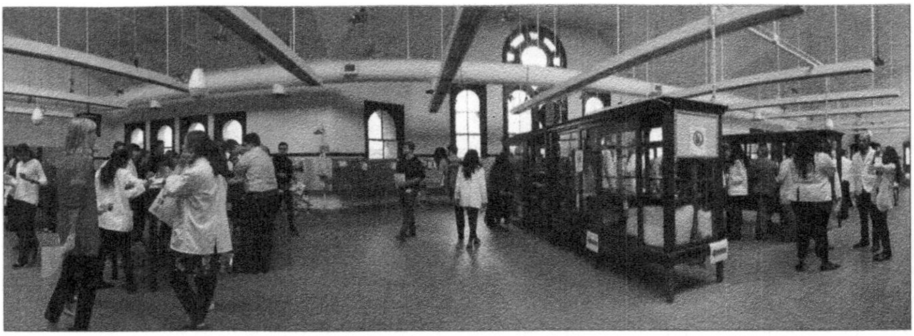

Fig. 11.2 IMH students and faculty working with interprofessional students attending the "Making Warren Matter" exhibit of specimens in the Old Red Medical Museum (Photo: J. Crowder 2019)

continuing) power of health professions to fragment, define, and display diseases and their carriers. In a future year, we plan to address the body politic with consultations and colloquium on vaccine hesitancy. Exactly as intended, the case study has been useful in encouraging the medical humanities, and the anthropologists among us, to define our roles and responsibilities in interprofessional education both to ourselves and to our fellow constituents.

Additionally, anthropology may prove useful in advancing and entrenching the broader mandate of interprofessional education. As Iveris Martinez (2015) points out, anthropologists are uniquely equipped to serve as interlocutors across the cultural worlds of varied health professions, bringing knowledges of enculturation, cultural differences, and skills in cross-cultural communication (p. 37). Several scholars note that ethnographic and/or qualitative methods may be particularly well suited to ascertaining the impact, effectiveness, and portent of interprofessional education and interprofessional collaboration (cf Gotlib-Conn 2010). Such methods have been used to investigate the impact of interprofessional education and practice on patient outcomes and medical error—two key rationales for the implementation of IPE (cf. Wilson et al. 2016; Rice et al. 2010; Jones and Jones 2011).

Anthropology may also be useful to interprofessional endeavors by observing and articulating the contexts that interprofessionalism is situated within and the social forces it responds to. DeMatteo and Reeves (2013) caution that the current regime of neoliberalism characterized by deregulation, flexibilization, the remodeling of public institutions along corporate lines, individual responsibilization and the "entreprenurializing" of the self, (p. 28) has profound impacts on the nature of professionalism generally and the current trend towards interprofessionalism specifically. Interprofessionalism, they argue, responds to the healthcare crisis of major cuts and underfunding not as issues of political economy, differential power, and inequality, but as a human resource issue—advocating a "flexible, team-oriented work force with broad, overlapping, professional 'scopes of practice'" (p. 28). The pervasive and growing 'enterprise culture' that is remodeling many public institutions "along corporate lines into sites of entrepreneurial activity" (p. 28) necessitates a particular kind of training, one more in line with the "efficient operation of health care facilities than with professional values and interests" (p. 28). Using qualitative methods, they point to discursive trends amongst IPE learners that solidify an "enterprise culture", albeit unwittingly: the tendency to view other professions as "resources"; the recalibration of physician from provider to professional manager; the slippage between patient as 'team member' and patient as 'consumer'; the rationale of economic "efficiency" for re-tooling as an "interprofessional"; the identification of deficiencies in cooperation and communication as the root cause of healthcare crises and the resultant responsibilization of the professional 'self'. "Without understanding the social context underlying the current shift toward interprofessionalism—and the powerful forces at play", they write in their concluding discussion, "interprofessional projects... as well as our public institutions, are at risk of becoming vehicles for advancing the global, neoliberal agenda to "privatize" and "corporatize" services" (p. 32).

Participant observation at my own institution underscores this unsettling possibility. Conversations with senior administrators of IPE have made clear that "eliminating redundancies" across the health schools is one of the key reasons for delivering "soft skills" training (teamwork, communication, collaboration, ethics) interprofessionally. Extensive curriculum mapping is the mechanism employed to discover such redundancies. Once identified and replaced by interprofessional initiatives, I was told that many faculty currently teaching such skills in their specific professional program can then be "released" to devote their time to clinical/research activity and the generation of revenue. The curriculum changes precipitated by interprofessional education also present an opportunity for enhancing "efficiencies" via online delivery of learning material, something senior IPE administrators have repeatedly voiced as desirable with little consideration of how such delivery methods actually enhance the interprofessional mandate. A tenured and senior pediatrician on campus related that his resistance to IPE was not the recalcitrance of an esteemed physician nostalgically longing for past days of privilege in a hierarchical medical arena (my original thesis!), but was instead closely aligned with the fears DeMatteo and Reeves (2013) articulate. Professional identity as a doctor, nurse, PT, OT, etc., he told me, is a bulwark against the enterprising culture of medicine that currently seeks to erect the more malleable identity of "health professional" to solidify its own neoliberal goals. The field of IPE seems ripe for the kind of critical, qualitative, discursive and contextual analysis that anthropology can bring.

However useful anthropology may prove to interprofessionalism, it behooves us to remember that interprofessionalism may also be useful to anthropology. In my optimistic moments, I am captured by the IPE vision of the health agenda diffused across a wide range of social actors—patients, policy makers, healthcare providers, first responders, social activists, pharmaceutical companies. It is a vision that intuitively recognizes that health is, at a minimum, socially orchestrated and dependent on respectful collaboration across domains of difference. Such an intuition foreshadows and legitimates more demanding anthropological understandings about the asymmetrical forces that define and determine health. In my idealist moments, I am swept up in imagining anthropologists as fully incorporated into this diffusive, inclusive understanding of partnering for health—wearing our own hat, and not solely employed to teach others how to better wear theirs.

Strategies of Legitimation: Crowder—The Role of the Arts in Medicine

Upon arrival at the Institute for the Medical Humanities (IMH), our role, and the expectations of us as social science scholars, was not clearly outlined nor well defined by the university, our director or our colleagues. Because of the prioritizing of the Humanist Self, it seemed like the faculty who hired us were most interested in our becoming "good citizens" and promoting ethical "values" to students, who would notice our behavior and follow our lead. They wanted us to become more like "them" and not conduct community advocacy, critical ethnography, nor teach contemporary social theory or qualitative methods. Instead we were encouraged to sit in on their classes that featured deep reading of the Western humanist classics, demonstrate good ethical behavior and focus on how doctors can become more empathetic, perhaps through reading narratives written by physicians. In essence, such behaviors reinforced our role to be handmaidens to medicine rather than "widening the sites and scales of 'the medical' beyond the primal scene of the clinical encounter" (Viney et al. 2015, 2) or offering a critical approach that probes the making, meaning and authority of health knowledges and practices. One senior medical school administrator commented that "the medical humanities are like the conscience of medicine, they remind us that we are human, too." Indeed, a particular type of human.

Trained as a medical anthropologist and visual researcher, I felt that my experience working with Aymara speaking migrants in urban Bolivia and Perú would directly relate to issues of access to health care, poverty, and medical literacy in Galveston. However, we had to develop a means for our own internal identity in the graduate teaching of the IMH, so we immediately began crafting complimentary syllabi that offered contemporary theory, methods, and comparative research to align with courses already being offered in the medical humanities department. For example, we developed a methods section for the medical historian's course in health disparities, teaching students how to conduct interviews and engage with island residents about the resources they access and care they receive. Geertz (1975) and Kleinman (1988) (among others) were also frequently "taught" out of context and any post-structuralist or critical writing (if offered) was used as a straw man in the medical humanities core courses, as more phenomenological and hermeneutical approaches were preferred. To counterbalance, we aligned our teaching to cover those same authors to broaden students' understanding of anthropological insights on the practice and epistemology of medicine and scientific research.

On the medical school side, we were given syllabi to teach and articles to discuss with first and second year medical students in their pre-clinical courses called

"Practice of Medicine 1" and "Practice of Medicine 2" (POM 1, POM 2), respectively; both "Humanities, Ethics and Professionalism" (HEP) courses were soundly based in classic medical humanities—most particularly bioethics. In HEP POM 1 (HEP1) for the first-year medical students, we "parachuted" into PBL small groups for an hour and helped the students and MD facilitator "unpack" the ethical issues of the case at hand. Our punctuated visits were not always welcomed by the small group facilitators as they were disruptive to the flow of their class and our intermittent presence deemphasized the everyday importance of ethics in all cases, signaling for students that there's some ethical component in a case they need special help to uncover or interpret. Such moments also made medical faculty feel like they were not capable of adequately discussing the case from an ethics perspective, creating an uncomfortable tension sensed by everyone in the small rooms.

Such visits went on for the following 3 years, until one year we were not invited back to participate in the course. The following year, new course directors took the helm of POM 1 and offered the Medical Humanities faculty five, 2-h sessions throughout the course for us to meet with students on Friday afternoons and discuss ethical and cultural issues. We, as a faculty, were then expected to develop materials to help students identify and unpack the issues taking place in the cases covered in their POM PBL small classes, while mapping content to the relevant competencies students would be tested on later (Englander et al. 2013; USMLE 2019). Again, we found our role being quite narrowly defined by the course directors (all MDs) and their expectations for when and how ethics and humanities issues should be addressed, disembodied from the medical discussions taking place in small groups, and relegated to Friday afternoons.

Similarly, in 2010, HEP POM 2 (HEP2), the course for second-year students was an intense 8-week course (met once a week for 2 h) offered in the middle of the summer, launching the second year of medical school and culminating in a five-page bioethics paper to demonstrate students' ability to "reason through" an ethical situation. In order to teach this class, the new faculty were expected to become "ethicists" while literally none of us were familiar with bioethics, its political history or its relationship with the medical humanities, much less medicine. We were also asked to take 2–3 classes per week. As a bilingual speaker, Crowder was asked to teach two of his three small groups in Spanish. We quickly learned that successful teaching required us to address the course materials from our academic strengths (e.g. medical/visual/Latin American anthropology, religious studies, political science), while incorporating our own interpretations into the material. For example, the curriculum included a 30 min clip from Bill Moyers' TV series *On Our Own Terms: Moyers on Dying* (Reisman 2000). The segment follows a young physician who cares for a privileged female patient dying of cancer. The doctor takes the time to visit the family at home, brief them on what her final moments of life may be like, and encourage them to be present with her—which they all can because of their flexible jobs and responsibilities. Once in the patient's home, the camera never enters the room of the dying woman, but "respectfully" remains outside her room, capturing the comments of the family, but not the patient. IMH faculty explained that this was an important segment to show young medical students as it may inspire them to think about a future career in palliative care.

However, when I showed it, I spoke to the intent of the video—to make viewers empathize with the white, upper-class family and normalize a "good death". Drawing on insights from visual anthropology, I broke the segment down by scene to show students how the filmmakers manipulated viewers' emotions through editing, mis-en-scène, and audio. Few students had never critically approached a visual piece and commented that they assumed what they were watching was "true" and "real" instead of intentionally constructed for a specific reaction. Many students identify with this segment because "it could be my family", which opens up a conversation about the privilege of professional education and the students' ability to identify with people different than themselves. The larger point was to help students recognize that "palliative care"—with all that it has to offer in caring for dying patients—is nevertheless steeped in white, upper class experiences of and assumptions about death.

Moreover, there is a sharp distinction between the choice of middle class, insured patients to elect palliative care, and the dispensing of palliation to uninsured and underinsured patients for whom other viable modes of treatment are precluded. Medical students needed a more balanced account of death in America; I asked the course director to make available to students and faculty an additional segment of the Moyers series in which he confronts the end-of-life struggles of the poor and uninsured in a southern city, providing students an example of how social disparities affect the way we die in the United States. Ultimately this second segment was made available to facilitators to use as complementary to the first, but was not required. As an anthropologist, I am regularly questioning assumptions people make, including myself, looking for alternative perspectives on a topic or issue. In this case, visual anthropology informed my viewing of the video and I asked the course-co-director for other relevant materials that would help support their intent for showing the video but would speak to other viewers' experiences.

Evolving the HEP2 Curriculum

Over the summers, as our involvement with HEP2 teaching became more routinized, we found ways of expanding upon the designated themes through our own specialties and interests. In 2015, I became POM 2 course co-director, and began to redesign the HEP curriculum to capitalize on our faculty's strengths as well as align with the biomedical issues students were addressing in their Problem-Based Learning (PBL) modules throughout the academic year (e.g. Cardiovascular Pulmonary, Renal, Gastro Intestinal, Psychiatry, etc.). Furthermore, the SOM expected us to expand the number of USMLE competencies we could address.

Working with the HEP POM 1 course co-director (another IMH faculty), we developed a trajectory for the HEP course (s) that considered all 11 meetings we would have with the students over the 2 years (HEP 1 = 5, HEP 2 = 6). Doing so allowed us to introduce basic ethical concepts in HEP 1 (along with a glossary of terms) and then explore them further in HEP 2, reinforcing the concepts and providing nuance not possible in year 1.

For HEP 2, I led the updating of the readings, drawing heavily on social medicine, graphic medicine and medical anthropology to complement the bioethics that remained central to its core. Focusing on ethical and social justice issues embedded in the PBL topic for each module, we developed larger socio-political themes throughout the course, and dove deeper into specific ethical concerns for each topic, including advance directives, conflicts of interest and professionalism, transplant, breaking bad news, artificial hydration & nutrition, and autonomy & patient's rights. We were asked to incorporate episodes from "Worlds Apart" (Grainger-Monsen and Haslett 2003), a four-part series on cross-cultural health care, into our HEP syllabus as the medical doctors in the PBLs were not interested in using it any longer. While appropriate to several of the themes, we found many more updated materials online to use to discuss intercultural dialogues in a clinic setting. Although we only teach the medical students for one 2-h period every 8 weeks, our goal is to provide students with enough contextual materials and expose them to relevant literature to expand their thinking and understanding of the ethical issues and anthropological concerns before each session. Faculty then facilitate a discussion within the small groups when students are expected to discuss the impact the readings had on them and personal experiences they may have had that dovetail with the week's theme. Essentially, we use the PBL theme as a platform from which to further explore socio-cultural issues through the lens of ethics and anthropology, establishing a set of references for them to return to when such issues appear in their clinical experiences during years 3 and 4.

For example, in the Renal module week, we selected "transplant" as an ethical theme, including blood transfusions, living donor and cadaveric donor situations. Transplant serves as an excellent opportunity to explore the socio-cultural issues of transplants in general and racial categories in medical practice (Braun et al. 2007; Kucirka et al. 2011). Specifically focusing on renal, we offer Scheper-Hughes "tyranny of the gift" dialog with a team of surgeons (Scheper-Hughes 2007; Hippen and Taylor 2007), or read Kaufman's ethnographic account of the growing social and medical imperative for adult children to donate kidneys to their aging parents, an effective transmutation of our forms of care precipitated by the forces that have made once-extraordinary treatments seem ordinary, necessary and desirable (Kaufman 2015).

For the social science faculty, we are assured that medical students are learning about the social determinants of health and the structural issues that affect patients who may otherwise be understood to be "non-compliant" or "bad patients" simply for how they present in the clinic, rather than thinking beyond the clinic door and recognizing the myriad of social variables that affect patient behavior, beliefs, and values before they enter. After years of cloaking our anthropological interests with ethics discourse, we feel our intentions can manifest in what and how we teach our students and share with our colleagues. Through our open presentation of method and theory, we are able to lower the cloak (a bit) and claim the hat of anthropology.

While what we “do” is far from appreciated at the highest levels of the university, our students experience the broadening of contexts and resolving of the structures of “professionalism” within which they are subject. When wearing our anthropological hat we also advocate for integrating materials and ideas across schools and curricula (e.g. IPE, HEP). Our continued survival depends upon our cloaking with bioethics to introduce ideas that would otherwise be ignored, dismissed or deprioritized for lack of scientific integrity, evidence-based research, or humanist ideals.

The Creative Expressions Project (2012–2015)

Moreover, between years 1 and 2, some students travel abroad on Short Term Experiences in Global Health (STEGHs) to learn about the delivery of biomedical care in underserved countries (e.g. Kenya, Uganda, Perú, Dominican Republic), experience cultures different from their own, and travel outside of the USA (Ventres and Wilson 2019). Usually, there is very little time between students’ return to the USA and the beginning of medical school coursework. Through the summer of 2015, one apparent immediate issue with this calendar was that returning students were not able to debrief and reflect on their experiences abroad before classes began. Instead, their discourse about their experiences often consumed in-class discussions in the HEP2 course and their final assignment in the HEP2 course, a five page “bioethics” paper. This sometimes made students stray off course to focus on their wrenching experiences with health disparities, suffering and structural violence they witnessed first-hand in clinics and villages around the world. Students were equally struck by the behaviors and actions of their colleagues, who expressed an ethnocentric subjectivity in light of those who had nothing. While a small group setting is a good place to have such conversations, HEP was not designed to accommodate those types of reflective discussions; neither the faculty in this team-taught course nor other students could completely relate and complained about the limited class time being consumed by “irrelevant” conversations.

When such “irrelevant” conversations did occur in my small groups, I asked the student(s) to elaborate on their experiences and identify how their observations and feelings aligned with the issues being raised in the course, or in their medical school education more broadly. Frequently STEGH students answered that they were not well “prepared” to deal with the politics, poverty and lack of resources they would find upon arrival. Further inquiry led to discussions about the role of international health organizations in providing care as well as their understanding about their relationships with ministries of health in these specific countries. What had initially begun as a comment about observations about differences in care throughout the world became a deeper questioning about the role medical students play in “alleviating” health disparities in far-away places. Inevitably, these “irrelevant” conversations returned to a reflection on similar issues found locally on Galveston island, in southeast Texas, as well as other parts of the United States. In my opinion, these were some of the most compelling moments in class, as students connected their experiences to the more abstract ethical concepts and cultural issues they may have read about before class.

Anthropologists are terrific at addressing the many forms of "culture shock" (cf Davis and Konner 2011) as our jobs traditionally require us to live cross-culturally in order to understand how (different) people's ethics, values and world-views manifest in their daily lives. Often we anthropologists experience the *shock* of integrating into a different culture than our own where the rules, customs, expectations, and language require long periods of time to learn and manage. Crowder offered HABLE sections of POM 2 in which Spanish was primarily spoken and Hispanic/Latinx cultural behaviors and beliefs discussed. STEGH participants, however, don't have this time scale and often disembark with expectations of impacting the lives of "others" through their limited knowledge of biomedicine, but witness the difference between health care system resources and knowledge in a short period of time. Historically students' preparation was limited to general understanding of the countries they were to visit and the locals' health care needs from a public health perspective. Little, if any, attention was given to the political history of the country or to the structural issues which produce health disparities in those populations. As was realized, upon their return there was not any forum offered to students to help them process their disjointed and stressful experiences.

In 2012 my concerns with STEGHs students coalesced with those in the Medical Education Office, worried about other types of structurally induced student distress, namely students' socialization into the culture of medicine. In their experience, students quipped that upon entering medical school, they "have to leave their creative selves at the door". Myself, a senior medical educator, and a physician artist colleague, developed a HEP2 companion course to facilitate reflection on stressful student experiences abroad or in medical school through art making and peer-to-peer conversation. We called this opportunity the Creative Expressions Project (CEP) and opened it to all second year medical students; their participation would be beyond that required of all students, they self-selected to be in CEP. That first year, six students volunteered to participate in this experiment we called CEP.

Our idea was to pair medical students with local artists so they could together develop an art project addressing what it means to be a doctor. Having an artist partner encouraged students to push beyond their "normal" and try an unfamiliar media, or format, in order to reflect on their experiences. Furthermore, we wanted to create a safe space void of medical faculty where students could experiment without suffering the consequences of failure. We encouraged the evolution of ideas, placing students in small groups to talk about their ideas and give each other feedback. CEP ran parallel with HEP, meeting on Friday mornings for the entire 8 weeks scheduled for HEP. Specialists in various artistic disciplines, including theater, sculpture, drawing, weaving, painting, photography, videography, music performance and composition, were available to advise students, listen to their ideas, and facilitate their projects. As director of CEP I wore multiple hats, that of visual anthropologist as well as "course" administrator while maintaining my cloak of ethics instructor; I could easily incorporate my knowledge and experience as a professional photographer to compliment those of other artists invited to help students explore their creative selves while reflecting upon their medical school education.

As the project evolved over the next few years, our understanding of CEP's purpose expanded to incorporate various types of reflection and feedback, which led to more profound engagement in the students' projects. Students were required to journal and blog each week about their progress and ideas and share images or files for others to see and comment on. Our weekly meetings began to include a didactic moment for teaching medical history or artistic practice and social science concepts (audience, intelligent eye, structural violence). Small group interactions, modeled off of story circles (Lambert 2013; Robin 2008), gave students the opportunity to share their project ideas for 2 min and receive direct peer feedback. Students were also asked to write an artist's statement, which summarized their inspiration and intent for their piece. Many of the STEGHs participants focused on their experiences abroad and developed projects subjectively witnessing inequities in care, substandard living conditions, unemployment, and the violence that so often dovetails with stress in a community. The small group sharing and journaling feedback pushed all of the participants to critically analyze their experience and demonstrate to an audience how and why they had been impacted.

After our initial year, we petitioned the SOM curriculum committee to formalize CEP as a part of HEP 2 and to grade the students writing project as a substitute for the heretofore requisite five-page bioethics paper. The following year, many more students joined CEP to avoid the paper (initially 22 students), but quickly realized that journaling was significantly more writing than the lengthy paper assignment for the course, so several resigned. For those with science backgrounds, writing in the first-person was not easy, for others it was a relief from the "objective" nature of medicine. As we reached the final weeks before the opening show, students presented their pieces to the entire group, explaining their intent and sharing an artist's statement, as well as to receive feedback from their peers and faculty. Each year we petitioned the Dean and other groups and individuals across campus for funds so CEP could reimburse students for the costs of their materials.

Frequently following these sessions, we overheard students commenting that they had no idea their peers were so creative, thoughtful, engaged or artistic, as they realized they only knew each other as medical students, not friends or individuals. Such insights, we thought, meant students were actively expanding their beliefs about why people want to become doctors and the many paths people follow in order to be one. More importantly, they had found a way to abate their stress, more openly spoke about their fears of becoming a physician, and explicitly recognized the structural violence in their own and others' lives.

From 2012 to 2014, the students' work was shown on campus, dedicating one night as an opening and inviting the university community to view it. In 2015, we partnered with the Galveston Art Center (GAC) to host a public opening of the students' work, including live performances, video screenings, sculpture, painting, and a tapestry. The GAC publicized the event through their distribution networks and we invited the university community. Over 150 persons attended the 3-h opening of the exhibit; each of the 12 students addressed the audience and explained

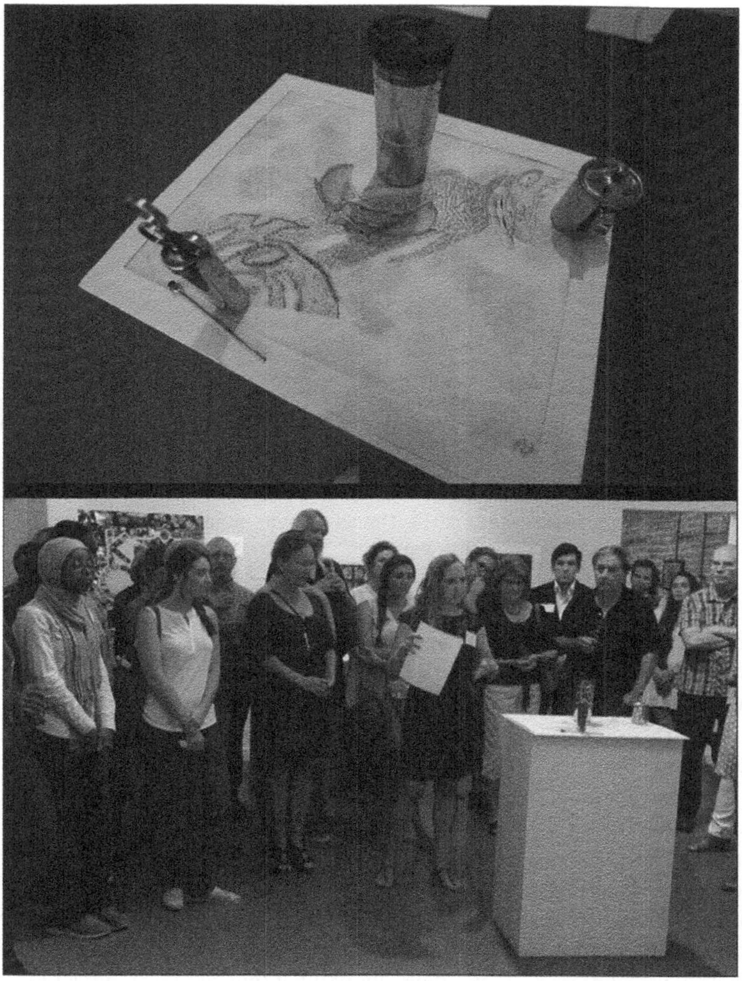

Fig. 11.3 "Life as a reflection of the dead". Joie Otto (MS2) explains her anatomical drawing as reflected in everyday objects during CEP reception, 2015 (Photo: E. H. Fletcher)

her/his piece, which significantly impacted the visitors. "I had no idea that medical school was so cool these days!", one guest exclaimed. One pathology professor commented on how impressed she was by students' in-depth knowledge of course materials and their ability to translate that knowledge into art (Fig. 11.3).

Excerpt of ethnographic influence from Otto's artist's statement,

> I saw death first as a student, eager to learn, looking for a perfect representation of what I had seen in the anatomical atlas: the Bible of GAR... As clumsily as I discovered the body, the pathologists navigated the organ systems like a familiar map. They knew where to look, they knew what to do, and most obviously to me: they did it reverently. They respected the life that was lost by making the death worth something.

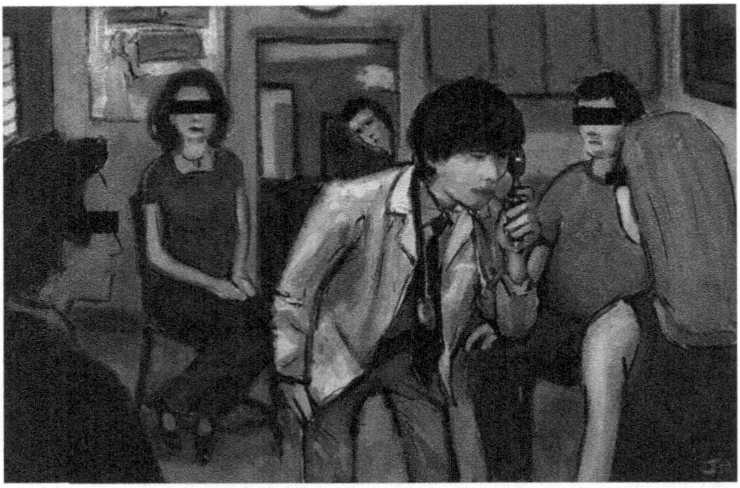

Fig. 11.4 "Eyes". Justin Hsu (MS2). 2014. Digital painting from series "Anonymous Visions". This is the last image in the series of five paintings

In their final reflections, CEP students explained the importance of sitting with their thoughts and experiences to develop a piece reflecting the stressful issues they address in medical school. Students commented on the importance of referring to their notes and documenting their process as a means for recognizing themes and issues in their work, alluding to the ethnographic fieldnotes mandate that one cannot remember everything they see, experience, or hear (Sanjek 1990). Amazing students create amazing projects and their ideas traversed the gamut, from life and work balance, mental health care, to structural violence, xenophobia and ethnocentrism, while recognizing their own role in affecting the lives of others and the growth they experienced by traveling abroad.

From an anthropological perspective, CEP borrows from field methods or participant observation and qualitative analysis by asking students to journal and document their work, conferring with others about what they are thinking, and presenting those ideas to larger groups for feedback and discussion. Students return to their journals to compose their personal statements in order to trace their steps and recognize the evolution in their thinking, the influences and multiple approaches to their project. Through this reflective process, medical students better understand their own issues and gain insight through the accounts of others. CEP is the product of employing ethnographic methods and analysis to produce art based upon a field experience (Fig. 11.4).

Excerpt of ethnographic influence from Hsu's artist's statement,

> Part of being a medical student is the stress and embarrassment of being watched by both faculties and patients as I clumsily interview and examine patients. However, this stress also urges me to move forward and to become a better, more knowledgeable doctor.

Conclusion: Obstacles and Opportunities

While there are certainly more hopeful and encouraging stories of anthropology in medicine, in our institution both 'cloaks' and 'many hats' have been necessary strategies to legitimate anthropology. We have made headway in incorporating social justice, cultural issues, qualitative data, and critical theory into the programs we are part of, but administrative hurdles, curricular debates, and disciplinary politics comprise a strong percentage of the structural forces we encounter every day. In conclusion, we would like to reflect on the obstacles that still loom, and the opportunities that beckon, in the incorporation of anthropology into medical education.

The current revisioning of the medical humanities to more inclusive and more critical renditions of "health humanities" and "critical medical humanities" is a real and welcomed opportunity for anthropological insights to be incorporated into medical education. Medical humanities is an established discipline in medical school curricula; the current challenges to its traditional disciplinary foci, its myopic focus on biomedicine, and its humanist understandings of self and sickness will increasingly make space for critical anthropological understandings of health to enter medical school curricula. It will be important for anthropologists to involve themselves in these critical movements from within medical humanities—both to solidify them and to challenge them to engage more directly with their ambivalent relationship with humanism.

But medical humanities (traditional or revisionary) is itself precariously positioned in the hierarchies of medical education. Whether as humanists or anthropologists, we encounter constant and consistent pushback from physicians who struggle to recognize how the historical, narrative, social, political and contextual issues we bring to bear on medical practice stand up to the scientific knowledge and clinical skills they teach and embody. "Remind me Jerome, are you a PhD or an EdD?" was a question asked by an MD peer who, even after years of working together on projects and teaching classes, needed to be reminded of our status on the academic ladder. The epistemic elitism embodied on medical campuses assumes that authoritative knowledge sports a long-white coat and a stethoscope around the neck. This is a persistent obstacle to more fully incorporating anthropology in medical school curricula.

The question of legitimacy in medicine is a perennial problem for all non-clinicians. Clinical ethicists, many of whom hold PhDs in philosophy, often sport white coats to signal their authority in clinic spaces and vis-à-vis the medical professionals they counsel. However, as several scholars have noted, the practice is fraught: what kind of legitimacy and authority do ethicists really want to embody (cf. Agich 1995), and—given their role as mediators and guides—how closely do they want to be identified with clinicians rather than patients (cf. Chambers 2008)? Anthropologists in medicine face a similar tension: what ought to be our demeanor, authoritative gestures, commitments, and contributions if we wish to be accepted as 'part of the team'? What ought to be our demeanor, authoritative gestures, commitments, and contributions if we wish to truly impart the insights of our discipline? This is exactly the dilemma Nancy Scheper-Hughes (1990) took up many years ago as she parsed the relative merits and demerits of an emerging "clinically applied anthropology". In typical fashion, her arguments were clarion and uncompromising. Clinically applied anthropologists who understood themselves to be "cultural brokers" between anthropological knowledge and the needs of health practitioners were, she declared, "putting anthropological knowledge at the service of the power brokers themselves" (p. 190) rather than putting anthropological knowledge to the tasks of questioning the "commonsense grounds and assumptions upon which biomedical knowledge is based [a traditional and intrinsic function of our method]" (p. 191). Rather than cultural broker, Scheper-Hughes advocated for the critically applied medical anthropologist as "court jester":

> The jester, the oppositional intellectual, works at the margins and sometimes (but not necessarily) from the outside, pulling at loose threads, deconstructing key concepts, looking at the world from a topsy-turvy position in order to reveal the contradictions, inconsistencies, and breaks in the fabric of the moral order without necessarily offering to 'resolve' them. (p. 191)

We have not had Scheper-Hughes audacity, although we too have resisted the accepted role of "cultural broker"—or what is similarly referred to in medical humanities as being the "handmaiden" to medicine (Bleakley 2015, 4; Macneill 2011). Perhaps we should have been more strident, but we settled for something more stealthy: we have worn our ethnographers' hats while cloaking ourselves as ethicists (sans white coats!). Bioethics stands as one of the few non-clinical or "non-scientific" (sic) disciplines to achieve legitimate status in medical culture. Our own methodologies are often referred to as "that stuff you do", or "the black box of qualitative methods", suggesting our work is not evidentiary and therefore not legitimate enough for science or medicine. Ethnographic research has significant levels of rigor built into it—our writing requires deep reflection and analysis, and we are often bilingual and multi-sited in our work—but because it is different, it is seen as inferior to an "evidence" which is often complicated by the socio-cultural issues we purport and teach. Such dismissive comments and constant scrutiny invoke the need to cloak ourselves in bioethical discourse and outwardly ignore our anthropological fundamentals for fear of being dismissed.

Ethical perspectives are also legitimated by the presence of "ethics questions" on USMLE tests (Step 1). The importance of these tests to students' future careers prioritizes an ethics focus, disincentives anthropology/humanities faculty to teach to their strengths, and offers students more than just what they will be tested on during the next shelf exam (and as a course director, I was not able to select, or see, the ethics questions on the Practice of Medicine "shelf" exam). Even as "ethicists", there are reactions within medical research teams and committees of MDs who fear being studied and scrutinized for their behaviors, or see us as "police" of sorts who report unethical instances to higher authorities (like the Institutional Review Board, or IRB). Nothing could be further from the truth for either of us, as we see the hierarchies and structural impediments within medicine as contributing to poor decisions or questionable behaviors by medical faculty, administrators, and students.

Within this 'cloaking' maneuver we have made or found opportunities to introduce important anthropological insights to the medical school curricula. The multilingual, multicultural experiences and research we bring to our individual teaching in POM 1 and POM 2 illustrates ideas and situations for students who have yet to encounter or understand the daily ethical situations clinics and hospitals create. How can we ask students to "break bad news" when so few of them have suffered a death or experienced a life-threatening illness themselves or within their families? Our ethnographic accounts bring ethical and cultural situations to life for students who tend to imagine a clinic where patients answer truthfully and completely, where "patient compliance" is a problem of patient education, and where people can be fixed. We identify with small victories like spending 8 weeks with 12 students to make art, or advising a medical student through an honors project investigating the role of race in emergency medicine. We have appreciated the opportunities we have had to formulate "professionalism" as not only the ethical practice of the profession one is entering, but also a reflexive and critical stance (anthropology's noted methodological stance) toward the profession one has the responsibility to shape. It is possible to work at the margins of medicine as an anthropologist and make a difference in the lives and perspectives of some of the students within.

Cloaking ourselves as ethicists has, however, created obstacles to our professional success in the academic health sciences and imperiled our paths to tenure. In an academic health sciences landscape, the process of educating peers, supervisors, administrators, tenure and promotion committees, grant writers and others about the methods, criteria, and contributions of anthropology is a monumental and incessant one. Each of us has experienced tremendous professional frustration from the misrecognition of the anthropological endeavor: fieldwork opportunities have been denied, grants to support fieldwork have been looked at askance, research questions have been seen as irrelevant to the mission of the institution, internal resources for anthropological research are non-existent, IRBs have been flummoxed by visual research methods, the production of films or books have been given insufficient weight in promotion and tenure evaluations, and APT committees have generally lacked expertise to evaluate the productivity or significance of anthropological research. These problems are endemic and the effort needed to overcome them is tremendous. When that effort is diverted into masking ourselves as "ethicists" we threaten our own ability to survive as anthropologists in medical education; as tenure-track faculty, at the time of this writing, the success of our tenure applications remain highly uncertain.

To paraphrase a wise, senior anthropologist before one of us accepted the tenure-track faculty position in medical humanities, "do NOT become bogged down in the trappings of administrative roles and committee work they will tell you is so important, as your own work will suffer and no one else is looking out for you and your work but you! Remember, humanities departments, like other social sciences at health science centers are nothing more than "pets", administrators will get rid of you when funds dry up. Unless you can bring in NIH funds and support yourself with grants, you won't be there long." More prescient words could not have been shared. Indeed, "service" to the institution is greedy, especially when medical faculty are encouraged to earn revenue value units (RVUs) in the clinic rather than FTEs in the classroom, responsibilities fall to those who are available and non-essential.

Finally, we believe there is opportunity for anthropologists to move outside medical education 'proper' and to establish their legitimacy in various community endeavors (such as public arts education) and pedagogical innovations (such as interprofessionalism). While it does necessitate wearing many hats, the terrain here feels a little less uphill, the ground newer and more receptive, the knowledges less established and thereby more open to anthropological insights. It may be that our legitimating experiences in these arenas will embolden us to "come out" more fully so that we can engage as anthropological researchers and instructors who bring culturally relevant, socially attuned, and critically informed knowledge to the education of diverse health professions students.

References

Abu-Lughod, L. 2002. Do Muslim women really need saving? Anthropological reflections on cultural relativism and its others. *American Anthropologist* 104 (3): 783–790.

Agich, G. 1995. Authority in ethics consultation. *Journal of Law, Medicine and Ethics* 23 (3): 273–283.

Albert, Mathieu, Elise Paradis, and Ayelet Kuper. 2015. Interdisciplinary promises versus practices in medicine: The decoupled experiences of social sciences and humanities scholars. *Social Science & Medicine* 126 (17–25).

Anderson, W. 2008. Teaching 'race' at medical school: Social scientists on the margin. *Social Studies of Science* 38 (5): 785–800.

Bishop, Jeffery. 2008. Rejecting medical humanism: Medical humanities and the metaphysics of medicine. *Journal of Medical Humanities* 29 (1): 15–25.

Bleakley, A. 2015. *Medical humanities and medical education: How the medical humanities can shape better doctors*. Routledge.

Braun, Lundy, Anne Fausto-Sterling, Duana Fullwiley, Evelynn M. Hammonds, Alondra Nelson, William Quivers, Susan M. Reverby, and Alexandra E. Shields. 2007. Racial categories in medical practice: How useful are they? *PLoS Medicine* 4 (9): e271.

Chambers, T. 2008. Good guys don't wear white. *American Journal of Bioethics* 8 (7): 8–11.

Chrisman, N., and T. Maretzki. 1982. Preface. In *Clinically applied anthropology: Anthropologists in health science settings*, ed. N. Chrisman and T. Maretzki. Dordrecht: Kluwer/D. Reidel Publishing.

Clifford, James. 1988. *The predicament of culture*. Cambridge: Harvard University Press.

Clifford, James, and George E. Marcus. 1986. *Writing culture: The poetics and politics of ethnography*. Berkeley: University of California Press.

Cole, T., N. Carlin, and R. Carson. 2015. *Medical humanities: An introduction*. New York: Cambridge University Press.

Crawford, P., B. Brown, C. Baker, V. Tischler, and B. Abrams. 2015. *Health humanities*. New York: Palgrave Macmillan.

Da Silva, S. 2018. Moral motivation and judgement in virtue ethics. *Philonsorbonne* 12: 107–123.

Davis, Sarah H., and Melvin Konner, eds. 2011. *Being there: Learning to live cross-culturally*. Cambridge: Harvard University Press.

De Frietas, E., and J. Paton. 2009. (De)facing the self: Poststructural disruptions of the autoethnographic text. *Qualitative Inquiry* 15 (3): 483–498.
DeMatteo, D., and S. Reeves. 2013. Introducing first-year students to interprofessionalism: Exploring professional identity in the “enterprise culture”: A Foucauldian analysis. *Journal of Interprofessional Care* 27: 27–33.
Dumit, J. 2004. *Picturing personhood. Brain scans and biomedical identity*. Princeton, NJ: Princeton University Press.
Englander, R., T. Cameron, A.J. Ballard, J. Dodge, J. Bull, and C.A. Aschenbrener. 2013. Toward a common taxonomy of competency domains for the health professions and competencies for physicians. *Academic Medicine* 88 (8): 1088–1094.
Fox, D. 1985. Who are we: The political origins of the medical humanities. *Theoretical Medicine and Bioethics* 6 (3): 327–341.
Geertz, Clifford. 1975. On the nature of anthropological understanding: Not extraordinary empathy but readily observable symbolic forms enable the anthropologist to grasp the unarticulated concepts that inform the lives and cultures of other peoples. *American Scientist* 63 (1): 47–53.
Gotlib-Conn, L. 2010. Using ethnographic methods to understand change in interprofessional practice. *Journal of Research in Interprofessional Practice and Education* 1 (3): 301–303.
Grainger-Monsen, Maren, and Julia Haslett. 2003. *World's apart: A four-part series on cross-cultural healthcare*. Boston, MA: Fanlight Productions.
Hippen, Benjamin E., and J.S. Taylor. 2007. In defense of transplantation: A reply to Nancy Scheper-Hughes. *American Journal of Transplantation* 7 (7): 1695–1697.
Interprofessional Education Collaborative Expert Panel. 2011. *Core competencies for interprofessional collaborative practice: Report of an expert panel*. Washington, DC: Interprofessional Education Collaborative.
Jones, T., M. Blackie, R. Garden, and D. Wear. 2017. The almost right word: The move from *medical* to *health* humanities. *Academic Medicine* 92 (7): 932–935.
Jones, Aled, and Delyth Jones. 2011. Improving teamwork, trust and safety: An ethnographic study of an interprofessional initiative. *Journal of Interprofessional Care* 25 (3): 175–181.
Jonsen, Albert R., Mark Siegler, and William J. Winslade. 2015. *Clinical Ethics. A practical approach to ethical decisions in clinical medicine*. 8th ed. New York: McGraw-Hill.
Kaufman, Sharon R. 2015. *Ordinary medicine: Extraordinary treatments, longer lives, and where to draw the line*. Durham: Duke University Press.
Kleinman, A. 1982. Clinically applied anthropology on a psychiatric consultation-liaison service. In *Clinically applied anthropology*, ed. N.J. Chrisman and T.W. Maretzki, 83–116. Dordrecht: Kluwer/D. Reidel Publishing.
———. 1988. *The illness narratives: Suffering, healing and the human condition*. New York: Basic Books.
Kucirka, Lauren M., et al. 2011. Association of race and age with survival among patients undergoing dialysis. *JAMA* 306 (6): 620–626.
Kutac, J., R. Osipov, and A. Childress. 2016. Innovation through tradition: Rediscovering the ‘humanist’ in medical humanities. *Journal of Medical Humanities* 37 (4): 371–387.
Lambert, Joe. 2013. *Digital storytelling: Capturing lives, creating community*. New York: Routledge.
Lock, Margaret. 2002. *Twice dead. Organ transplants and the reinvention of death*. Berkeley: University of California Press.
Macneill, P.U. 2011. The arts and medicine: A challenging relationship. *Medical Humanities* 37: 85–90.
Mahmood, Saba. 2001. Feminist theory, embodiment, and the docile agent: Some reflections on the Egyptian Islamic revival. *Cultural Anthropology* 16 (2): 202–236.
———. 2005. *Politics of piety. The Islamic revival and the feminist subject*. Princeton, NJ: Princeton University Press.
Marcus, George E., and Michael J. Fischer. 2014. *Anthropology as cultural critique: An experimental moment in the human sciences*. 2nd ed. Chicago: University of Chicago Press.

Martinez, Iveris L. 2015. Integrating anthropology in medical education: Opportunities, challenges, and lessons. *Practicing Anthropology* 37 (1): 35–39.
Mattingly, Cheryl. 2012. Two virtue ethics and the anthropology of morality. *Anthropological Theory* 12 (2): 161–184.
Nelson, S., M. Tassone, and B. Hodges. 2014. *Creating the health care team of the future: The Toronto model for interprofessional education and practice*. Ithaca, NY: Cornell University Press.
Peabody, F. 1927. The care of the patient. *JAMA* 88 (12): 877–882.
Purcell, T. 1998. Indigenous knowledge and applied anthropology: Questions of definition and direction. *Human Organization* 57 (3): 258–272.
Reisman, D. 2000. *On our own terms: Moyers on dying*. New York: Public Affairs Television.
Rice, K., M. Zwarenstein, L. Gotlib Conn, C. Kenaszchuk, A. Russell, and S. Reeves. 2010. An intervention to improve interprofessional collaboration and communications: A comparative qualitative study. *Journal of Interprofessional Care* 24 (4): 350–361.
Robin, Bernard R. 2008. Digital storytelling: A powerful technology tool for the 21st century classroom. *Theory into Practice* 47 (3): 220–228.
Rose, Nikolas. 1998. *Inventing ourselves: Psychology, power, and personhood*. Cambridge, UK: Cambridge University Press.
Rowen, J., Shell, E. J., Smith, S., Ashmore, K., Arcari, C., & Rudkin, L. (2016). *What's wrong with Warren? An interprofessional case study to learn roles and responsibilities*. Poster presentation, American Academy of Medicine Annual Meeting, Seattle, WA.
Sandor, K., V. Sierpina, H. Vanderpool, and S. Owen. 2006. Spirituality and clinical care: Exploring developmental changes in nursing and medical students. *Explore* 2 (1): 37–42.
Sanjek, Roger. 1990. *Fieldnotes: The makings of anthropology*. Ithaca, NY: Cornell University Press.
Scheper-Hughes, N. 1990. Three propositions for a clinically applied anthropology. *Social Science & Medicine* 30 (2): 189–197.
———. 2001. Commodity fetishism in organs trafficking. *Body & Society* 7 (2–3): 31–62.
———. 2007. The tyranny of the gift: Sacrificial violence in living organ donors. *American Journal of Transplantation* 7: 507–511.
Scheper-Hughes, N., and M. Lock. 1987. The mindful body: A prolegomenon to future work in medical anthropology. *Medical Anthropology Quarterly* 1 (1): 6–41.
Sharp, Lesley A. 2006. *Strange harvest. Organ transplants, denatured bodies, and the transformed self*. Berkeley: University of California Press.
———. 2007. *Bodies, commodities, and biotechnologies: Death, mourning, and scientific desire in the realm of human organ transfer*. New York: Columbia University Press.
Smith, K. 2012. From dividual and individual selves to porous subjects. *The Australian Journal of Anthropology* 23: 50–64.
Strathern, M. 1992. *After nature. English kinship in the late 20th century*. Cambridge, UK: Cambridge University Press.
Taylor, C. 2007. *A secular age*. Cambridge: Harvard University Press.
United States Medical Licensing Examination. 2019. USMLE Physician Tasks/Competencies. Federation of State Medical Boards of the United States, Inc. (FSMB) and National Board of Medical Examiners (NBME). https://www.usmle.org/pdfs/tcom.pdf. Accessed 2 July 2018.
Ventres, W., and B. Wilson. 2019. Rethinking goals: Transforming short-term global health experiences into engagements. *Academic Medicine*. https://doi.org/10.1097/ACM.0000000000002841.
Viney, W., F. Callard, and A. Woods. 2015. Critical medical humanities: Embracing entanglement, taking risks. *Medical Humanities* 41: 2–7.
Whitehead, A., and A. Woods, eds. 2016. *The Edinburgh companion to the critical medical humanities*. Edinburgh: Edinburgh University Press.

Wilson, A.J., L. Palmer, T. Levett-Jones, C. Gilligan, and S. Outram. 2016. Interprofessional collaborative practice for medication safety: Nursing, pharmacy, and medical graduates' experiences and perspectives. *Journal of Interprofessional Care* 30 (5): 649–654.

Arlene L. Macdonald, PhD is Assistant Professor, Institute for the Medical Humanities, University of Texas Medical Branch, Galveston. She teaches required and elective courses on humanities, professionalism, ethics and social medicine to undergraduate medical students. She has been integral in bringing these topics into interprofessional education, serving on the institution's Interprofessional Education and Practice Advisory Committee and Interprofessional Curriculum Advisory Committee. She trains graduate students at the Institute for the Medical Humanities, an interdisciplinary program granting the MA, PhD, and MD/PhD degree in Medical Humanities; she jointly developed a graduate-level curricular concentration in Social Medicine. Her research draws on critical qualitative methods and social theory to illuminate the intersections of religion and health. A prominent focus of her research has been organ transplantation and donation; she serves on the President's Advisory Council of the Children's Organ Transplant Association, a national service organization. More recently, she has been investigating the challenges and opportunities associated with religious diversity. She was a postdoctoral fellow for the Religion & Diversity Project, a research initiative housed at the University of Ottawa, and a Fellow with the Engaged Scholars Studying Congregations Program, funded by the Lilly Endowment. She holds a PhD in Religious Studies from the University of Toronto.

Jerome W. Crowder, PhD is Associate Professor in the Department of Social and Behavioral Sciences at the University of Houston College of Medicine. From 2010 to 2019 he taught Humanities, Ethics and Professionalism to first and second year medical students at University of Texas Medical Branch (Galveston, Texas), and served as co-director of the Practice of Medicine course for second year medical students since 2015. Concerned with student burnout and dedicated to integrating arts practices in medical education, Crowder developed the Creative Expression Project for second-year medical students to reflect on their reasons for becoming a physician and to learn how to maintain creativity throughout their practice. Trained as a medical and visual anthropologist, Crowder's applied work has appeared in journals, books, and museums throughout the Americas. He co-edited an issue of Medical Anthropology (2017) on the role of images in medical anthropology research, and was photo editor for the *Handbook of Medical Anthropology* (Routledge, 2016). Supported through federal and state sponsored agencies (e.g. AHRQ, NSF, NEH and Humanities Texas) his community-driven research spans conducting dialogues on patient-centered outcomes, to health care decision making and continuity of care, to the role of photography in ethnographic research and issues of representation. He has offered courses on visual analysis for the National Science Foundation (NSF) and the University of Florida, health and migration for Pan-American Health Organization (PAHO) and made a film about Dax Cowart, patients' rights activist, which is distributed by Alexander Street Press. He is the current President of the Society for Visual Anthropology.

Chapter 12
Inclusivity in Medical Education: Teaching Integrative and Alternative Medicine in Kentucky

Lee X. Blonder

Introduction

Anthropologists have made valuable contributions to American medical education and medical research over the last century, most notably in the areas of anatomy, human evolution, forensic pathology, pediatric growth and development, nutrition, doctor-patient communication, health disparities, ethnomedicine, and patient-centered medicine. While the value of anthropology in medical education is evident to those in the field, its relevance is often under-appreciated by healthcare college administrators as well as basic science and clinical faculty. This may be related to lack of familiarity with the discipline, misconceptions regarding what anthropologists do, or because biomedicine and anthropology have different histories and, in some respects, divergent philosophies. Biomedicine, also referred to as conventional medicine or allopathic medicine, aligns itself with the biological sciences and the scientific method. Anthropology, on the other hand, has mixed roots, with differing views regarding its endorsement of science and the scientific method.

The 2015 revision of the Medical College Admission Test (MCAT) by the Association of American Medical Colleges (AAMC) includes assessment of the impact of behavioral and sociocultural factors on health outcomes. Yet the MCAT revision emphasizes preparation in psychology, sociology, and biology, but not anthropology. In particular, the AAMC website states that the Psychological, Social, and Biological Foundations of Behavior section of the revised MCAT will "test concepts taught at many colleges and universities in first-semester psychology and sociology courses." Further, they estimate that the exam content draws 65% from introductory psychology, 30% from introductory sociology, and 5% from

L. X. Blonder (✉)
Sanders-Brown Center on Aging and Department of Behavioral Science, University of Kentucky, Lexington, KY, USA
e-mail: lxblond@uky.edu

I. L. Martinez, D. W. Wiedman (eds.), *Anthropology in Medical Education*,
https://doi.org/10.1007/978-3-030-62277-0_12

introductory biology. Assessment of material covered in introductory anthropology courses like hominid evolution and human biological and cultural variation, is absent. Taken together, these notable omissions in medical school admission testing underscore the need for anthropologists appointed in medical schools to advance an anthropological perspective.

I am a tenured professor in the Department of Behavioral Science in the College of Medicine at the University of Kentucky (UK), with joint appointments in the departments of Neurology and Anthropology (College of Arts and Sciences). I trained as a biomedical anthropologist, a subfield that "combines the theoretical and methodological aspects of physical anthropology and medical anthropology in the study of disease and health among human populations" (Johnston and Lowe 1984). The Department of Behavioral Science, where I hold my primary appointment, is one of a handful of stand-alone behavioral science departments in medical schools nationally. The department was founded in 1959 by Robert Straus, a Yale-trained medical sociologist who was instrumental in establishing the UK College of Medicine in 1960. Current faculty members include anthropologists, psychologists, sociologists, social workers, an epidemiologist, a psychiatrist, and others. Faculty in Behavioral Science teach, perform clinical and service activities, and engage in scholarly pursuits and extramurally funded research. The department offers masters and doctoral degrees and a graduate certificate in clinical translational science, as well as an undergraduate certificate in medical behavioral science. The department is also engaged in the teaching of medical students, and directs *Introduction to Clinical Medicine*, a year-long course required of all first-year medical students.

During my three decades in the College of Medicine at UK, I have served as a preceptor in first-year medical student courses. These courses typically have directors that organize and design the classes, and a dozen or more faculty who teach small groups of students. As a preceptor, I have taught "Communication and Interviewing" as well as "Physicians, Patients, and Society" and "Introduction to Clinical Medicine." The design and content of these courses reflects the behavioral science and clinical background of the course directors and preceptors and their expertise in medical education, as well as the educational requirements set forth by the Liaison Committee for Medical Education (LCME) accrediting body and the competencies assessed by the United States Medical Licensing Examination (USMLE) Step 1 Board exam.

These courses have employed a variety of pedagogical techniques, including small groups (8–9 students), team teaching involving physician and behavioral scientist dyads, problem-based learning, experiential or service learning, and mock interviews with simulated patients. For example, "Introduction to Clinical Medicine" is a year-long course currently required of all first-year (M1) medical students at UK and its regional campuses. The course is co-directed by faculty in the department of Behavioral Science and Internal Medicine and the M1 classes are divided into groups of approximately nine students. Each small group has a physician and a behavioral science preceptor who meet regularly and engage in activities such as small group discussions and presentations on various topics (e.g. medical ethics, the placebo effect, behavior change, health literacy, health disparities, grief and loss, addiction, nutrition and obesity, depression). Students read articles, online modules, and view videos in preparation for small group meetings.

We also have sessions devoted to practice interviews in which community actors and trained volunteers pose as patients. Students learn to elicit the patient's chief concern, history of the present illness, past medical and family history, review of systems, and social history. We emphasize verbal and nonverbal communication skills and students attend "labs" during which they engage in one-on-one practice interview sessions with a standardized patient. The interview sessions are not designed to teach diagnostic skills or treatment planning, but rather train students to interact with and motivate patients, obtain pertinent health information, display empathy and active listening behavior, and handle sensitive topics. We also emphasize the importance of asking patients their thoughts on the possible cause of their illness or symptoms and what they hope to gain from the visit. This line of questioning emanates from the explanatory model approach pioneered by Arthur Kleinman (1988). Students engage in shadowing and community service and they are required to complete activities of their choosing such as reading books related to medicine, attending grand rounds or medical interest group sessions, listening to medical podcasts, or watching relevant TED talks. Students write portfolio reflections that they upload to Canvas, the online learning management system. Preceptors give written feedback and entries are graded complete/incomplete. The course itself is graded pass-fail, consistent with a nationwide trend in medical education (AAMC).

Throughout the last several years, I have sought to apply my experience and interests as a biomedical anthropologist and faculty member in a medical school to curriculum development. I embarked on a mission to teach integrative and alternative medicine, a subject that, although recognized, currently falls outside mainstream medical education. This is unfortunate given that approximately 50% of consumers in the U.S. use dietary supplements or some form of "complementary" or "alternative" therapy (Kantor et al. 2016; Clarke et al. 2015; Eisenberg et al. 1993). In particular, Eisenberg et al. (1993) found that 34% of 1539 adults surveyed reported using some form of unconventional medical therapy during the prior year, and that most of these treatments were paid out of pocket. In a follow-up study, Eisenberg et al. (1998) showed that the use of unconventional therapies had increased from 34% in 1990 to 42.1% in 1997. More recently, Clarke et al. (2015) analyzed data collected by the National Health Interview Survey of 88,962 U.S. adults and showed that the percent who used some form of complementary health approach (e.g., yoga, chiropractic, meditation, homeopathy, acupuncture, non-vitamin, non-mineral dietary supplements, etc.) was 32.3% in 2002, 35.5% in 2007, and 33.2% in 2012. Kantor et al. (2016) investigated dietary supplement use among approximately 28,000 U.S. adult participants in the National Health and Nutrition Examination Survey (NHANES) and found that 52% of respondents used some form of dietary supplement in 2011–2012. Despite Eisenberg et al.'s (1993) conclusion that the use of unconventional medicine has "an enormous presence in the U.S. healthcare system," conventional medicine has made little effort to incorporate education in complementary and alternative practices into the standard curriculum and has largely ignored their widespread use by patients.

To the extent that integrative and alternative medicine includes non-Western, non-European traditions that in some cases are philosophically at odds with biomedicine, its lack of incorporation into mainstream allopathic medical education reflects both the ethnocentrism and paternalism that underlies "scientific medicine," as practiced in the U.S. and as promulgated by the American Medical Association (AMA), the American Association of Medical Colleges (AAMC), and the LCME. This belief in the absolute authority of conventional medicine reflects the underlying assumption that science transcends culture. Anthropologists and others have criticized that view (Singer 2009). Hans Baer et al. (2013:9) state that "Even though physicians in industrial societies purport to practice a form of science-based health care that is distinct from magic, religion, and politics, in reality their endeavors are intricately intertwined with these spheres of social life."

As an anthropologist and preceptor in the College of Medicine, I became increasing cognizant of the circumscribed training—philosophically, historically, and practically, that medical students receive, in both medical school and in the pre-medical curriculum—and the unrecognized bias that underlies some of the teaching. Given the statistics cited above regarding the widespread use of complementary and alternative medicine (CAM) by the U.S. population, it is pedagogically unacceptable that (1) mainstream medical practitioners have little to no formal training in these modalities and (2) by virtue of the training they do receive, are tacitly encouraged to harbor biases that would not hold up if subjected to proper scrutiny using all available evidence: historical, cross-cultural, evolutionary. I therefore decided to offer a three-credit elective on integrative and alternative medicine to UK undergraduates, as well as one-credit electives to first and second-year medical students. To further my goal of promoting integrative and alternative medicine in medical education, I teamed up with a UK family physician, fellowship-trained and board certified in integrative medicine. We received grants from the Weil Foundation to expand integrative medicine offerings to fourth year medical students, residents, and faculty members.

The courses that I have developed provide students with an introduction to integrative and alternative medicine as practiced in the U.S. They are designed to illuminate Western cultural biases inherent in conventional medicine that often masquerade as science, and to educate students regarding: 1) mechanistic vs holistic approaches, 2) the socio-cultural, political, historic, and economic drivers that influence medical education, practice patterns, and healthcare beliefs, 3) the role of evidence-based medicine in promoting pharmaceuticals and medical procedures while at the same time marginalizing integrative and alternative medical approaches that may be less profitable; and 4) the various prevention and treatment strategies used by integrative and alternative medicine that have proven efficacious but are rarely taught in the conventional medical curriculum. These courses are not simply a "smorgasbord" of possible "complementary" treatments that might be used in stress management or lifestyle medicine. Rather, I have sought to develop courses that expose the historical and philosophical influences that have generated the constructs of complementary, alternative, functional, and integrative medicine in the U.S. today. Further, these courses are designed to teach students approaches to diagnosis, treatment, and healing that are currently employed by integrative, functional, and alternative medicine practitioners.

In this chapter, I will discuss key topics included in the courses I have developed and their relevance to medical education and practice. These experiences and lessons learned serve as a window into the role of anthropologists in medical education and the avenues for future contribution.

Medical Education and the Standard Curriculum

The Liaison Committee for Medical Education (LCME) is recognized by the U.S. Department of Education as the accrediting body for medical education programs leading to the MD degree in the United States and Canada. The LCME is jointly sponsored by the AMA and the AAMC. To receive and maintain accreditation, medical schools must meet the standards set forth by the LCME in its document "Functions and Structure of a Medical School" (LCME 2018). This document is available on the LCME website and Standard 7 outlines Curricular Content (p. 10). The outline includes (1) content from biomedical, behavioral, and socioeconomic sciences, including "mastery of contemporary scientific knowledge;" (2) organ systems, life cycle, clinical experiences, primary, rehabilitative, and end of life care; (3) scientific method and clinical translational research; (4) critical judgment and problem solving skills; (5) societal problems; (6) cultural competence and health care disparities; (7) medical ethics; (8) communication skills; and (9) interprofessional collaborative skills.

The LCME Curricular Content standards emphasize instruction in or mastery of scientific knowledge and the scientific method. Medical schools are not expected or required to teach the philosophical and historical context within which biomedicine has developed. Further, there are no requirements to educate students in indigenous and traditional medical systems as practiced around the world. These gaps in the curriculum likely reflect the positions of the AMA and the AAMC that "conventional" or "science-based" medicine is medicine, and all other medical traditions and treatment modalities are "alternative" unless subjected to rigorous study involving randomized clinical trials and "proof" of efficacy. Key partners in promoting this approach, including the "diagnose and dispense" model of patient care, are the insurance and pharmaceutical industries that are driven by the profit motive and influence both healthcare policy and practice in the U.S. (Kemper 2016; Starr 2017; Baer 2001).

Elective Courses in Integrative and Alternative Medicine

Anthropologists are uniquely poised to educate students regarding the socio-historical context of biomedicine as well as other systems of healing around the world (Baer 2001; Baer et al. 2013). The electives on integrative and alternative medicine that I have developed address these topics. I began by creating a course entitled *Frontiers in Integrative and Alternative Medicine* that I first taught to undergraduates in the Honors Program (now Honors College) at UK. This course attracted pre-medical students and those from diverse majors, including health sciences, nursing, engineering, business, English, and the social sciences. I then created a fully online version of this course that I offered to junior and senior undergraduates in the following year. Recently I designed a hybrid Honors adaptation of this course to target junior and senior undergraduates, including but not limited to those enrolled in the Honors College at UK. The conversion of the course from face-to-face to fully online and hybrid has resulted in additional enrollment by pre-medical and pre-health students who prefer the online format or find it easier to fit online courses into their packed schedules. At the same time, I began offering a one credit face-to-face version of the elective to first and second-year medical students, as well as a three-credit elective rotation to fourth-year medical students.

These electives consist of several modules, available through Canvas, the online learning management system used by the University of Kentucky. The material covered includes variations on the following topics: Introduction and Western Historical Context, Global Traditions and Influences, Integrative and Alternative Medicine in the U.S., Evidence and Efficacy in Conventional and Alternative Medicine, Personal Genomics and the Future of Medicine, Micronutrient and Botanical Supplementation, Diet and Nutrition, and Mind Body Medicine. Students listen to short lectures, read articles, chapters, blogs and material posted on websites, watch TED talks and videos, engage in discussion and written reflections, both face-to-face and online. In face-to-face and hybrid versions of the courses, I invite integrative and alternative practitioners to give guest lectures to class to engage in discussions and lead mind-body practices with students (e.g. guided imagery, meditation). To tailor the content to medical students, I co-teach with a Board-certified fellowship-trained integrative medicine physician colleague and present case studies in integrative medicine, clinically relevant readings, and lessons on motivational interviewing, treatment planning, and the use of botanicals and mind-body approaches in the clinical setting. In the fourth-year rotation, students shadow integrative and alternative practitioners in the community and apply integrative medicine motivational interviewing and treatment planning in the care of specific patients seen in the Family Medicine clinic at our university.

Three to four medical students tend to enroll in the integrative and alternative medicine electives. By contrast, I cap the undergraduate courses at 20–25 students and there is often a waitlist. The undergraduate electives have received excellent reviews and students comment that the material was interesting, that it was one of their favorite classes, and some lamented that they had wished they had taken it earlier because they had not realized there were so many "alternative" career paths available. Some students state that a class like this ought to be required of all pre-health students.

I have encountered some skepticism from medical students enrolled in the electives, but student feedback indicates that the elective introduced them to interesting and useful material not covered in the standard curriculum. Nevertheless, medical students are very focused on clinical application, and request more of that and less emphasis on socio-cultural, historical and philosophical background. This suggests that we miss an opportunity to educate pre-medical students on these topics if we do not target them at that stage, as once students arrive in medical school they are transformed into "practitioners in the making" and desire that their education be clinically-oriented to prepare them for their role as physicians.

To illustrate the ways in which an anthropological perspective has the potential to enhance medical education and ultimately the way students think and practice, I will review select topics in integrative and alternative medicine that students study in these electives. The topics I focus on include (1) Historical Background, (2) the Flexner Report, (3) Global Perspectives, (4) Evidence-Based Medicine, (5) Personalized Medicine and Genomics, and (6) Career Opportunities. Given the strong adherence to and insistence on "staying on message", i.e. scientific medicine as "truth" and the scientific method as the means to acquire such, I feel somewhat heretical in teaching what I am about to describe. I succeed in part because integrative medicine is recognized at our institution and nationally. For example, the University of Kentucky Markey Cancer Center houses an Integrative Medicine in Health Program that consists of a physician director and staff who offer various CAM therapies to patients as well as programs on meditation, yoga, and culinary medicine directed to staff and students. In addition, the university belongs to the Academic Consortium for Integrative Medicine, an organization that advances integrative medicine within academic institutions across the U.S. At the national level, integrative medicine has been recognized by the American Board of Physician Specialties. Beginning in 2005, the American Board of Integrative Holistic Medicine (ABIHM) began offering a peer-reviewed, psychometrically validated board certification exam for medical doctors and osteopathic physicians. There is also growing support for integrative and alternative medical education by healthcare and college administrators who recognize the value and popularity of these approaches and that medical students and physicians lack training. Lastly, College of Medicine faculty members are encouraged to offer medical students electives. Principles of academic freedom and respect for the expertise and professional autonomy of the professoriate prevail, such that curriculum committees tasked with reviewing and approving electives tend to focus on student learning outcomes, assessment methods, required expectations, and overlap with other courses, rather than the micromanagement of course content.

The Nineteenth Century American Medical Landscape

To facilitate understanding of the philosophical and historical context within which designations such as "complementary," "alternative" and more recently "integrative" and "functional" medicine evolved, my first goal as an anthropologist is to provide students with a basic introduction to the history of medical education and medical practice in the United States. I begin by teaching students about medical practice and education in frontier America during the late eighteenth to the mid-twentieth centuries, and the significance of the Flexner report (Ludmerer 2011). Most students have little to no knowledge of Abraham Flexner or his report, although they may have heard of the Flexner Master Educator awards for teaching, offered in many medical schools including ours. This lesson also includes information regarding socio-cultural, economic, and political forces that came together, including the role of the AMA and philanthropists like Carnegie and Rockefeller, in implementing and funding the standards in medical schools in accordance with Flexner's recommendations.

Over the last 100 plus years, biomedicine has become the predominant medical system in the United States and many parts of the world. During the same period, American anthropology came into prominence with the seminal work of Franz Boas and his followers who pioneered the four fields approach, ethnographic studies of diverse cultures, and the concept of cultural relativism (Stocking 1982). The deeply rooted holistic approach characteristic of American anthropology has distinguished it from other disciplines. As anthropology has developed, various sub disciplines have emerged and contributed to our understanding of health and healing, including biomedical anthropology, ethnomedicine, and critical medical anthropology (Alexandrakis 2001). Critical medical anthropology adds an important perspective in the understanding of biomedicine such that it recognizes the influence of global capitalism on health practices and outcomes (Singer and Baer 1995). Few medical students have exposure to the development of anthropological knowledge or theory as related to medicine, or to concepts and findings in the anthropological literature. Nor are they typically aware of the fact that nineteenth century American medicine was pluralistic, and medical training was highly variable (Beck 2004; Starr 2017; Baer 2001). Modalities practiced in nineteenth century America included Thomsonianism, homeopathy, chiropractic, osteopathy, naturopathy, and eclectic medicine. Eighteenth and nineteenth century "heroic" medicine, the predecessor to conventional or allopathic medicine, used treatments such as blood-letting, leaches, the dispensing of heavy metals, opium, and other potentially harmful regimens. A famous case is that of George Washington, who likely died from blood loss due to the "heroic" treatments he received, rather than pharyngitis, his presenting illness. The shift toward scientific medicine, accelerated by the Flexner Report of 1910, began in the late nineteenth and early twentieth centuries with the development of Louis Pasteur's germ theory and advances in diagnostic technologies (e.g., the stethoscope and microscope), public sanitation, vaccination, surgery—as well as discoveries like penicillin and insulin (Rothstein 1972; Starr 2017; Baer 2001).

Events that occurred more than 100 years prior to this shift, set the stage for the ensuing battle between conventional medicine and alternative practices. During the late eighteenth century, German physician Samuel Hahnemann became disenchanted with the harsh treatments of his day. In 1796 he coined the term "homeopathy," to refer to the medical practice he described in his writings (Hahnemann and Boericke 1922). Homeopathy means "similar suffering/pathos" in ancient Greek. Hahnemann chose this term to reflect his treatment philosophy that includes three principles: (1) the law of similars (like cures like); (2) the law of individuation (every individual is unique): and (3) the law of minimal doses involving serial dilutions with water or alcohol. Hahnemann contrasted homeopathy with what he labeled "allopathy," or the harmful practices employed during his time. In ancient Greek "allopathy" means opposite suffering. Hahnemann considered "allopathic" treatments as antagonistic, in that, unlike homeopathy, they produced effects that did not mimic the disease or condition. The term "allopathy" is no longer used as Hahnemann intended. Currently, allopathy commonly denotes the Doctor of Medicine degree (M.D.) in contrast to the Doctor of Osteopathy degree (D.O.). Osteopathy is a manipulative practice that originated in the late nineteenth century and has since transformed itself to conform to current biomedical standards.

The American Institute of Homeopathy was founded in 1844, 3 years prior to the founding of the AMA, and became the first national medical association in the U.S. Homeopathy was particularly appealing to women and attracted them as practitioners, patients, and mothers—who sometimes preferred these treatments for their children (Squier 1995). There is some evidence that homeopathic remedies were efficacious in the treatment of infectious diseases like yellow fever (Coulter 1982).

The AMA, founded in 1847, has a long history of opposing homeopathy and seeking its demise (Coulter 1982). Nevertheless, in 1938, homeopathy was incorporated into the Food, Drug, and Cosmetic Act thanks to the efforts of U.S. Senator Royal Copeland. This act recognized the Homeopathic Pharmacopeia of the United States and instituted the regulation of homeopathic treatments as drugs (Junod 2000). The FDA continues to review homeopathic treatments and reconsider regulatory guidelines (Servick 2015). Population surveys suggest that about 2–3% of U.S. adults use homeopathic remedies (Dossett et al. 2016), however, conventional medicine does not recognize homeopathy as evidence-based. Thus, twenty-first century American medical students have no formal training in homeopathy or its history and are often surprised to learn that the British Royals, including Her Majesty Queen Elizabeth II, use homeopathy. In particular, Queen Elizabeth's personal physician, the late Peter Fisher, was a renowned homeopath (Illman 2018). While homeopathy is dismissed by the AMA and the National Center for Complementary and Integrative Health as lacking scientific validity, the practice is recognized by the governments of India and several other countries, particularly in Europe, South America, and the Middle East (de Barros and Galhardi 2008; Ghosh 2010). Many countries offer professional education and credentialing in homeopathy, as well as statutory or private insurance coverage for homeopathic treatments. In the U.S., the regulation of homeopathy varies from state to state, but a handful of states license medical doctors and osteopaths to practice homeopathy, provided they have post-graduate training.

By familiarizing American pre-medical and medical students with homeopathy, they are exposed to its tenets and remedies, and encouraged to scrutinize the historical, political, economic, and philosophical forces that shape conventional medicine today. In teaching this lesson, I use several strategies. After I give a brief introduction, students are assigned readings and videos on the topic, construct questions directed towards their peers based on the material, and discuss them online or face-to-face. This multi-faceted approach is well-received and facilitates student engagement. It also sets the stage for students to understand the events of the early twentieth century, the rise and eventual dominance of scientific medicine, and the recasting of ancient, non-conforming, and traditional or indigenous healing modalities as complementary or alternative. Given that scientific medicine is just over a century in the making, historian William Bates' (2000) aptly poses the following question in his seminal article by the same title: "Why not call Modern Medicine 'Alternative?' His answer underscores the dominance of biomedicine today: "Because we can't."

The Flexner Report

The pluralistic landscape of the nineteenth century changed dramatically during the first two decades of the twentieth century. A major catalyst was the Flexner report of 1910, which transformed medical education in the United States and aligned it with biomedical science (Flexner and Carnegie Foundation for the Advancement of Teaching 1972; Janik 2014). The impetus for the Flexner report came about in 1904, when the AMA created the Council on Medical Education (CME). The CME sought to promote the restructuring of medicine in the U.S. in accordance with the AMA's goals. The CME requested that the Carnegie Foundation for the Advancement of Teaching conduct a survey of medical schools in the U.S. and Canada. Henry Pritchett, President of the Carnegie Foundation, chose Abraham Flexner, an educator from Louisville, Kentucky, to do so (Halperin et al. 2010). Flexner visited 155 medical schools over a 1-year period and wrote a detailed report that is currently available online. Flexner's model was that of Johns Hopkins, and his recommendations included reducing the number of poorly trained physicians and medical schools, increasing the pre-requisites, aligning medical schools with universities, training physicians to practice in a scientific manner, and engaging the faculty in research (Flexner and Carnegie Foundation for the Advancement of Teaching 1972).

The Flexner Report contributed to the standardization of medical education in the U.S. In the years following the report, 70 of 155 medical schools closed, including 13 out of 15 homeopathic medical schools, five out of seven African American medical schools, and six out of seven women's medical colleges (Thomas 2001; Burrow and Burgess 2001; Sullivan and Suez Mittman 2010). Many of these schools closed because they were unable to secure the funds needed to meet the standards that Flexner recommended, or because they failed to satisfy increasingly stringent state licensing and accreditation rules championed by the AMA and the Federation of State Licensing Boards, founded in 1912. In some states, practitioners of "alternative" medicine such as chiropractic and naturopathy were prosecuted for practicing medicine without a license. State licensing boards succeeded in restricting "alternative" practices and enforcing the adoption of biomedical curricular standards (Baer 2001).

Flexner's recommendations have continued to influence medicine over a century later due to support from philanthropists such as Rockefeller and Carnegie, medical educators, the AMA, and licensing and accrediting bodies (Duffy 2011). The American medical school curriculum, with basic sciences in the first 2 years and clinical training in the last 2 years has been modified to some extent, but the 4-year curriculum and the pre-medical requirements that were championed by Flexner, remain today. In addition, the alliance of allopathic medical schools with universities, and the archetype of the academic physician engaged in biomedical research endures, although tenure eligible positions for physician scientists are vanishing and the new generation of physicians who work in university systems tend to be clinical faculty on year-to-year contracts. Such faculty often engage in teaching, however a loss of autonomy coupled with an increased emphasis on income-generating activities, has eroded the ideal of the physician scientist that Flexner envisioned.

The Flexner report placed great emphasis on the teaching of basic laboratory sciences including anatomy, physiology, biochemistry, and pharmacology as well as pathology and bacteriology. The structure of most medical schools includes departments or divisions devoted to these subjects and Ph.D. basic scientists, traditionally appointed in these departments, are integral contributors to medical education and basic and translational research. In contrast, the only subject on Flexner's list that truly dovetails with anthropological expertise is anatomy. Physical anthropologists have secured faculty positions in U.S. medical schools by teaching gross anatomy to first-year medical students. In recent years, the financial pressures that academic health centers in the U.S. face have fostered the expectation that all medical school faculty participate in revenue generating activities to cover varying portions of their salaries. Anthropologists who also have a medical degree are at a distinct advantage in this regard, given their capacity for clinical activity and their possession of the credentials that advanced training in basic and clinical sciences confer. For anthropologists employed in U.S. medical schools who do not have a clinical degree, it is increasingly important to stress one's contributions, often by teaching in the standard medical curriculum or by conducting extramurally funded research that provides salary reimbursement, benefits, and institutional overhead. This usually involves securing highly competitive National Institute of Health grants to fund "science-based" medical research on topics of programmatic interest to the funding agency.

Positive outcomes attributed to the Flexner report include the following: medical students received uniform training in the basic and clinical sciences; medical education became standardized and regulated; the alignment with science eliminated any vestiges of heroic medicine as practiced in the eighteenth and nineteenth centuries; and the affiliation with universities upgraded teaching and fostered research as well as the translation of findings into clinical practice. Nevertheless, the report, which bolstered the power and authority of the AMA, also fostered an elitism that endures to this day. Women, minorities, residents of rural and poor areas, and alternative medical approaches have suffered from a lack of support or marginalization and the definition of what constitutes "medicine" in the U.S. narrowed. Clinical practice guidelines are the norm now in conventional medicine and medical malpractice cases have shaped the definition of standard-of-care. This further constrains physician behavior, particularly with respect to using unconventional treatments (Moffett and Moore 2011).

One of my goals as an instructor of undergraduates and medical students is to develop critical thinkers who question mainstream views. As such, it is important that students understand this history and how it has impacted their education and curricula, as well as the positive and negative outcomes associated with Flexner's recommendations. I teach this by providing background via lecture, slide presentations, and videos on heroic medicine and the nineteenth century medical landscape. Students read articles, have access to the original Flexner report, and engage in online and face-to-face discussions. They also write reflection essays synthesizing and analyzing the material.

Flexner's recommendations, coupled with philanthropic support, the rise of the pharmaceutical and health insurance industries during the early to mid-twentieth century, as well as the discoveries and innovations noted above (antiseptic surgery, vaccination, pasteurization, public health measures, antibiotics and insulin), consolidated biomedicine's sovereignty and rebranded other healing modalities as "alternative." More recently, "evidence-based-medicine," and its hierarchical taxonomy in which randomized clinical trials (RCTs) represent the gold standard, further disadvantages alternative medicine. The National Center for Complementary and Integrative Health (NCCIH), originally established in 1998 as the National Center for Complementary and Alternative Medicine, funds RCTs on natural products and "alternative" treatments to address the need for scientifically valid evidence. Yet NCCIH and the mainstream medical establishment aim to selectively incorporate "alternative" practices, secularized and "evidence-based," to "complement' the pharmaceutical and surgical management of illness. At the same time, an increasing number of patients and practitioners question biomedicine's "pill for an ill" and "one size fits all" approaches (Kemper 2016). Associations like the Academic Consortium for Integrative Medicine and the Academy of Integrative Health and Medicine are making inroads. Yet to achieve a paradigm shift in the healthcare enterprise as well as in medical education and practice, scholars, clinicians, and educators must work for further integration and expose unconscious bias and industry interests in biomedicine that serve as barriers.

Global Perspectives

In contrast to this post-Flexnerian model of medicine as practiced in the U.S., the United Nations and the World Health Organization (WHO) have recognized the importance and widespread use of traditional and indigenous medicine. The United Nations Declaration on the Rights of Indigenous Peoples, initially adopted in 2007, includes the recognition of traditional medicine and healers, and the WHO 2014–2021 strategic plan addresses traditional medicine world-wide (World Health Organization 2013). The significance of this global perspective is key to student learning—as it exposes students to: (1) the myriad healing systems that have evolved throughout the world and the steps taken by WHO member states to understand and regulate these modalities and integrate them into healthcare, (2) the ways in which indigenous plants and their components have been used by traditional healers and studied, synthesized, and monetized by the pharmaceutical industry, sometimes to the detriment of native people and their lands, and (3) the implicit ethnocentrism in biomedical education that they had not heretofore appreciated. Such bias, unexamined, is key in promoting and maintaining the belief that conventional medicine is unrivaled.

The WHO Strategic Plan represents a good introduction to how member nations are integrating traditional and conventional medicine. Some of the most compelling examples come from Africa and China, where traditional healers work alongside conventional medical doctors in hospital settings to treat patients. An important topic that students explore in this module on global perspectives is the traditional medicinal value of indigenous plants. This topic has long been the subject of inquiry by anthropologists, ethnobotanists, and ethnopharmacologists (Hsu and Harris 2010; Cox and Balick 1994). The standard medical curriculum emphasizes pharmaceutical drug mechanisms and prescribing standards. What is often omitted is the fact that historically, the pharmaceutical industry has exploited compounds in nature and in traditional healing that are isolated, synthesized, patented, subjected to the Food and Drug Administration (FDA) approval process, and marketed as the next blockbuster drug.

To educate students on global perspectives as well as colonialism in biomedicine, students read the WHO Strategic plan, watch WHO videos on the integration of traditional and conventional medicine in Africa, view presentations on traditional remedies that have inspired pharmaceuticals, and watch the TED talk, "What the People of the Amazon Know that You Don't," by ethnobotanist and conservationist Mark Plotkin. Medical students find this material enlightening, as they realize that the origin of some drugs they are learning about in the standard curriculum derive from native plants and animals used by traditional healers. They are also made aware of issues surrounding property rights of indigenous peoples and the negative impact of drug discovery, production, and use on the environment.

Recently in the U.S., the opioid crisis has led to interest in non-pharmaceutical pain remedies and as a result, many conventional practitioners and hospitals now incorporate Eastern modalities such as acupuncture, meditation, yoga, and botanicals, as well as chiropractic in the care of patients. The American College of Physicians now recommend non-pharmacologic treatments such as massage, acupuncture, or spinal manipulation for low back pain (Qaseem et al. 2017). In January of 2018, the Joint Commission non-profit that accredits healthcare institutions, began to require that hospitals provide education and treatment for pain using acupuncture, chiropractic and other non-pharmacologic modalities.

The generation of medical students we are currently instructing have been exposed to practices like yoga and meditation and some have utilized chiropractic and acupuncture. Baer (2001) attributes the increasing acceptance of these heterodox modalities in part due to the rise of the Holistic Health Movement in the 1970s. According to the WHO, acupuncture is the most widely used modality in traditional medicine, with some 80% of 129 reporting countries recognizing it (World Health Organization 2013). Despite this, few medical students are familiar with the philosophies or principles of Chinese or Ayurvedic medicine, or have in-depth exposure to integrative, functional, or naturopathic medicine. Thus, teaching these modalities prepares them for interprofessional clinical care and collaboration. As explained below, there are pathways available for medical students and physicians to become credentialed in integrative and functional medicine. In contrast, the Doctor of Naturopathic Medicine degree (N.D.) in the U.S. is a 4-year degree that constitutes an alternative to the MD or D.O. degrees and is notable in its incorporation of traditional medical modalities and its focus on primary care. Currently naturopathy is licensed or regulated in 22 states as well as the District of Columbia, Puerto Rico, and the U.S. Virgin Islands. There is overlap between the Doctor of Naturopathic Medicine curriculum and the conventional medical curriculum. Yet unlike allopathic training, naturopathy incorporates global, traditional, and indigenous approaches including homeopathy, Ayurveda, traditional Chinese medicine, botanical medicine, and other modalities considered quackery by many proponents of conventional medicine.

Evidence-Based Medicine

One of the principal barriers to the acceptance of integrative, traditional, indigenous, and alternative medicine by medical students and conventional healthcare providers is the concern that such treatments are not "evidence-based." It is vital to address this view as it is pervasive and is used to justify premature dismissal of unconventional medical modalities. There are several ways to confront these concerns pedagogically. I have found that a multi-faceted approach works best in which students are educated about evidence-based medicine (EBM), then exposed to research design issues, the profit motive, and strategies used in conventional pharmaceutical drug development, analysis, approval, and marketing (Goldacre 2014). Finally, students examine the criticisms leveled at EBM by integrative and alternative practitioners (Jagtenberg et al. 2006).

The phrase "evidence-based medicine" was coined in 1991 by Gordon Guyot, however many consider David Sackett the father of EBM (Sackett et al. 1996; Guyatt 1991). In Sackett's original formulation, EBM is "the conscientious, explicit and judicious use of current best evidence in making decisions about the care of the individual patient. It means integrating individual clinical expertise with the best available external clinical evidence from systematic research" (Sackett et al. 1996). In its most recent formulation, EBM uses a combination of scientific evidence derived from meta-analyses and randomized clinical trials (RCTs), practitioner judgment, and patient values and preferences, to decide if a treatment is appropriate. EBM education is an important component in the enculturation of medical students, as evidence-based practice is an expectation in healthcare decision-making (Djulbegovic and Guyatt 2017).

While EBM principles that utilize practitioner judgment and patient values and preferences are consistent with the treatment philosophies of integrative and alternative medicine, reliance on RCTs and meta-analyses in determining whether an integrative or alternative approach meets criterion for use is problematic for several reasons (Jagtenberg et al. 2006). First, RCTs are very costly and often conducted by pharmaceutical companies that invest billions of dollars in drug development and stand to profit from FDA approval and the sale of patented medicines. Second, the design of RCTs typically targets patients who possess a disease or condition defined by the International Classification of Diseases (ICD). ICD codes are tied to payment for healthcare services around the world. The National Center for Health Statistics in the U.S. is responsible for updating the ICD to adapt it to American healthcare (Topaz et al. 2013). American physicians must use ICD codes to collect clinical revenue. ICD categories may not overlap with diagnoses in traditional medicine, however. Thus, when a clinical trial tests the safety and efficacy of a non-conventional or "alternative" treatment using ICD diagnostic criteria, the results may be invalid. For example, a RCT may study the efficacy of acupuncture in treating "migraine," as defined by the ICD. In contrast, Traditional Chinese Medicine (TCM) practitioners diagnose patients presenting with migraine-like symptoms according to TCM theory and methods refined over centuries, not ICD codes. Because proper TCM diagnosis is critical in determining acupuncture points, studying a disease or condition based on ICD diagnostic criteria may lead to improper treatment and erroneous, uninterpretable, or negative results. It has long been a topic of discussion in medical and psychological anthropology as to the universality of Western diagnostic criteria and whether indigenous or "culture bound" illnesses map onto Western diagnoses (see Farmer 1988). "Culturally appropriate" RCT designs, although uncommon at this time, recognize the importance of alternative diagnostic classifications and medical philosophies, rather than simply focusing on promising treatments taken out of context. The ICD-11 includes a chapter on traditional medicine, defined by the WHO as "disorders and patterns which originated in ancient Chinese Medicine and are commonly used in China, Japan, Korea, and elsewhere around the world." Nevertheless, the use of this chapter is optional, and it is not to be employed for mortality reporting (Morris et al. 2012).

A third reason why EBM's principles and methods are problematic reflects what has been termed a "one size fits all" approach that continues to inform clinical trial designs, meta-analyses, and prescribing practices. With the advent of precision or personalized medicine, the concept that each person is unique, genetically and with respect to the metabolism of food, dietary supplements and drugs—has begun to take hold in the U.S. Nevertheless, from a conventional perspective, precision medicine is largely employed in cancer diagnosis and treatment at this time. On the other hand, traditional medicine, integrative medicine, and functional medicine are often highly personalized and based on extensive examination of the patient by a knowledgeable practitioner. The fields of pharmacogenetics and nutrigenetics recognize the importance of interpersonal genetic variation in the metabolism of drugs, supplements, and food. As of this writing, conventional medicine and RCT designs are slow to consider these factors, although some integrative, functional, and naturopathic practitioners use available personalized testing in treatment planning (Liu et al. 2011).

In the module that I teach on nutrigenomics, I emphasize that patients' response to a prescription drug, dietary supplement, or micronutrient may vary depending upon polymorphisms in cytochrome P450 genes or in the genes responsible for the breakdown of nutrients (e.g. folate, beta carotene), requiring tailored therapy or personalized dietary supplement regimens. Recent discoveries in the field of epigenetics have shown that genetic expression can be "turned on" or "turned off" based on lifestyle and dietary modifications. This underscores the importance of integrative and alternative medicine's personalized, preventative, and "holistic" approach versus the outdated "one size fits all" models used by the pharmaceutical industry, RCT design, and conventional treatment guidelines (Kanherkar et al. 2017). Moreover, variation in immune responses to foods, or even in real-world adherence to treatment protocols, often addressed in integrative and alternative care, may impact RCT results. Lastly, although EBM is the standard to which conventional practitioners are expected to adhere, many healthcare providers prescribe drugs "off-label"—i.e., for uses that are not FDA approved or validated—rendering questionable any claim that treatment decisions in conventional medicine routinely adhere to EBM standards.

Although there is much to be gained from rigorously conducted clinical research, particularly in assessing the safety and efficacy of novel pharmaceutical drugs, medical devices, and procedures, the process that treatments must undergo to be considered "evidence-based' are costly, often impersonal, and narrowly focused on RCTs as the gold standard. Centuries of historical use and experimentation are not recognized as high quality evidence in the EBM hierarchical model. An example that I use to illustrate the shortcomings of this approach is the work of Nobel laureate Tu Youyou, who combed through ancient Chinese texts to uncover not only the medicinal plant, artemisinin to use in the treatment of malaria, but the proper method of extraction to achieve efficacy (Kong and Tan 2015). Evidence-based medicine is a key paradigm that informs standard of care and insurance reimbursement in the U.S. In practice however, data may be manipulated, study designs flawed, profit prioritized, and providers non-compliant or uninformed (Goldacre 2014).

The medical school curriculum typically does not include a sociocultural or historical analysis of EBM. Rather, courses focus on EBM principles, the scientific method, clinical trial design, basic biostatistics, and drug development. These topics are important components of conventional medical education, in part due to the risks associated with administering new and powerful synthetic compounds, implanting newly invented devices, performing complex surgical procedures, and running potentially harmful diagnostic tests. Well-designed RCTs offer some reassurance of safety and efficacy and medical students need training in the evaluation of biomedical research to optimize clinical decision-making. Nevertheless, EBM promotes bias and serves the healthcare industry more than is acknowledged, via its narrow definition of what constitutes quality evidence that supports the pharmaceutical and medical device industries, the FDA approval process, and those individuals who serve on hospital boards and regulatory panels yet have conflicts of interest (Pham-Kanter 2014).

Anthropologists have the knowledge and ability to teach medical students to consider these factors including the role of EBM in dismissing many ancient and "alternative" treatments as quackery or worse, unsafe. Critical medical anthropology in particular emphasizes "the importance of political and economic forces, including the exercise of power, in shaping health, disease, illness experience, and healthcare" (Singer and Baer 1995:5). Even though the medical profession sounds repeated alarms regarding the damaging effects of alternative treatments, the actual statistics document far more adverse events associated with prescription and over-the-counter medication (Alliance for Natural Health 2012). Further, it is apparent that the public desires alternative treatments, yet conventional medicine is doing little to educate students and providers in their judicious selection and use.

The ever-increasing diversity of U.S. medical students, residents, and faculty has advanced interest in and acceptance of integrative and alternative medicine. Students from varied ethnic backgrounds and countries of origin often have exposure to traditional and indigenous medicine practiced in their culture or by their kin. Approaches that have personal relevance for the students and residents I have taught include TCM, Ayurveda, African healing traditions, homeopathy, and Appalachian herbal remedies. The conventional curriculum does not provide students the opportunity to learn about non-conventional healing modalities, apart from mind-body approaches such as meditation and yoga—stripped of their Eastern religious heritage and deployed to reduce the epidemic of stress and burn-out in the United States (West et al. 2018). Once learners study these traditions and modalities, they often have renewed excitement about their profession, enhanced tools to use in patient care, and possible declines in "burn-out." I have personally witnessed this renewed excitement among the students I educate.

Personalized Medicine and the Direct to Consumer Movement

As noted above, conventional medicine is slowly beginning to adopt a personalized or precision approach, mainly in the areas of tumor genomics and pharmacogenetics. This has been made possible by the revolutionary achievements of the Human Genome Project that enabled newfound opportunities to personalize healthcare using genomic sequencing. In 2015, President Obama launched the precision medicine initiative, with a goal of developing models of individualized care by enrolling participants in federally-funded studies that assess genes and other biomarkers as well as, lifestyle, environment and health conditions. Thus, it is likely that in the future, a precision approach will become standard-of care in medicine.

In the meantime, the Direct-to-Consumer (DTC) movement, fueled by entrepreneurial companies like *23andme* that provides ancestry reports including reporting on health predisposition, wellness, carrier status and traits, has empowered individuals to explore personal genetic data without the need for referral or prior approval by a healthcare practitioner or insurance company (Allyse et al. 2018). DTC genetic testing is increasingly incorporated into integrative, functional, naturopathic, and alternative care, as it represents a logical extension of the personalized approach that these practitioners provide. DTC genetic analysis allows individuals to examine genetic polymorphisms that impact enzymatic activity and health risks and to personalize diet and supplementation to modify gene expression. *23andme* is one of several privately held personal genomics companies that also affords consumers direct access to their raw genetic data. Thus, customers may take a deeper dive into findings, either directly or by uploading results to third party interpretation sites (e.g. Promethease, LiveWello), to learn more about "actionable" single nucleotide polymorphisms that may impact disease risk or drug or supplement response (Badalato et al. 2017).

Despite growing consumer use of DTC genetic technology, most medical schools have not instituted curricular modifications to address the trend pedagogically. In contrast, many integrative, functional, and alternative practitioners including naturopaths and chiropractors have self-educated and attended workshops and conferences on this topic and have recommended DTC genetic testing to patients. Moreover, DTC genetic testing has spawned as an alternative healthcare consulting industry, largely web-based, that is operating outside of conventional medicine. Various online forums now exist for carriers of select genetic polymorphisms to share information and seek support. This grass roots movement in patient driven healthcare has been characterized as "disrupting the translational pipeline" as it poses a threat to the medical establishment that is built on expertise, credentialing, and hierarchical control of access to information, testing, and treatment (Williams 2015).

Given the widespread use of DTC genetic testing, it is important that students understand the challenges and opportunities it presents and be able to counsel patients who seek advice in interpreting DTC test results. To educate students on this topic, I use lectures, discussions, videos, articles and links to websites. We focus on issues such as privacy and data security, the Genetic Information Discrimination Act, the personal and familial implications associated with the discovery that one possesses one or more genetic polymorphisms associated with a disease, and the current state of knowledge regarding lifestyle, diet, and supplement choices that may alter gene expression and that as practitioners they might recommend. As an anthropologist, I also point out that interpersonal and interpopulation variation in human genetic polymorphisms evolved in response to differences in subsistence strategies, diet, climate, altitude, isolation, and other factors. By exposing students to this information, they gain knowledge and perspective as well as the foundation needed to pursue additional training in the application of these tools.

Career Pathways for Medical Students

It is somewhat challenging teaching medical students as an anthropologist because anthropologists typically do not have clinical experience and must overcome any negative assumptions held by medical students related to perceived lack of credibility. For this reason, I have found it important to establish an identity as an anthropologist by presenting a cross-cultural, evolutionary, and historical perspective on this material, and by emphasizing socio-political context and biases that may have not been considered or encountered in prior education. Furthermore, as described previously, I have teamed up with a Board-Certified integrative medicine physician in Family and Community Medicine at my university who teaches students clinical approaches using patient cases and encounters. I have also found it important to engage additional practitioners, some in the community, to give guest lectures, interact with students, and provide shadowing opportunities. Providers have included integrative and functional medicine physicians, a chiropractor, an integrative dietician/nutritionist, and a licensed acupuncturist. Medical students also have had the opportunity to observe art, pet, and music therapy, as well as Jin Shin Jyutso and narrative medicine offered by the Integrative Medicine and Health Program at our medical center. Lastly, I feel a responsibility to provide in-depth information on the professional path forward, which I shall explain below, should students wish to pursue and eventually practice integrative, functional, or non-conventional medicine.

While there are many opportunities for residency, fellowship, and continuing educational training in traditional or alternative treatment modalities, the two approaches that are most accessible to allopathic and osteopathic physicians in the U.S. are integrative medicine and functional medicine. Andrew Weil, M.D. is largely credited as being the "father" of integrative medicine. He founded the Center for Integrative Medicine at the University of Arizona in 1994 (Maizes et al. 2015). This center was recently renamed the Andrew Weil Center for Integrative Medicine following major philanthropic donations by Dr. Weil. The Andrew Weil Center for Integrative Medicine provides online and face-to-face training to medical students, residents, fellows, and other health professionals. Some of their programs, including the Integrative Medicine in Residency program, are offered by site coordinators at medical schools and healthcare organizations across the country, including ours. In 2016, the Academy of Integrative Health & Medicine launched the Interprofessional Fellowship Program, a 2-year hybrid program designed for clinicians from various backgrounds (Riley et al. 2016). Several universities in the U.S. have established integrative medicine programs, among them the Osher Centers for Integrative Medicine at UCSF, Vanderbilt, and Northwestern, the Marcus Institute of Integrative Health at Thomas Jefferson, and the Goldring Center for Culinary Medicine at Tulane. The Society for Medical Anthropology sponsors an interest group on Complementary, Alternative and Integrative Medicine and members conduct applied research in a variety of settings including universities, tribal communities, and the Veterans Administration Medical Center.

Functional medicine, a cousin to integrative medicine, was originally conceived by Susan and Jeffery Bland, Ph.D. in the 1980s to promote a personalized, systems-based approach to medicine through their company HealthComm International. They founded and funded the Institute for Functional Medicine (IFM) in 1991, which over the years has grown into a non-profit organization that supports practitioner education through online courses and certification programs. David Jones, M.D. served as president of the organization from 1999 to 2013 and during his tenure the IFM obtained accreditation as an educational institute by the Accreditation Council for Continuing Medical Education (Jones et al. 2013). There are several centers for functional medicine across the U.S. One of the most well-known is the Center for Functional Medicine at the Cleveland Clinic, established in 2014 with the support of Cleveland Clinic President and Chief Executive Officer Delos Cosgrove. Mark Hyman, M.D., who was instrumental in gaining President Cosgrove's backing, is a contract physician at this center and a well-known practitioner of functional medicine. He gave a widely viewed TED talk on functional medicine in 2009.

Integrative and functional medicine are similar in approach and to varying extents, emphasize the following:

- Personalized medicine as opposed to a one-size-fits-all approach.
- Holistic versus mechanistic medicine, including the use of mind-body modalities.
- Identifying and treating the root cause rather than symptoms.
- Recommending a variety of conventional and unconventional diagnostic tests and practices including dietary supplements not typically used by conventional practitioners.
- Strategic use of pharmaceuticals versus what some refer to as the "pill for an ill" approach.
- Emphasis on the importance of diet and nutrition in preventing and treating illness.
- Belief in and support for the body's capacity to heal itself.

Providers of integrative and functional medicine work in a variety of settings including academic medical centers, outpatient clinics, and private practices. While many accept health insurance that may reimburse for patient visits and diagnostic testing, some do not. In addition, some tests and treatments that are recommended by integrative and functional medicine practitioners may require sizable co-payments or may not be covered by insurance at all. Practitioners may also advise patients to pay out of pocket for DTC personal genetic testing (e.g. 23andme) or laboratory analyses, and to purchase dietary supplements and devices to support health maintenance, illness prevention, and treatment. Lack of insurance reimbursement for many recommended procedures and therapies may restrict not only how a physician practices, but also patient demographics, as only well-off individuals with disposable income are able to pay out of pocket for procedures and products. Among insured patients in the U.S., prescription medications are often cheaper than dietary supplements, although in some cases the latter may have proven benefit with fewer side effects. Physicians who work for large organizations such as academic medical centers often have productivity targets and are restricted in how much time they can spend with patients and what tests and treatments they can order. This constrains physicians' ability to use a full range of integrative or functional medicine diagnostic tools and treatment protocols. It is important that students understand these issues so that they can make informed career decisions based on consideration of both the rewards and the challenges they may face in practice.

Final Thoughts

The emphasis on biomedical science as a standard in medical education was uniformly adopted in the decades following the Flexner report of 1910, commissioned by the Carnegie Foundation and the AMA. The implementation of Flexner's recommendations, along with socioeconomic developments and efforts by the AMA to discredit alternative medicine over the years, contributed to the closing of many medical schools and the decline of "alternative medicine," e.g., herbal medicine, native American medicine, and homeopathy. In the U.S. osteopathy survived by transforming its curriculum to meet "scientific standards", and chiropractic waged a successful legal battle against the AMA to achieve parity and eventual acceptance, but this took decades. Thus, we have in the U.S., a status hierarchy in which biomedicine occupies the top position and traditional and indigenous medicine that has not been subjected to "scientific" scrutiny, is considered "complementary" at best. The curricular content promulgated under these standards does not require formal education in "alternative," "integrative," or functional medicine and training in diet and nutrition is limited. The medical curriculum does incorporate education on diversity, cultural competence, and health care disparities. Yet the underlying philosophy, that biomedicine represents scientific truth and the scientific method is superior to other means of obtaining evidence, compels non-conventional medical approaches to undergo proper "scientific" verification (e.g. randomized clinical trials), to be incorporated into conventional medical treatment planning. To the extent that indigenous and traditional medicine emanate from non-Western cultures and peoples, conventional medical student training promotes ethnocentrism and implicit bias.

Anthropologists are in a unique position to expose these issues and educate the next generation of healthcare practitioners to appreciate them. The difficulty we face is to find ways to infuse conventional medical pedagogy with a uniquely anthropological perspective that is palatable to this population of learners as well as the faculty and administrators involved in approval of and support for pedagogical innovation. Our role is not simply to impart relevant information, but to inspire learners to identify prejudices in science-based medicine that may prevent them from investigating traditions and modalities that would otherwise be of value in practice. Teaching at any level should encourage students to think critically and creatively. To accomplish this, anthropologist educators need to expose medical students to divergent views that may oppose "the party line" and the messages embedded in mainstream culture or the medical curriculum. With respect to biomedicine in the U.S., that means imparting awareness of and respect for intra and inter-cultural variation in medical traditions, and reflecting on the role of history, economics, culture, and politics in shaping "science-based medicine." Once students understand these influences and the myriad ways in which they constrain conventional medical practice, they are well-equipped to choose a different path, a path that may afford them the opportunity to further the integration of multiple medical approaches, to avert disillusionment and "burn-out," and to enhance patient care and optimize health.

References

AAMC. Number of medical schools using selected grading systems. https://www.aamc.org/initiatives/cir/406418/11.html. Accessed 9 Oct 2019.

Alexandrakis, O. 2001. Medical anthropology: The development of the field. *Totem: The University of Western Ontario Journal of Anthropology* 9 (1).

Alliance for Natural Health. 2012. *Natural health products ultra-safe and drugs as dangerous as war*. https://www.anhinternational.org/2012/07/11/anh-exclusive-natural-health-products-ultra-safe-and-drugs-as-dangerous-as-war/. Accessed 9 Oct 2019.

Allyse, Megan A., David H. Robinson, Matthew J. Ferber, and Richard R. Sharp. 2018. Direct-to-consumer testing 2.0: Emerging models of direct-to-consumer genetic testing. *Mayo Clinic Proceedings* 93 (1): 113–120. https://doi.org/10.1016/j.mayocp.2017.11.001.

Badalato, Lauren, Louiza Kalokairinou, and Pascal Borry. 2017. Third party interpretation of raw genetic data: An ethical exploration. *European Journal of Human Genetics* 25 (11): 1189–1194. https://doi.org/10.1038/ejhg.2017.126.

Baer, Hans A. 2001. *Biomedicine and alternative healing systems in America: Issues of class, race, ethnicity, and gender*. Madison, WI: The University of Wisconsin Press.

Baer, Hans A., Merrill Singer, and Ida Susser. 2013. *Medical anthropology and the world system: Critical perspectives*. 3rd ed. Santa Barbara, CA: Praeger.

Bates, Donald G. 2000. Why not call modern medicine alternative? *Perspectives in Biology and Medicine.* 43 (4): 502–518.

Beck, Andrew H. 2004. STUDENTJAMA. The Flexner report and the standardization of American medical education. *Journal of the American Medical Association.* 291 (17): 2139–2140. https://doi.org/10.1001/jama.291.17.2139.

Burrow, Gerard N., and Nora L. Burgess. 2001. The evolution of women as physicians and surgeons. *The Annals of Thoracic Surgery* 71 (2 Suppl): S27–S29.

Clarke, Tainya C., Lindsey I. Black, Barbara J. Stussman, Patricia M. Barnes, and Richard L. Nahin. 2015. Trends in the use of complementary health approaches among adults: United States, 2002-2012. *National Health Statistics Report* 79: 1–16.

Coulter, Harris L. 1982. *Divided legacy: The conflict between homeopathy and the American Medical Association*. Vol. 3. Washington, DC: North Atlantic Books.

Cox, Paul A., and Michael J. Balick. 1994. The ethnobotanical approach to drug discovery. *Scientific American* 270 (6): 82–87.

de Barros, N.F., and Wania M. Galhardi. 2008. National Policy on Integrative and Complementary Practices in the Brazilian Health System: Steps towards the expansion of homeopathy. *Homeopathy* 97 (1): 53. https://doi.org/10.1016/j.homp.2007.09.003.

Djulbegovic, Benjamin, and Gordon H. Guyatt. 2017. Progress in evidence-based medicine: A quarter century on. *Lancet* 390 (10092): 415–423. https://doi.org/10.1016/S0140-6736(16)31592-6.

Dossett, Michelle L., Rodger B. Davis, Ted J. Kaptchuk, and Gloria Y. Yeh. 2016. Homeopathy use by US adults: Results of a National Survey. *American Journal of Public Health* 106 (4): 743–745. https://doi.org/10.2105/AJPH.2015.303025.

Duffy, Thomas P. 2011. The Flexner Report–100 years later. *Yale Journal of Biology and Medicine* 84 (3): 269–276.

Eisenberg, David M., Rodger B. Davis, Susan L. Ettner, Scott Appel, Sonja Wilkey, Maria Van Rompay, and Ronald C. Kessler. 1998. Trends in alternative medicine use in the United States, 1990-1997: Results of a follow-up national survey. *Journal of the American Medical Association* 280 (18): 1569–1575.

Eisenberg, David M., Ronald C. Kessler, Cindy Foster, Frances E. Norlock, David R. Calkins, and Thomas L. Delbanco. 1993. Unconventional medicine in the United States. Prevalence, costs, and patterns of use. *New England Journal of Medicine* 328 (4): 246–252. https://doi.org/10.1056/NEJM199301283280406.

Farmer, Paul. 1988. Bad blood, spoiled milk: Bodily fluids as moral barometers in rural Haiti. *American Ethnologist* 15 (1): 62–83.

Flexner, A., and Carnegie Foundation for the Advancement of Teaching. 1972. *Medical education in the United States and Canada; A report to the Carnegie Foundation for the Advancement of Teaching, Medicine & society in America*. New York: Arno Press.

Ghosh, Ajoy K. 2010. A short history of the development of homeopathy in India. *Homeopathy* 99 (2): 130–136. https://doi.org/10.1016/j.homp.2009.10.001.

Goldacre, Ben. 2014. *Bad pharma: How drug companies mislead doctors and harm patients. First American Paperback*. edition. ed. New York: Faber & Faber, Inc., an affiliate of Farrar, Straus and Giroux.

Guyatt, Gordon H. 1991. Evidence-based-medicine. *ACP Journal Club* 114 (2): A-16.

Hahnemann, Samuel, and William Boericke. 1922. *Organon of medicine*. 6th ed. Philadelphia: Boericke & Tafel.

Halperin, Edward C., Jay A. Perman, and Emery A. Wilson. 2010. Abraham Flexner of Kentucky, his report, Medical Education in the United States and Canada, and the historical questions raised by the report. *Academic Medicine* 85 (2): 203–210. https://doi.org/10.1097/ACM.0b013e3181c88506.

Hsu, Elisabeth, and Stephen Harris. 2010. *Plants, health and healing: On the interface of ethnobotany and medical anthropology, epistemologies of healing*. New York: Berghahn Books.

Illman, John E. 2018. Peter Fisher: Homeopathic physician to the Queen. *British Medical Journal* 362: k3611.

Jagtenberg, Tom, Sue Evans, Airdre Grant, Ian Howden, Monique Lewis, and Judy Singer. 2006. Evidence-based medicine and naturopathy. *Journal of Alternative and Complementary Medicine* 12 (3): 323–328. https://doi.org/10.1089/acm.2006.12.323.

Janik, Erika. 2014. *Marketplace of the marvelous: The strange origins of modern medicine*. Boston: Beacon Press.
Johnston, Francis E., and Setha M. Lowe. 1984. Biomedical anthropology: An emerging synthesis in anthropology. *Yearbook of Physical Anthropology* 27: 215–227.
Jones, David S., Sheila Quinn, and Leo Galland. 2013. Functional medicine. In *Textbook of natural medicine*, ed. J.E. Pizzorno and M.T. Murray, 8–16. London: Churchill Livingstone.
Junod, Suzanne W. 2000. An alternative perspective: Homeopathic drugs, Royal Copeland, and federal drug regulation. *Food and Drug Law Journal* 55 (1): 161–183.
Kanherkar, Riya R., Susan E. Stair, Naina Bhatia-Dey, Paul J. Mills, Deepak Chopra, and Antonei B. Csoka. 2017. Epigenetic mechanisms of integrative medicine. *Evidence-Based Complementary and Alternative Medicine* 2017: 4365429. https://doi.org/10.1155/2017/4365429.
Kantor, Elizabeth D., Colin D. Rehm, Mengmeng Du, Emily White, and Edward L. Giovannucci. 2016. Trends in dietary supplement use among US adults from 1999-2012. *Journal of the American Medical Association* 316 (14): 1464–1474. https://doi.org/10.1001/jama.2016.14403.
Kemper, Kathi J. 2016. Diagnose and dispense vs. envision and empower-integrating yang and yin in health care. *Complementary Therapies in Medicine* 26: A1–A2. https://doi.org/10.1016/j.ctim.2016.05.001.
Kleinman, Arthur. 1988. *The illness narratives: Suffering, healing, and the human condition*. New York: Basic Books.
Kong, Ling Y., and Ren X. Tan. 2015. Artemisinin, a miracle of traditional Chinese medicine. *Natural Product Reports* 32 (12): 1617–1621. https://doi.org/10.1039/c5np00133a.
LCME. 2018. *Functions and structure of a medical school*. http://lcme.org/publications/. Accessed 9 Oct 2019.
Liu, Liang, Elaine L. Leung, and Xiaoying Tian. 2011. Perspective: The clinical trial barriers. *Nature* 480 (7378): S100. https://doi.org/10.1038/480S100a.
Ludmerer, Kenneth M. 2011. Abraham Flexner and medical education. *Perspectives in Biological Medicine* 54 (1): 8–16. https://doi.org/10.1353/pbm.2011.0009.
Maizes, Victoria, Randy Horwitz, Patricia Lebensohn, Hilary McClafferty, James Dalen, and Andrew Weil. 2015. The evolution of integrative medical education: The influence of the University of Arizona Center for Integrative Medicine. *Journal of Integrative Medicine* 13 (6): 356–362. https://doi.org/10.1016/S2095-4964(15)60209-6.
Moffett, Peter, and Gregory Moore. 2011. The standard of care: Legal history and definitions: The bad and good news. *Western Journal of Emergency Medicine* 12 (1): 109–112.
Morris, William, Stacy Gomes, and Marilyn Allen. 2012. International classification of traditional medicine. *Global Advances in Health and Medicine* 1 (4): 38–41. https://doi.org/10.7453/gahmj.2012.1.4.005.
Pham-Kanter, Genevieve. 2014. Revisiting financial conflicts of interest in FDA advisory committees. *Milbank Quarterly* 92 (3): 446–470. https://doi.org/10.1111/1468-0009.12073.
Qaseem, Amir, Timothy J. Wilt, Robert M. McLean, Mary A. Forciea, and Clinical Guidelines Committee of the American College of Physicians. 2017. Noninvasive treatments for acute, subacute, and chronic low back pain: A clinical practice guideline from the American College of Physicians. *Annals of Internal Medicine* 166 (7): 514–530. https://doi.org/10.7326/M16-2367.
Riley, David S., Robert Anderson, Jennifer C. Blair, Seroya Crouch, William Meeker, Scott Shannon, Nancy Sudak, Lucia Thornton, and Tieraona Low Dog. 2016. The academy of integrative health and medicine and the evolution of integrative medicine practice, education, and fellowships. *Integrative Medicine (Encinitas, California)* 15 (1): 38–41.
Rothstein, William G. 1972. *American physicians in the nineteenth century: From sects to science*. Baltimore: Johns Hopkins University Press.
Sackett, David L., William M. Rosenberg, J.A. Gray, R.B. Haynes, and W.S. Richardson. 1996. Evidence based medicine: What it is and what it isn't. *British Medical Journal* 312 (7023): 71–72.
Servick, Kelly. 2015. FDA takes a new look at homeopathy. *Science* April 21.

Singer, Merrill. 2009. *Introduction to syndemics: A critical systems approach to public and community health*. New York: Wiley.

Singer, Merrill, and Hans A. Baer. 1995. *Critical medical anthropology*. New York: Baywood Publishing.

Squier, Harriet A. 1995. Women in nineteenth century homeopathic medicine. *Journal of Medical Humanities* 16 (2): 121–131.

Starr, Paul. 2017. *The social transformation of American medicine*. Updated edition. New York: Basic Books.

Stocking, George W. 1982. *Race, culture and evolution: Essays in the history of anthropology*. Chicago: University of Chicago Press.

Sullivan, Louis W., and Ilana S. Mittman. 2010. The state of diversity in the health professions a century after Flexner. *Academic Medicine* 85 (2): 246–253. https://doi.org/10.1097/ACM.0b013e3181c88145.

Thomas, P. 2001. Homeopathy in the USA. *British Homeopathy Journal* 90 (2): 99–103.

Topaz, Maxim, Leah Shafran-Topaz, and Kathyrn H. Bowles. 2013. ICD-9 to ICD-10: Evolution, revolution, and current debates in the United States. *Perspectives in Health Information Management* 10: 1d.

West, Colin P., Liselotte N. Dyrbye, and Tait D. Shanafelt. 2018. Physician burnout: Contributors, consequences and solutions. *Journal of Internal Medicine* 283 (6): 516–529. https://doi.org/10.1111/joim.12752.

Williams, Marc S. 2015. Is the genomic translational pipeline being disrupted? *Human Genomics* 9: 9. https://doi.org/10.1186/s40246-015-0032-4.

World Health Organization. 2013. *WHO traditional medicine strategy. 2014-2023*. Geneva: World Health Organization.

Lee X. Blonder, PhD received her doctorate in Anthropology from the University of Pennsylvania in 1986, and subsequently completed a 2-year postdoctoral fellowship in Behavioral Neurology at the University of Florida. She is a biomedical anthropologist and a tenured professor in the Department of Behavioral Science in the College of Medicine at the University of Kentucky (UK). Dr. Blonder is also a faculty associate of the Sanders-Brown Center on Aging and the Lewis Honors College at UK. She has joint appointments in the Departments of Neurology and Anthropology. Her research has focused on cognitive and emotional processing in patients with stroke and Parkinson's disease. Dr. Blonder has taught the courses: "Communication and Interviewing", "Patient's Physicians and Society", and "Introduction to Clinical Medicine" to first-year medical students. In addition, she developed and has taught electives in "Integrative and Alternative Medicine" to first, second, and fourth year medical students. She has served as a co-site leader for the Integrative Medicine in Residency online program through the Andrew Weil Center for Integrative Medicine at the University of Arizona. Dr. Blonder has also taught graduate students and undergraduates and has been active in University faculty governance and served as University Senate Council Chair and one of two faculty representatives on the UK Board of Trustees.

Part IV
Addressing Socio-cultural Determinants of Health and Health Disparities

Chapter 13
Anthropology in the Implementation of a New Medical School in South Florida

Iveris L. Martinez

Introduction

Where we find ourselves is not always where we intended to be. However, this is not necessarily a bad thing, as I have learned throughout my career. I never envisioned myself as a founding faculty in a new medical school. In fact, I had not studied medical anthropology. However, I was able to apply the skills I gained through my anthropological training and applied experiences in both academic and government positions to my multiple roles in medical education. The purpose of this chapter is to reflect on the challenges and accomplishments made in my role as a founding member of a new medical school tasked with developing and teaching courses on "medicine & society," as well as the training and experiences that led me to this unique opportunity.

In September 2007, I joined the founding faculty of what would become the Herbert Wertheim College of Medicine at Florida International University (FIU). The school was approved by the Florida legislature in 2006 in order to train physicians that represented the diversity of the South Florida community and meet the unique medical needs of this community. Accordingly, the school's mission is to prepare "Socially accountable, community-based physicians. . .uniquely qualified to transform the health of patients and communities."

Without Dennis Wiedman's background in medical anthropology and experience as a clinical medical anthropologist in the 1980s in Miami, the community-based medical school he helped envision as a strategic planner may not have come to fruition. It was this focus on community that made it natural fit for another anthropologist (me) to be hired as one of the founding faculty and to hold a key role in

I. L. Martinez (✉)
Center for Successful Aging, College of Health and Human Services, California State University – Long Beach, Long Beach, CA, USA
e-mail: iveris.martinez@csulb.edu

I. L. Martinez, D. W. Wiedman (eds.), *Anthropology in Medical Education*,
https://doi.org/10.1007/978-3-030-62277-0_13

curriculum development. (See Wiedman 2016; Wiedman and Martinez 2017, and also Wiedman's Chap. 6 in this volume on the planning of the medical school at FIU.)

I was trained as a cultural anthropologist, but my interest in aging and well-being among immigrants led me to complete a joint PhD in anthropology and public health at Johns Hopkins University. This interest and degree propelled me into a health-oriented career rather different from the interests in ethnicity and expressive culture that brought me to the field of anthropology. My original goal post-graduation was to be a practicing anthropologist working on aging issues in government agencies. However, my career has taken many twists and turns, all of them unexpected, but likewise valuable. My first position after receiving my doctoral degree was at the State of Oregon Department of Health and Human Services working on a care coordination program for transitioning older adults between acute and long-term care. I also worked pre and post-graduation on various health promotion projects in aging and health throughout Latin America at the Pan American Health Organization (PAHO) based in Washington, DC.

My desire for more experience in working within community settings, which I deemed important to be more effective in my work at PAHO, led me to pursue post-doctoral training in community-based participatory research (CBPR) at the Johns Hopkins University's School of Public Health with support from the Kellogg Foundation. While closely akin to participatory action research, this training gave me a beginning vocabulary with which to later translate many anthropological concepts to a public health setting and medical school curriculum. During my post-doctoral training I worked to assess the health needs of the recently arrived Central American population in Baltimore City in conjunction with Centro de la Comunidad, a local community-based organization (Martinez and Carter-Pokras 2006; Martinez et al. 2009).

After completing my post-doctoral training in 2003, I joined the faculty of the Johns Hopkins Center on Aging and Health first as a research associate in order to help coordinate some of the ongoing population-based research at the center. I was later promoted to assistant professor, with an appointment in the Department of Geriatrics and Gerontology at the Johns Hopkins School of Medicine, where I remained for 4 years. The center director was looking for someone with experience working with communities to assist in the expansion and evaluation of a community-based intervention to promote physical, cognitive, and social engagement among the city's older adults through voluntarism while seeking to improve school outcomes (Martinez et al. 2006). I eventually became the director of evaluation for the program's clinical trial funded by the National Institute on Aging (NIA) to evaluate this intervention (Fried et al. 2013). In this role, I gained valuable experience working across various health disciplines including medicine, nursing, neuropsychology, epidemiology, and school health. In this position, I also received my own NIA grant on social pathways to disability as a supplement to a grant on cognitive pathways to disability. I also received a Macarthur Foundation grant to study the socio-economic and ethnic barriers to health promoting social activities working largely with African-American older adults (Martinez et al. 2009, 2010, 2011).

In early 2007, as a BA in Anthropology/Sociology alumna of FIU, I learned of the new community-based medical school at FIU and was intrigued by the possibilities. After several conversations with the founding deans about their vision to create a Medicine & Society Program, which included placing students in underserved communities to emphasize the social determinants of health disparities, I was hired as course director for Medicine & Society in August 2007. My transferable skills in community research and cross-cultural perspectives was key in this decision. Medicine & Society was one of five curricular "strands" in the new school intended for horizontal and vertical integration of content (Dambach et al. 2010). Medicine & Society was intended to prepare medical students to work in communities as part of interprofessional teams. As Course Director, I assisted the strand leader, a physician, in envisioning and develop the content of the coursework in the strand that was to include ethics, cultural competency, health disparities, and interprofessional teamwork, household visits, as well as a community practicum.

Those first 2 years went quickly! There were towers of accreditation documents to develop in order to obtain preliminary accreditation prior to enrolling students. There was little time for reflection as to my role and contributions as an anthropologist nor real formal preparation for my role. Meeting Dennis Wiedman (circa 2011) gave me the opportunity to reflect on my role in the medical school. I started sharing my experience as an anthropologist in medical education with his students in a Medical Anthropology course. I learned that the strategic plan he spearheaded in the 1990s provided the vision for a community-based medical school in South Florida—a medical school that was not based in a hospital-system, but where medical students were embedded in the community through rotations and experiences in neighborhood homes, community organizations, and clinics. The longevity of this vision and the power of anthropological theory and methods in this process is documented in the journal Human Organization (Wiedman and Martinez 2017). We compared the 1996 University Strategic Plan compared to the 2015 FIU Medical School plan. Using longitudinal content analysis of the words and phrases in these plans, we identified the themes that continued over these 20 years. The majority of initial concepts continued, demonstrating the influence of anthropologists at the time of conceptualization to implementation and routinization. Through our conversations and collaborations on the aforementioned journal article, we started exploring the history of anthropologists in medical education, while reflecting on and discussing our own career experiences. In this chapter, I detail further my role in the development and implementation of the medical curriculum at FIU, other contributions I was able to make to the medical school, as well as lessons learned from the challenges I faced in my role as a member of the medical school faculty.

Development and Implementation of the Medicine and Society Curriculum

Because the Herbert Wertheim College of Medicine was brand new and intended to focus primarily on education (as opposed to research), in the first 2 years there were very few traditional medical school departments. We were organized instead as curricular "strands." Medicine and Society was one curricular "strand" among others that encompassed more traditional subject matter: 1) Human Biology, 2) Disease, Illness and Injury, 3) Clinical Medicine, 4) Professional Development, and 5) Medicine and Society. The Medicine and Society Strand focused on the social determinants of health and disparities, interprofessional teamwork, and medical ethics, with a strong emphasis on the social contract of medicine with society, and engaging students in experiential service learning through conducting household visits in local underserved communities. The household engagement would eventually be termed NeighborhoodHELP™ (Health Education Learning Program). Furthermore, Professional Development focused on other non-biological aspects of medicine, such as medical jurisprudence, professionalism, clinical epidemiology, and health systems. Clinical experiences were introduced in the first year through coursework on history taking, emergency room rotations, and primary care preceptorships. I was invited on occasion to provide a lecture on working with interpreters for clinical medicine, or to help develop an assignment to integrate reflective thinking into the primary care preceptorship.

Early clinical and community-based engagement was notably innovative at the time of the school's opening since traditionally medical school students do not have contact with patients until their third year. The idea of exposing students early to community experiences came in part from Dr. Pedro Jose Greer, Jr., a gastroenterologist and hemotologist, who had started providing care to the homeless in Miami, as well as establishing clinics for undocumented immigrants in the 1980s. Dr. Greer completed his medical studies in the Dominican Republic where medical students are required to provide services early in their training to underserved communities. It also grew out of my experience in community health and anthropological research, which helped elucidate the connections between community experiences and health outcomes. However, early conversations of systematically integrating non-biological competencies across the more traditional coursework of foundational science courses and organ systems courses through a more innovative patient case-based approach never came to fruition. Innovations promoted by newer faculty were often vetoed by the more traditionally trained physicians who formed the leadership.

With only 43 medical students in the first two cohorts, and a vision that was slowly taking shape to embed students in our local medically underserved communities, my initial responsibilities included developing all the course syllabi for the Medicine & Society strand, setting the groundwork for what would become the NeighborhoodHELP program, and serving as Course Director, under the supervision of a physician known for his work with the underserved. The courses I developed and oversaw included "Ethical Foundations of Medicine" (later taught by an ethicist from another local university), "Introduction to Social Medicine," "Interprofessional Teamwork" for first year medical students, as well as a three-course series on community health in the second year, and a fourth year capstone course intended to address a community-level health issue identified by students in consultation with community partners. I was responsible for the creation and teaching of all the courses to the first two cohorts of medical students. As the school grew, the second year courses were assumed by Family Medicine faculty and the fourth year capstone was overseen by a PhD in Public Health that I hired.

The first iteration of the "Introduction to Social Medicine" course was not well-received. It was perhaps too theoretical for a medical student audience, and given the conservative political environment of Miami, discussions of equity and disenfranchisement without clear connections to clinical medicine became interpreted as pushing a liberal political agenda rather than legitimate or important and applicable learning material based on scientific evidence. Therefore, I recreated the course as "Introduction to Socio-economic and Cultural Aspects of Health: Addressing Health Disparities," adding clinical case studies and exercises to each lesson. I also started co-teaching with a physician who would provide the clinical "pearls" that are central to medical education (Lorin et al. 2008), in order to better illustrate the relevance of the material by providing the type of clinical examples that medical students expected. This helped them better understand how population-based data may be reflected in individual clinical encounters. This introductory course was intended to give students the basic information they needed to be prepared to interpret what they would see and hear when they started visiting households in the most medically underserved communities in Miami.

There was no textbook on the topic when I started teaching this material in 2009, nor were there guidebooks on how to best convey anthropological knowledge to a medical audience as far as I knew at the time. Through student feedback, self-training, attending faculty development offerings on campus and at other institutions, working towards a certificate in Instructional Methods in Health Professions Education from the University of Michigan, and drawing deeper from my community-based research and applied experiences, I refined the course throughout the years. I presented at medical education meetings and later published on my lessons learned in both anthropology and medical teaching (Martinez et al. 2014; Martinez 2015). My first presentation at such a medical education conference was titled "How not to teach the social determinants of health in medicine," a title which several remarked as brave.

The topics covered in this introductory course were a basic introduction to health disparities and social determinants, cultural humility, the historical basis of health disparities, sex and gender, structural violence, infectious disease, and how to work with a medical interpreter. Through the years, I refined the course, incorporating case-based and other hands-on activities to drive home complex topics in a short amount of time. For example, I developed a case of a pre-diabetic adolescent female and challenged students to explore the neighborhood levels factors as they related to her health and her opportunities for implementing their recommendations of diet and exercise. I found it helped to incorporate constructive feedback from students whenever possible and to involve the students themselves in the revision of sessions and assignments. Other cases I found through the medical literature, but elaborated on them by developing or modifying the case discussion guides. For one such case, students were to draw a concept map (or a diagram relating concepts) to better understand the complexities of poorly controlled hypertension in an African-American male patient (Cooper 2009). This case followed my lecture on the historical basis of health disparities, which focused largely on racism in medicine, giving students a historical context that most students were lacking. They were also prepared with pre-readings critiquing the use of "race" in medical studies and debunking the notion that hypertension is associated with biological "race" as would appear in standard medical literature (Cooper 2013). As part of the case, students were able to identify not only the usual "familial risk factors" but also identify systemic societal issues contributing to the patient outcomes. Another case, on taking an inclusive sexual history (Eckstrand et al. 2012), was included as part of a lecture on Gender and Health, including LGBT health. This session made the distinction between sex and gender (which many seemed unfamiliar with), as well as highlighted some of the disparities faced by women and the LGBT community. In this case, I also challenged students to think how they could address these disparities in their future medical practice.

In addition to efforts to integrate social determinants of health and social science competencies (Cuff and Vanselow 2004; AAMC 2011) into medical education, another important trend in medical and health professions education more broadly is the quality improvement movement and its emphasis on interprofessional teamwork and communication skills. The Interprofessional Education Collaborative (IPEC), a joint effort of the various associations of colleges of Nursing, Osteopathic and Allopathic Medicine, Pharmacy, Public Health and Dentistry, released a seminal report outlining competencies for interprofessional teamwork and collaboration (IPEC 2011, 2016). These reports cited several reasons for interprofessional education, including the needs of an aging and diverse population, as well as the Affordable Care Act, which includes new financial incentives that reward care coordination, chronic disease management, and reductions in readmissions, all of which can be realized through effective care teams. Furthermore, the Affordable Care Act has caused a peaked interest in community health.

A Note on Teaching Cultural Competency

Anthropologists are often called upon to teach "cultural competence" to future physicians. In the early years of the course I developed, a geneticist who happened to be the medical school dean of academic affairs, insisted that the Medicine & Society course must include sessions on the culture of specific ethnic groups that were most populous in the region of the school. This, of course, would only serve to reinforce stereotypes, especially among students from less diverse regions of the state. In fact, the term "cultural competence" has received quite a bit of criticism since its popularity in the 1990s and its peak with the introduction of accreditation standards for cultural competency in 2000, and the Tool for Assessing Cultural Competency Training (TAACT) in 2006 by the American Association of Medical Colleges. https://www.aamc.org/initiatives/tacct/ The standard on "Cultural Competence and Health Care Disparities," as well as the TAACT have been revised in subsequent years. The standard currently reads:

> The faculty of a medical school ensure that the medical curriculum provides opportunities for medical students to learn to recognize and appropriately address gender and cultural biases in themselves, in others, and in the health care delivery process. The medical curriculum includes instruction regarding the following:
>
> - The manner in which people of diverse cultures and belief systems perceive health and illness and respond to various symptoms, diseases, and treatments
> - The basic principles of culturally competent health care
> - The recognition and development of solutions for health care disparities
> - The importance of meeting the health care needs of medically underserved populations
> - The development of core professional attributes (e.g., altruism, accountability) needed to provide effective care in a multidimensional and diverse society
>
> (AAMC, March 2018 http://lcme.org/publications/#Standards)

The notion of being able to teach cultural competence in medicine has been critiqued by many, including Kleinman and Benson (2006) who point out the concept of cultural competency suggests culture can be reduced to a technical skill, portrays culture as static, and makes culture synonymous with ethnicity, race, or language, i.e. "Chinese believe X. . .Mexicans believe Y..." Furthermore, they note that it excludes a discussion of the culture of the provider. In fact, as Weaver noted as far back as 1968, "The provision of an understanding of culture and not cultures is the real contribution which the anthropologist can make." (Weaver 1968, 6).

I therefore tried to convey an understanding of culture, within the limited amount of curricular time that was available, through the concept of cultural humility. Cultural humility is a set of principles that guide thinking, behavior and actions (Tervalon and Murray-Garcia 1998). These principles are: 1) lifelong learning and critical self-reflection, 2) recognizing and changing power imbalances, and 3) holding institutions accountable. In other words, to be culturally humble is to recognize and take responsibility for what one does not know about others and its consequences in the practice of medicine. To achieve this, students need to reflect on their own cultural beliefs and the culture of medicine into which they are being enculturated.

I found Kluckholn and Strodbeck's *Value Orientation Theory* (1961) to be a useful tool for reflection. This framework posits that there are five basic questions that all human societies must answer. These concerns include: 1) human nature (evil, mixed, or good); 2) man-nature relations (subordinate to nature, in harmony, or dominant); 3) time sense (past, present, or future oriented); 4) activity (being, becoming, or doing), and 5) the nature of human relations (hierarchical, collateral, or individual). I provided students with a matrix based on these concerns and potential responses. After observing a role play of a gastrointestinal patient case (based on Shields et al. 2009), I asked students to imagine where their patient may fall on this rubric and where their own belief system aligns. I then had them reflect on how any differences in these beliefs may affect their ability to communicate with and treat the patient effectively. I then challenged them to think of strategies to improve communication and arrive at the correct diagnosis.

These types of exercises deconstructing complex concepts and asking students to reflect on their own beliefs and assumptions help students better understand how their perspectives may vary from that of their patients, and in particular, how culture impacts patients' understanding of disease and disease treatment, as well as how physicians communicate with their patients. As Kagawi-Singer et al. (2014) succinctly explained, "Each population group has devised unique solutions to their common problems over time and space, such as adequate nutrition or family structures, as well as religious or spiritual practice. . .within their particular circumstances and available resources." Our challenge is this respect is to convey the concept of culture with both simplicity and nuance, and highlight its impact on health practices and healthcare.

Interprofessional Teamwork

In my first year teaching, I was asked to teach an Interprofessional Teamwork Course in conjunction with Nursing. This posed some logistical challenges, particularly around space, since enrollment with both disciplines raised the number of students to over 200 students and space was not readily available on campus to facilitate weekly team-based work. The interprofessional course was an opportunity to experiment with creative ways of introducing medical students to other health disciplines with which they would intersect in practice. For example, I organized a "speed dating" session between medical students and members of different divisions of the local health department to introduce them to the public health field and resources available for the local population. From this course also emerged the "Interprofessional Clinical Workshop" that I convened and led for 9 years and that was probably one of the most popular sessions in the Medicine & Society strand. For this one afternoon workshop, medical students were paired with nursing, social work, dietetics, speech therapy, physical therapy, and occupational therapy to observe experienced clinicians hold an interprofessional case discussion, and later work together at roundtables on their own case (Martinez and St. Prix 2013). I ran the workshop by consensus with equal representation on the committee from each participating discipline to ensure that the learning needs of all students were met. Over the years, we worked together for continuous improvement, meeting several times a year to review the session, and vote on any major changes. Over the 9 years I led the event, nearly 4000 students participated. In the last 2 years, we added students from our new Physician Assistant program.

As noted earlier, the field of interprofessional education has grown rapidly in the last decade (IPEC 2016). The development and implementation of interprofessional learning and practice often poses challenges for the health professions. However, my training as an anthropologist helped me bridge long-standing cultural divides among health disciplines and successfully facilitate the process. From student feedback, participation in these interprofessional sessions were some of the most enriching experiences I was able to create for students. This is a role that I believe anthropologists are uniquely prepared for as we are trained to recognize and navigate cultural differences, as well as communicate across cultures. In this case, I was equipped to navigate professional cultures. Although I was based in medicine, as a non-physician I did not represent the established hierarchy of the health professions where the physician assumes the unquestioned role of leader. Moreover, as a trained researcher, I implemented evaluative measures from the beginning that were used as objective measures of the impact of the workshop on student learning as a means of refining the curriculum.

The interprofessional course was one of the first times I faced challenges around my authority as a medical educator. The course was cancelled after 2 years when medical students who had failed to successfully complete a team-building task of creating a balloon tower complained to the Dean of Curriculum that they did not go to medical school to build balloon towers. Students were unfamiliar with and some were disinterested in the body of pedagogical strategies on team building that is applied across fields and the importance of teamwork in medicine. The fact that nobody spoke to me, as the Course Director, about the decision to cancel the course before the action was taken, and that there was no opportunity to discuss the exercise in question and course content with the Dean of Curriculum, was perhaps my first experience of the power dynamics of medical education that I was now enmeshed in.

I realized then that influencing the medical curriculum as an anthropologist required persistence and creativity. When the interprofessional course was dissolved, the workshop was integrated into my social determinants of health course. I continued to introduce medical students to other disciplines in a variety of ways. I created another session within the social determinants course where medical students were to review a hypothetical case of a household they might visit in NeighborhoodHELP and then had them meet with social work faculty in small groups to revisit the case, therefore benefiting from the social work perspective. Through this experience students obtained an appreciation of the insight that social workers have about family dynamics and the wealth of knowledge they have about resources (Martinez et al. 2014). I also worked with the Medical-Legal Clinic, which had been established to support NeighborhoodHELP households with legal issues as well as to take on broader policy issues impacting communities we served. I worked with students on raising awareness of those left behind when Florida did not expand Medicaid under the Affordable Care Act (Martinez et al. 2016). The latter was part of the Community Practicum for five medical students whom we paired with law students. Again, it was my experience and ethnographic skills as an anthropologist that helped teach students how to collect patient narratives and work with community members to tell their stories. Students took their patient's stories to the state capital and to local legislators. One student told me that this experience changed how they intended to practice medicine.

Transitions and Alternative Roles in Medical Education

One of the reasons I was hired was to develop a household visitation program where students would visit medically underserved and ethnically diverse communities as part of interprofessional teams. In this program, now known as NeighborhoodHELP (Rock et al. 2014), medical students make household visits as part of a team with social work and nursing students. It has become the flagship of the medical school curriculum. As the program developed, it became clear that more people were needed to implement it, so we hired a Public Health professor to develop the community arm of the program, and a Family Medicine physician to supervise the medical students in the field. Because the Medicine and Society program was part of a "strand" and not a department, I noted to my supervisor, the Strand Leader, that the program may be easily eliminated, and recommended that we organize as a department both for a more permanent presence in the school as well as a mechanism for organizing the growing faculty. Hence, the Department of Humanities, Health, and Society was established in 2009. When the department was created, I was promoted to Chief of the Division of Medicine and Society within the department. The other two divisions were "Family Medicine" and "Community Engagement". As Chief, I was able to hire an ethicist to develop the ethics and humanities program, as well as another faculty member with a doctorate of public health and background in community based participatory research to lead the fourth year "Community Practicum" course and assist in teaching. With the growth of the student body, so did the faculty of the division of Family Medicine and the staff of the division of Community Engagement.

However, my footing in the department and the college, which I now realize was precarious to start with, diminished through the years, especially with the growth of the family medicine faculty, some of whom claimed to be capable of fulfilling the role of teaching the material I was hired to teach. I often heard the expression that innovating an established medical curriculum was like moving a battleship in a pool. With a clean slate, there was ostensibly more room for innovation, though the majority of those involved in curriculum development were trained in very traditional medicine and found a certain discomfort with dedicating too much time to the "non-science" courses. And in fact, the original four credit hours dedicated to Medicine & Society in the first Period (August to March) was soon cut back to two credit hours. The Interprofessional Teamwork course was eliminated. Emphasis on the social determinants of health and the root causes of disparities were essentially removed from the second year. The course became lecture-based and focused on the diseases students would encounter during their household visits instead of the social roots of the disease disparities that they were facing. The third year consisted of a traditional Family Medicine clerkship with continued responsibilities for households, but without time in the curriculum for visits and debriefings. The dedicated time for the Community Practicum course in the fourth year was also eliminated, but the course requirement was not. This created substantial challenges to executing the Practicum that was now more of a longitudinal independent study for all medical students with no time allotted to it. And while I presented and advocated for existing models for the community practicum in medicine, the course never garnered the support and resources required for it to be a robust student experience.

As a non-physician and non-basic scientist, I clearly did not have equal footing and was not invited to the table on some key roles despite my founding faculty role. I did not have a vote on the Curriculum Committee despite being tasked with developing the core of the curriculum for the Strand. The Medicine & Society program was poorly funded despite its scholarly productivity, good evaluations, and my advocacy. As one of the only women on the faculty early on (and the only social scientist), the intersection of gender and expertise in relation to my relative lack of power is now quite evident to me. The role of gender in academic medicine has been well documented (Pololi et al. 2013; Bates et al. 2016). Eventually the Division of Medicine and Society was dissolved despite innovations, publications, and other successes. The Department of Humanities, Health and Society, continued to grow, however, with two more traditional divisions added—ethics and internal medicine.

I transitioned to a role in geriatric research and I continued to teach the first year course on social determinants of health and led the interprofessional workshop. I also started focusing more on grant writing. While I was unable to integrate very much anthropological knowledge beyond the second year, with funding from the Komen Foundation, I was able to develop a learning module on breast health disparities, in partnership with a community partner that was integrated into the second year course (Martinez et al. 2016). I also started teaching in the university's Honors College undergraduate course, "Challenges in Healthcare I & II," designed as a pipeline for medical students. My sessions in the Honors College courses on cultural competency, social determinants of health, and gender were well-received and recognized as an innovative and example of global learning at the university (Landorf and Doscher 2015). Global Learning is defined by the American Association of Colleges and Universities as ". . . a critical analysis of and an engagement with complex, interdependent global systems and legacies (such as natural, physical, social, cultural, economic, and political) and their implications for people's lives and the earth's sustainability" (AACU 2014).

I also had the opportunity to influence other aspects of the new medical school beyond curriculum development for the Medicine & Society Strand. The second year at the College I was asked by the Dean to help with the planning process of a Geriatric Research and Education Center. Having come from the Johns Hopkins Center on Aging and Health, and conducted research on aging for several years, I had the experience and connections to assist with this process. In addition to conducting several site visits to existing centers, one of my first actions was to draw their attention to embedding the Hartford Competencies in geriatrics into the curriculum (Leipzig et al. 2009; Martinez and Mora 2012). This was based on my experience in the Department of Geriatrics and Gerontology at Hopkins, as well as my involvement in the Association of Anthropology, Gerontology, and the Life Course (AAGE) of which I would eventually serve as President.

In addition to my role in curriculum development and implementation, I served as Vice-Chair (for 1 year) and then Chair (for 4 years) of the medical school's Admissions Committee, which put me in a position to shape the early student body. Our mission was to have a diverse student body that represented and would serve the local community. My anthropological perspective gave me a unique voice in promoting diversity and advocating for students with complex social backgrounds.

Challenges and Strategies for More Effectively Teaching in Medicine

> These problems have involved difficulties in accommodating his materials and teaching methods to medical curriculum requirements, in resolving methodological and conceptual differences between himself and the medical field, in adjusting to a different social and academic environment, and in compensating for the inadequate development of his own science.—Thomas Weaver (1968)

As early as 1968, Weaver astutely summarized some of the core challenges anthropologists face in medical education. Unbeknownst to me when I embarked on my journey as a medical teacher, others had already documented some of the similarly challenging experiences of anthropologists in medical school and provided some useful recommendations on how to be more effective (Benjamin 1956; Weaver 1968; Read 1970). However, many of these gems are buried in the literature, such as the insightful work of Johnson (1991) found in a special publication by the American Anthropological Association called *Training Manual in Applied Medical Anthropology*. Drawing upon this literature and my experience in medical education, I attempt to share some of the lessons learned and strategies implemented to counter some of these shared challenges.

Philosophical Isolation and Its Antidote

Anthropologists may experience a "philosophical isolation" vis-à-vis "utilitarian case study approach" of medical education (Weaver 1968, 6). As noted earlier, I had to adapt my approach to the subject matter I was introducing and "take it down a notch" in order to effectively communicate with an audience with little background in the social sciences. However, case studies gave me the vehicle and the freedom to elaborate on these concepts in a way that made an impact on student understanding of complex issues. And while there is rarely room for in-depth philosophical discussion in a medical classroom, conversations did sometimes achieve such depth. The latter really depends on the quality of the case assignments as well as the facilitation of the discussion. Other times it depends on the unique composition of the small group, their member's experience and insight, and willingness to engage. The latter often depended on the competing demands medical students faced, i.e. whether they are preoccupied by the pharmacology exam or pathology lab deadline.

The other type of isolation I faced, as do many others anthropologists teaching in medicine, is that from one's own field of anthropology. This is due to several reasons, including the all consuming demands of teaching in medicine, expectations to publish in medical journals, as well as criticisms from within anthropology of those of us who chose a more "practice-oriented" career. Anthropologists in medicine are often absorbed by their roles as medical teachers and may stop participating in anthropological associations or conducting anthropological research. This may be an issue of time, resources, funding streams, and general support from medical schools for such activities. Furthermore, it can also be difficult to find fellow anthropologists and anthropological contributions in medicine because the task of teaching and publishing in medical education can be all-absorbing. Most of my publications during my period as faculty in a medical school were in biomedical journals. And I, as I suspect many other anthropologists employed in medical schools, lost my identity as an anthropologist.

I found that if I was to succeed as an anthropologist in medicine, I needed to stay connected to both medicine and anthropology. However, it was not always easy to find a home in anthropology. Beyond the critical medical anthropology perspective, I wanted to connect with anthropologists that were trying to influence medicine from within. One strategy for combating this "isolation" is continued engagement in anthropological research, associations, and joint appointments (Weaver 1968), as well as fieldwork and ethnography (Johnson 1991). It was when I reconnected with the field of anthropology, that I was most effective in teaching and scholarly productivity. I was isolated from anthropology for many years and it was very stressful. Once I started writing in anthropology, attending meetings again, and connecting with colleagues in anthropology, especially in the Society for Applied Anthropology, my role in medicine was more rewarding and manageable. Our power comes in applying anthropology theory and methods daily. Staying rooted in our anthropological networks allows us to step back from our roles as medical teachers and not lose sight of this.

Thriving Within the "Status Gap"

The "status gap" of anthropology in medical education has been noted by several scholars (Weaver 1968, 6–7; Johnson 1991, 135; Read 1970). Read noted that anthropology was associated with "lower grade" subjects within the hierarchy of medical subfields (Read 1970), namely preventive and community medicine, family medicine, and psychiatry. Furthermore, anthropologists are at the bottom of the hierarchy in a medical setting after other basic science faculty (PhDs) who are themselves under clinician faculty (MDs). In this environment, students may resist an anthropological perspective and are empowered to criticize anthropology material

(Weaver 1968). Anthropological knowledge may be dismissed as "common sense" and not "science."

This was certainly my experience as the Medicine & Society courses were often referred to by my colleagues and students alike as the "soft" sciences or the "non-science" courses. This attitude may have emboldened students to complain directly to the college's leadership regarding the content of the courses if they did not themselves feel it was important, and in certain instances, I was told by persons with no content knowledge how I should teach the material to be covered under the courses I was hired to teach because of my expertise. These situations required much patience and diplomacy, and keeping the end goal of improving medical education and patient care in mind. On a few occasions students complained that the material I was presenting to them was "common sense" and therefore a waste of time. My response on this, which I tried to deliver with humor, was that either it was not common sense, or if it was, they themselves lacked common sense given their poor grades on the quizzes.

Over the years, I learned that grounding my lecture and course activities in the scientific literature, always citing the source of the ideas presented, demonstrating their relevance to clinical practice, and establishing myself as the content expert, contributed to lessening the resistance. Most importantly, we need to translate anthropological knowledge and skills to lived experiences and applied settings. We need to devote time to getting other medical faculty on board with the importance of an anthropological perspective, co-developing lectures and small group activities with them. Engaging physician faculty as co-lecturers and small group leaders is important as it serves as validation and can provide the clinical integration that anthropologists alone cannot always accomplish.

Working with Increasingly Diverse Medical Students

Some of the few existing publications offering strategies and guidelines for teaching anthropology in medical school were published in the 1960s and 1970s, when medical students were largely male, White, and with backgrounds in the biological sciences. However, medical students today are more ethnically diverse and have more varied educational backgrounds. Some may have in fact studied anthropology or other social sciences as undergraduates. They may have master's degrees in public health and be familiar with social epidemiology. The great majority, nonetheless, have a more narrow focus on traditional pre-medical training background, many having majors of biochemistry and biology and thus possessing limited exposure to social and behavioral sciences. Therefore, the challenge is presenting material in a manner that can be grasped by the range of students in a class with different levels of knowledge and experience in thinking critically about the role of social and cultural factors in health and healthcare. One tactic I utilized was to incorporate those with more experience strategically across small groups for discussion. Another is to encourage those with this background to share their expertise in the large classroom setting. And of course, there is the general approach that there are no wrong questions, making students comfortable in asking for clarification by posing questions and comments as long as they do so in a respectful manner. Because many of the topics I introduced could be perceived as sensitive topics, such as the historical basis of race disparities, continued racial inequities, non-binary gender and sexual identities, and distribution of healthcare access, to name a few, it was important to encourage respectful dialogue.

Developing Empathy for Medical Students

As an anthropologist in medical education, I found that I needed to better understand the implicit culture of medical education, while being able to function within it. This required learning and adapting to a new terminology, and trying to see things from the student perspectives (Johnson 1991). Truth be told, learning empathy for what medical students go through as they are initiated into the world of medicine, helped me become a better teacher. Success as a teacher of medicine came with a better understanding of the culture of medicine and speaking more "like a physician." Once I eased up on or changed my expectations (though not my standards) of what medical students needed to grasp of complex social phenomena, I was more successful as a teacher. In other words, I learned it was not about teaching them all there is to know about the social determinants of health and the role of culture, but to give them the basic tools they needed to start thinking about these issues. Lectures were not always helpful nor necessary. I challenged myself to find creative ways to communicate with medical students and present the material using various strategies that would be more memorable and were more hands on to fit the medical approach.

Focusing on Clinical Relevance

Johnson (1991) cautioned that we must, among other things, demonstrate clinical relevance of material through cases, and establish teaching presence in third year clinical clerkships, going beyond the classroom setting typical of the first 2 years of education. He also suggests anthropologists should consider dual training in a clinical professional field. Using clinical cases is extremely helpful, though tricky when one does not have a clinical background. Johnson recommends participating actively by attending rounds at least three times a week (Johnson 1991, 141) and seizing "teaching moments" to encourage students to incorporate psychosocial data in their presentation and progress notes (Johnson 1991, 140). I was rarely invited to participate in educational activities in clinical sites, and I myself, was uncomfortable with the prospect of it. Because of my lack of clinical training, I found it difficult to find a footing in the third and fourth year when students are rotating through hospitals.

Establishing a Common Language

I learned early on to reflect on my challenges to effectively reach my medical students, and turn these into lessons for teaching (Martinez et al. 2015). Some of these tips for effective teaching in medical schools are quite simple, such as defining key terms. It is important to find a common language and not assume that students understand the terminology you are familiar with which may derive from anthropology or public health. Instead, you must always define key terms and sometimes find related concepts that they can relate to. This could be something as basic as defining the distinction between sex and gender (Krieger 2003), or more complex things like finding biological models of the impact of stress on organ systems (Sapolksy 2004), to relating food insecurity to diabetes management at a biological level (Seligman et al. 2010).

Conveying Complex Ideas Simply

One of the biggest challenges was to introduce complex ideas in the simplest manner and work backwards from expected outcomes. Instead of my original starting point of all the things that I thought were important for medical students to know, I found myself asking: "what do I want students to walk away from in this lesson?". The topics that anthropologists may find themselves teaching, such as gender, inequality, racism, etc., require self-reflection. However, students must be guided in this self-reflection. They also need a historical context for their beliefs and understandings of race, gender, and other categories of inequality. I tried to incorporate history lessons into discussions of disparities having found that many students did not have a historical perspective on the inequalities we see in society today. For example, I engaged students in critically appraising the use of "race" in modern science and medicine, given that race is one of the categories in medical research that is not usually scientifically defined but relies on lay understandings of what race may popularly mean.

In order to accommodate different learning styles, develop different student skill sets, and to challenge students to tackle issues from various perspectives, I found it useful to implement diverse modalities of teaching. I had students work with population data for the neighborhoods that they were rotating through. For example, for the previously mentioned diabetes case, I had the students use local health statistics available online, as well as mapping, to better understand the resources and challenges faced by a hypothetical patient—a pre-diabetic adolescent girl—depending on the neighborhood she lived in. Students then compared their findings across neighborhoods and discussed the differences through the online chat function of the course's learning management system page. They were also asked to pose hypothetical questions relevant to the hypothetical patient's health to hypothetical community partners (persons working in non-profit, government, and other sectors that are engaged in addressing the social determinants of health). Different groups of students were assigned different local zip codes so that they could compare the possibilities of their fictive patient succeeding in maintaining their health while residing in different areas. This helped students think beyond common arguments of "free will" and helped them see how patient choices are often shaped by their environment. We also created service-learning opportunities in order to immerse students in communities and challenge them to provide answers both at the household level and at the community level. It is important to not only expose students to the social issues that impact health, but also to give them examples of existing solutions and engage them in being part of the remedies in order for them not to be overwhelmed or disheartened by the obstacles their patients may face.

Conclusions

In 2018, after 10½ years in medical education, I moved on to a position outside of medicine, but still in the health sciences. I am now the director for the Center for Successful Aging within the College of Health and Human Services at California State University, Long Beach. I do, however, hope that my anthropological perspectives during my time as a professor of medicine had some impact on positively influencing medical students to consider and integrate social and cultural perspectives in addressing their patient's health, as well as being more collaborative partners in delivering healthcare. The exchanges I had with certain students and the feedback from my courses certainly tells me that I did to some extent. In particular, I was able to have the greatest impact on interprofessional education through the activities I spearheaded. I believe that it was my training in anthropology that helped me convene faculty from across diverse health disciplines and bridge the cultural gaps that exist between them to develop the workshop and implement it seamlessly year to year, as well as find other vehicles of interprofessional collaboration (Martinez 2015).

In some ways, anthropology is the unrecognized other profession in interprofessional medical education, and perhaps we would succeed more if we interjected ourselves explicitly as such. I can only speak to this impact from personal reflection, and data I embedded in some of my learning activities, since an evaluation of the curriculum and the role of social sciences in it was not established and rarely is done. Moreover, it is difficult to quantify the impact of anthropology and anthropologists on the medical school. We are perhaps too immersed in what we are doing to evaluate and publicize the impact of our contributions. This is a task we should be better prepared to do by purposively embedding evaluation of learning and change in attitudes in our efforts and pinpointing the uniquely anthropological contributions that contribute to these changes.

Finally, to be an anthropologist in medical education one must learn to thrive in ambiguity and expect transitions in one's position and roles and within the medical schools themselves. This was certainly my experience and one of my greatest lessons. I had to learn to be flexible, take on new and unexpected roles, especially when decisions and transitions were out of my control. Opportunities may vary at different times of one's career between different practice roles in the medical school, university administration, anthropology, and other roles. The path is rarely the straight line one expects in academic anthropology roles, and it is definitely not for everyone. However, maintaining my identity as an anthropologist while holding the role of medical faculty helped me thrive and I believe will solidify anthropology's presence and sustained impact in medical education by strengthening our ability to make the unique and much needed anthropological contributions that the field of medical education both needs and is requesting.

References

American Association of Medical Colleges (AAMC). 2011. *Behavioral and social science foundations for future physicians*. Washington, DC: Association of American Medical Colleges.

Association of American Colleges and Universities. 2014. *Global Learning VALUE Rubric*. www.aacu.org/value/rubrics/globallearning.cfm. Accessed 11 Mar 2014.

Bates, Carol, Lynn Gordon, Elizabeth Travis, Archana Chatterjee, Linda Chaudron, Barbara Fivush, Martha Gulati, Reshma Jagsi, Poonam Sharma, Marin Gillis, Rebecca Ganetzky, Amelia Grover, Diana Lautenberger, and Ashleigh Moses. 2016. Striving for gender equity in academic medicine careers: A call to action. *Academic Medicine: Journal of the Association of American Medical Colleges* 91 (8): 1050.

Benjamin, Paul. 1956. Anthropology and public health. In *Some uses of anthropology: Theoretical and applied*, 49–57. Washington, DC: Anthropological Society of Washington.

Cooper, Lisa A. 2009. A 41-year-old African American man with poorly controlled hypertension: Review of patient and physician factors related to hypertension treatment adherence. *Journal of the American Medical Association* 301 (12): 1260–1272.

Cooper, Richard S. 2013. Race in biological and biomedical research. *Cold Spring Harbor Perspectives in Medicine* 3 (11): a008573.

Cuff, Patricia A., and Neal Vanselow, eds. 2004. *Improving medical education: Enhancing the behavioral and social science content of medical school curricula*. Washington, DC: National Academies Press.

Dambach, George, Joe Leigh Simpson, and John A. Rock. 2010. Florida International University Herbert Wertheim College of Medicine. *Academic Medicine 85* (9): S140–S143.

Eckstrand, Kristen, Kimberly Lomis, and Lisa Rawn. 2012. An LGBTI-inclusive sexual history taking standardized patient case. *MedEdPORTAL* 8: 9218.

Fried, Linda P., Michelle C. Carlson, Sylvia McGill, Teresa Seeman, Qian-Li Xue, Kevin Frick, Erwin Tan, Elizabeth K. Tanner, Jerry Barron, Constantine Frangakis, Rachel Piferi, Iveris Martinez, Tara Gruenwald, Barbara K. Martin, Laprisha Berry-Vaughn, John Stewart, Kay Dickersin, Paul R. Willging, and George W. Rebok. 2013. Experience corps: A dual trial to promote the health of older adults and children's academic success. *Contemporary Clinical Trials*. https://doi.org/10.1016/j.cct.2012.05003.

Interprofessional Education Collaborative. 2016. *Core competencies for interprofessional collaborative practice*. Washington, DC: Interprofessional Education Collaborative. 2016 update.

Interprofessional Education Collaborative Expert Panel. 2011. *Core competencies for interprofessional collaborative practice: Report of an expert panel*. Washington, DC: Interprofessional Education Collaborative.

Johnson, Thomas M. 1991. Anthropologists in medical education: Ethnographic prescriptions. In *Training manual in applied medical anthropology*, ed. C.E. Hill. Washington, DC: American Anthropological Association.

Kagawi-Singer, Marjorie, William W. Dressler, Sheba Mariam George, and William N. Elwood. 2014. *The cultural framework for health: An integrative approach for research and program design and evaluation*. Bethesda: National Institutes of Health, Office of Behavioral and Social Sciences Research.

Kleinman, Arthur, and Peter Benson. 2006. Anthropology in the clinic: The problem of cultural competency and how to fix it. *PLoS Medicine* 3 (10): e294.

Kluckhohn, Florence R., and Fred L. Strodtbeck. 1961. *Variations in value orientations*. Oxford: Row, Peterson.

Krieger, Nancy. 2003. Genders, sexes, and health: What are the connections—and why does it matter? *International Journal of Epidemiology* 32 (4): 652–657.

Landorf, Hilary, and Stephanie P. Doscher. 2015. Defining global learning at Florida International University. *Diversity and Democracy* 18 (3): 24–25.

Leipzig, Rosanne M., Lisa Granville, Deborah Simpson, M. Brownell Anderson, Karen Sauvigné, and Rainier P. Soriano. 2009. Keeping granny safe on July 1: A consensus on minimum geriatrics competencies for graduating medical students. *Academic Medicine* 84 (5): 604–610.

Lorin, Martin I., Debra L. Palazzi, Teri L. Turner, and Mark A. Ward. 2008. What is a clinical pearl and what is its role in medical education? *Medical Teacher* 30 (9-10): 870–874.

Martinez, Iveris L. 2015. Integrating anthropology in medical education: Opportunities, challenges and lessons. *Practicing Anthropology* 37 (1): 35–39.

Martinez, Iveris L., and Jorge Camilo Mora. 2012. A community-based approach for integrating geriatrics and gerontology into undergraduate medical education. *Gerontology and Geriatrics Education* 33 (2): 152–165.

Martinez, Iveris L., Isis Artze-Vega, Alan L. Wells, Jorge Camilo Mora, and Marin Gillis. 2015. Twelve tips for teaching social determinants of health in medicine. *Medical Teacher* 37 (7): 647–652.

Martinez, Iveris L., and Olivia Carter-Pokras. 2006. Assessing health concerns and barriers to health in a heterogeneous Latino community. *Journal of Healthcare for the Poor and Underserved* 17 (4): 899–909.

Martinez, Iveris L., Olivia Carter-Pokras, and Pamela Bohrer Brown. 2009. Addressing the challenges of Latino health research: Community-based approaches in an emergent urban community. *Journal of the National Medical Association* 101 (9): 908–914.

Martinez, Iveris L., Natalie Castellanos, Casey Carr, Christopher J. Plescia, Andres L. Rodriguez, Sairah Thommi, Lynn Zaremski, David Weithorn, Peggy Maisel, and Alan L. Wells. 2016. Increasing awareness on health care access in Florida: A community-based medical-legal practicum project. *Progress in Community Health Partnerships: Research, Education, and Action* 10 (1): 141–147.

Martinez, Iveris L., Donneth Crooks, Kristen S. Kim, and Elizabeth Tanner. 2011. Invisible civic engagement among older adults: The role of informal volunteering. *Journal of Cross-Cultural Gerontology* 26 (1): 23–37.

Martinez, Iveris L., Kevin Frick, Thomas A. Glass, Michelle Carlson, Elizabeth Tanner, Michelle Ricks, and Linda P. Fried. 2006. Engaging older adults in high impact volunteering that enhances health: Recruitment and retention in the Experience Corps™ Program in Baltimore. *Journal of Urban Health* 83 (5): 941–953.

Martinez, Iveris L., Kevin D. Frick, Kristen S. Kim, and Linda P. Fried. 2010. Older adults and retired teachers in address teacher retention in urban schools. *Educational Gerontology* 36 (4): 263–280.

Martinez, Iveris L., Kumar Ilangovan, Ebony B. Whisenant, Maryse Pedoussaut, and Onelia G. Lage. 2016. Breast health disparities: A primer for medical students. *MedEdPORTAL* 12: 10471. https://doi.org/10.15766/mep_2374-8265.10471.

Martinez, Iveris L., Kristen Kim, Elizabeth Tanner, Linda P. Fried, and Teresa Seeman. 2009. Ethnic and class variations in promoting social activities among older adults. *Activities, Adaptation and Aging* 33 (2): 96–119.

Martinez, Iveris L., Lourdes Martin, Mary Helen Hayden, and Valeria Balmaceda. 2014. Incorporating social work perspectives into interprofessional health teams: Engaging students in a biopsychosocial assessment of family. *MedEdPORTAL* 10: 9915. https://doi.org/10.15766/mep_2374-8265.9915.

Martinez, Iveris L., and C. Rose-St Prix. 2013. A hybrid educational experience training future health professionals to work together to improve patient outcomes. *MedEdPORTAL* 9: 9304.

Pololi, Linda H., Janet T. Civian, Robert T. Brennan, Andrea L. Dottolo, and Edward Krupat. 2013. Experiencing the culture of academic medicine: Gender matters, a national study. *Journal of General Internal Medicine* 28 (2): 201–207.

Read, Margaret. 1970. Some problems in teaching medical anthropology. *Social Science & Medicine* 4 (1): 163–167.

Rock, John A., Juan M. Acuna, Juan Manuel Lozano, Iveris L. Martinez, Pedro J. Greer Jr, David R. Brown, Luther Brewster, and Joe L. Simpson. 2014. Impact of an academic-community partnership in medical education on community health: Evaluation of a novel student-based home visitation program. *Southern Medical Journal* 107 (4): 203–211.

Sapolsky, Robert M. 2004. Social status and health in humans and other animals. *Annual Review of Anthropology* 33: 393–418.

Seligman, Hilary K., Terry C. Davis, Dean Schillinger, and Michael S. Wolf. 2010. Food insecurity is associated with hypoglycemia and poor diabetes self-management in a low-income sample with diabetes. *Journal of Health Care for the Poor and Underserved* 21 (4): 1227.

Shields, Helen M., Vinod E. Nambudiri, Daniel A. Leffler, Chitra Akileswaran, Edith R. Gurrola, Rachel Jimenez, Amy Saltzman, et al. 2009. Using medical students to enhance curricular integration of cross-cultural content. *The Kaohsiung Journal of Medical Sciences* 25 (9): 493–502.

Tervalon, Melanie, and Jann Murray-Garcia. 1998. Cultural humility versus cultural competence: A critical distinction in defining physician training outcomes in multicultural education. *Journal of Health Care for the Poor and Underserved* 9 (2): 117–125.

Weaver, Thomas. 1968. Medical anthropology: Trends in research and medical education. In *Essays on medical anthropology*, 1–12. Athens: University of Georgia Press.

Wiedman, Dennis. 2016. Strategic planning. In *History of the Florida International University Medical School*, ed. Thomas Breslin and Barbra Roller. Gainesville: University of Florida Press.

Wiedman, Dennis, and Iveris L. Martinez. 2017. Organizational cultural theme theory and analysis of the strategic planning for a new medical school. *Human Organization* 76 (3): 264–274.

Iveris L. Martinez, PhD is Professor, Archstone Foundation Endowed Chair in Gerontology, and Director of the Center for Successful Aging at California State University, Long Beach. She was a founding faculty member of the Herbert Wertheim College of Medicine (HWCOM) at Florida International University where she served as chief of the Division of Medicine & Society and chaired the admissions committee for the college for 5 years. Between 2007 and 2018, she taught the first year introductory course and other course content on health disparities, cultural competency, and social determinants of health at HWCOM, as well as led an annual interprofessional clinical workshop across the health sciences. An applied anthropologist, she has received funding from the National Institutes of Health, the Macarthur Foundation, and others for her community-based research on social and cultural factors influencing health, with an emphasis in aging, Latinos, and minority populations. Her current research interests include improving services for caregivers of persons with Alzheimer's, reducing social isolation in aging, as well as interprofessional efforts to create age-friendly communities. She previously served as the Chair of the Board of the Alliance for Aging, Inc., the local area agency on aging for Miami-Dade and Monroe Counties, and President of the Association for Anthropology, Gerontology, and the Life Course. She holds a joint Ph.D. in Anthropology and Population & Family Health Sciences (Public Health) from Johns Hopkins University.

Chapter 14
Anthropologists on Interprofessional Health Education Teams: A Model from Upstate New York

Robert A. Rubinstein and Sandra D. Lane

Introduction

Anthropologists have long maintained that the methods and insights of their discipline have much to contribute to the education of health professionals. Of anthropology's many potential contributions to health education and training three are often offered as particularly salient: recognizing and responding to the social determinants of health (e.g., Macgregor 1961; Marmot 2005), cultural competence in health care practice (e.g., Clark 1983), and understanding the importance of teams in health practice (e.g., Solimeo et al. 2016). Many have worked for the inclusion of anthropology in the curricula of medical schools, nursing schools, schools of public health, and in the training of other health professionals. The results of their advocacy have been mixed; some schools have integrated anthropology into their teaching and training, while others have not. In Central New York, Syracuse is the home of three institutions of higher education for medical and other health professionals: Upstate Medical University (Upstate) of the State University of New York, Le Moyne College, and Syracuse University. Upstate includes a medical school, a nursing school, a graduate college, and a college of allied health professions (including physical therapy, and medical technology programs, among others). Le Moyne's Purcell School of Professional Studies houses physician assistant, occupational therapy, and nursing programs. Syracuse University includes undergraduate and

R. A. Rubinstein (✉)
Department of Anthropology, Syracuse University, Syracuse, NY, USA
e-mail: rar@syr.edu

S. D. Lane
Department of Public Health and Department of Anthropology, Syracuse University, Syracuse, NY, USA

Department of Obstetrics and Gynecology, Upstate Medical University, Syracuse, NY, USA
e-mail: sdlane@syr.edu

I. L. Martinez, D. W. Wiedman (eds.), *Anthropology in Medical Education*,
https://doi.org/10.1007/978-3-030-62277-0_14

graduate education, including doctoral training in anthropology, and professional study of public health, social work, and marriage and family therapy.

This chapter reviews the history of educational collaborations by both authors in Syracuse, New York, with a variety of health professional disciplines. We describe work we have done from 1994 to the present, in a chronological sequence. As context, we begin this chapter by describing our arrivals in Syracuse and relate our positionality as anthropologists working with the medical and health sectors in the city. The next section describes an early collaboration that predated our work that provided an additional context for our work. We then describe a model of collaboration that we have developed to facilitate the work of community members and university based researchers. The model, which we call Community Action Research and Education (CARE), provides the modes of interaction through which our work is accomplished. We then relate how the CARE model both contributed to and then elaborated work on the social determinants of health using research we conducted in Syracuse. Among the things that we describe is the use of the CARE model to apply and evaluate the *Framework for Educating Health Professionals to Address the Social Determinants of Health*, and which resulted from the work of a National Academies of Science, Engineering, and Medicine committee chaired by Sandra Lane. This is followed by a section describing the creation of an inter-university collaboration that links faculty from universities along the New York State Thruway, and which takes its name from that route: *The Route 90 Collaborative*. Finally, we conclude this chapter with reflections on what we have learned working as anthropologists to enhance the education of health professional students while working with community members and colleagues from a variety of medical and health disciplines.

In 1994, Rubinstein was hired by the Maxwell School of Syracuse University, where he joined the department of anthropology, and became the director of the Program on the Analysis and Resolution of Conflicts. He was invited at that time to join the Black Leadership Commission on AIDS. Lane joined the Onondaga County Health Department as a behavioral scientist in 1996. There she was responsible for developing strategies to address infant mortality disparities. She was the founding director of Syracuse Health Start, a federally funded intervention project to reduce infant mortality, which she led for 6 years. In 2001, she joined the faculty of the Department of Obstetrics and Gynecology at Upstate Medical University. In 2005, she was recruited by Syracuse University to start an undergraduate program in public health.

When we arrived in Syracuse, anthropology had only a passing presence in health professional education programs in the region. A few anthropology classes were available through the Consortium for Culture and Medicine (described below), a program that allows students from Le Moyne College, Syracuse University, and Upstate Medical University to enroll in classes at one another's campuses, and anthropologists contributed to medical humanities teaching. For instance, at the Le Moyne Physician Assistant program, the medical humanities course was for a time coordinated by an anthropologist. Yet, it would be fair to say that there was very limited representation of anthropology in health professions education and training programs in Syracuse.

Bringing anthropology into the educational and training life of health professionals was not our initial goal; instead, we focused on understanding and addressing health inequalities in our community through community action research (Lane 2008). As our work developed, we found that through the model of research and community engagement that we were using for our research, we were able to make anthropology more present in health professional education in Syracuse, and we began to pay explicit attention to that goal. As we will describe below, our model of research is team-based involving faculty and students from a variety of programs in the investigation of health, together with the collaboration of community members and representatives of government agencies (e.g., the county department of public health and the city police department), and from community based agencies (like, a clinic for low income and uninsured people, and several community centers). The results of this research got noticed and led to invitations to present our research results at Grand Rounds in various departments of the medical school (including, Obstetrics and Gynecology, Psychiatry, and Preventive Medicine), at community presentations, consultations with local government staff, and through *pro bono* advocacy at the request of community leaders. These activities led in turn to the incorporation of our research activities—neighborhood violence and trauma (Lane et al. 2017a), health of the uninsured (Lane et al. 2017b), food insecurity (Lane et al. 2008b), lead poisoning (Lane et al. 2008a)—into some educational programs. Our articles and books reporting our research were adopted as required readings at each of the three universities. The Le Moyne Physician Assistant Program adopted Lane's (2008) *Why are our Babies Dying?: Pregnancy, Birth, and Death in America* as a core reading for their curriculum.

In addition, shortly after we began our community collaboration, in 2001 we began to work with health professional students directly. Lane, for instance, in her capacity as a research professor in the Department of Obstetrics and Gynecology, served as the faculty supervisor for 12 obstetrical residency capstone projects. Together we have supervised numerous students from all of the health professional education programs in the city. As well, those schools have supported some of their students with summer grants to allow them to participate as research collaborators on our projects. As anthropologists, we were able to bring unique perspectives to the college of medicine and other health professional disciplines, by presenting cross-cultural, comparative, and ethnographic information on diverse issues taught at the schools. For example, Lane is in the second year of co-teaching an engaged learning course on refugee health that is conducted by pairing Upstate medical students with students from anthropology and public health at Syracuse University; each pair of students is matched with a newly resettled refugee family with whom the students make home visits and attend clinical appointments. Lane taught for several years the human sexuality lecture to medical students and Obstetrics and Gynecology residents. In addition to Grand Rounds and other presentations at the college of medicine, including to the departments of Public Health, Obstetrics and Gynecology, Psychiatry, Humanities and Bioethics, and Pediatrics, we have also made such presentations at the SUNY College of Nursing and the Le Moyne Physician Assistant Program. We have also brought together collaborations among community agencies, community leaders, and the universities. Our group has been unique in maintaining collaborative relationships over-time, rather than establishing and ending project focused work in the community. We are in the community whether or not we are doing a particular project. Thus, like long-term ethnographers, we stay in the community even when not specifically conducting data collection. We see our roles as long-term fieldworkers in our own community maintaining relationships with our community partners, and regularly crafting engaged learning activities as well research to benefit our students and the community.

More recently, we have extended this work beyond Syracuse by creating a collaborative health professional education innovation network focused on the social determinants of health (National Academies of Sciences Engineering and Medicine 2016), that spans New York State from Albany to Buffalo. In this paper, we describe our experiences and offer these as one way of keeping anthropology present in health professional education.

Consortium on Culture and Medicine: Institutional Infrastructure

The right environment can facilitate the contributions of anthropologists to the health professions. We are fortunate to have an organizational structure that links Syracuse University, Upstate Medical University, and Le Moyne College, called the Consortium for Culture and Medicine (CCM). CCM was founded in 1978 by psychiatrist at Upstate Medical University, Dr. Robert W. Daly and two colleagues (see, e.g., Daly 1967, 1981). The creation of the Consortium was associated with efforts throughout the country to develop educational, research, and clinical programs in the medical humanities. The Consortium "focuses on the cultural, ethical, social and psychological dimensions of medicine and health care by, as described on their website:

- offering accredited courses linking the humanities and social sciences to the practice of medicine and healthcare
- sponsoring faculty seminars and community events
- encouraging interdisciplinary research in health care

> Faculty members from the three cooperating institutions represent academic disciplines such as anthropology, economics, health policy, history, law, literature, medicine, medical ethics, philosophy, political science, public health, psychology, social work, and sociology (see, http://www.upstate.edu/ccm/).

Offering courses through CCM adds a diversity of disciplinary backgrounds to the student cohort. The basic design of CCM eliminates otherwise nearly insurmountable bureaucratic obstacles to students taking courses on a campus that is not their home institution. The decision to have a course be part of the CCM offerings is made through a process that involves the initiating instructor submitting a syllabus to CCM. That syllabus is then reviewed by the CCM coordinators (one from each cooperating institution), who suggest any changes they see as essential. The course syllabus is then submitted to the curricula committees of each of the cooperating schools for approval. By including students from nursing, physician assistant, medical and other health professions into medical anthropology courses, undergraduate and graduate students are exposed to the clinical and other perspectives and knowledge that the clinical students bring. Similarly, the health professions students are exposed to the critical and conceptual discourses of medical anthropology, meeting new concepts like syndemics, structural violence, and the importance of cultural contexts in health care. In our experiences, the practical effects of this interaction are to expose health professional students to social science research methods, ethical concerns, and the writing of research papers, things to which they ordinarilly have less exposure. The non-clinical undergraduate and graduate students get exposed to the language, concepts, and culture of the biomedical professions, and thus better understand the constraints and imperatives to which clinicians respond in their practice. This gives the non-clinical undergraduate and graduate students a more grounded and balanced view of the health care field.

The variety of disciplinary backgrounds of students in our CCM courses is reflected in the variety of students whom we had over the years in class, from undergraduate and graduate nursing, medical students, marriage and family therapy students, environmental biology majors from the SUNY College of Environmental Sciences and Forestry, and graduate and undergraduate students from public health, biology, anthropology, policy studies, public administration, international relations, Middle East studies, writing, magazine journalism, and social work. To accommodate the students from the various institutions, as well as the mature students who often work full time, the courses are held once per week in a 3-hr evening block. Our recent article (Lane et al. 2019) describes the experience of two CCM courses—Global Health and Reproductive Health—into which we integrated social determinants of health and engaged learning strategies.

Initially much of our work with health professional education took place through CCM. We designed classes specifically to bring anthropological concepts and data to the professional school students. As we approached the design of classes that we would offer through CCM, we kept in mind the prerequisites for culture change articulated by anthropologists (e.g., Goodenough 1963), principally that the changes sought must make sense to the community being engaged. Therefore, since anthropology still was seen as exotic, we framed our courses in terms of the connections between anthropological literature and public health. The fact that both of us are Ph. D. anthropologists with public health degrees gave us professional standing in the two communities. Thus, we ensured that the CCM courses we developed were cross-listed at the graduate and undergraduate levels in both public health and anthropology; that is, they "count" toward the major and minor requirements for student in the anthropology and the public health departments at Syracuse University, or as regular distribution courses for students.

We developed three medical anthropology courses for the consortium: 1) Global Health, 2) Culture and Reproductive Health, and 3) Public Health Ethics. Global Health and Reproductive Health have as their primary home and course prefix anthropology, and each is cross-listed with public health; Public Health Ethics is accepted as a course for the medical anthropology minor. We designed the Global Health class offered by any of the three consortium member institutions. In designing this class, we sought to ensure that anthropological insights about power, politics, and poverty were woven throughout the curriculum. And, we wanted to ensure that the core anthropological principle of comparative analysis was represented. This meant, for us, emphasizing that the social and cultural contexts of health internationally are experienced in similar ways in the United States as they are abroad. Thus, for example, in designing the unit on structural violence we linked, Paul Farmer's (1999) work on how health decisions and behavior in Haiti and elsewhere are constrained by structural and cultural factors with an examination of similar constraints on health behavior among poor people, and people of color in Syracuse.

In the Culture and Reproductive Health class, the curriculum was designed with similar intention. The class includes anthropology's nuanced attention to gender, sexuality, patriarchy, and power, as well as readings on the clinical perspective on sexually transmitted infections, pregnancy, childbirth, and other topics. For example, this course pairs discussion of the acceptance of and access to new reproductive technologies globally with the realities of their use in the United States by juxtaposing Marcia Inhorn's (2003) work in the Middle East with work we have done in Syracuse. Considered are the ways in which power and patriarchy constrain and shape attitudes towards infertility and towards the use of new reproductive technologies, and explores the reasons that people have differential access to those technologies.

The Public Health Ethics class uses the anthropological focus on the importance of population-level health issues in contrast to individual rights. Covered are units on food stamps and health insurance, immunizations, the Tuskegee syphilis experiment, legal and policy responses to infectious diseases and epidemics, the right to clean water, and the role of religious and social values in setting health policy, among others. It approaches these topics with an emphasis on how social and cultural factors contribute to ethical decision making. In the course, for example, we link Goffman's (1963) concept of stigma with both the treatment of Mary Mallon (the woman infamously known as Typhoid Mary) and recent prosecutions of HIV positive men of color whose actions resulted in HIV transmission to others.

In all three courses, we make use of web-based teaching support, like Blackboard, using it as a computer repository for all readings, the syllabi, discussion boards, and for students to post their work. This allows courses to be nearly "paperless," with no materials passed out to students (except the in class evaluation) and no assignments submitted in paper form. The three courses adapted the "flipped classroom" approach (e.g., Cheng et al. 2017), in that students were required to undertake assigned readings prior to class and to post responses to the readings on Blackboard, which was set up so that students could read each other's posts. Rather than aiming to impart "facts", the course content emphasizes concepts grouped into weekly modules. In class, the students apply the assigned readings, the key concepts, and literature they research to address problems, such as, disproportionate infant mortality among communities of color (Lane et al. 2004b). In this regard, we draw on a long history of developing innovative teaching strategies, including Lane's collaboration with the Le Moyne College Physician Assistant Program in securing a federal Health Resources and Services Administration grant (2005–2008) to develop problem based modules for teaching cultural competence to health professional students.

In addition, the Upstate Center for Bioethics and Humanities has sponsored events featuring CARE research (described below) done in collaboration with our community colleagues, the Street Addiction Institute, Inc. and the Trauma Response Team. This inclusion of community members of our research team presenting to medical and nursing students about health disparities that affect their families and neighborhoods helps promote social science and humanities approaches to the social determinants of health in the curriculum at Upstate.

Community Action Research and Education: Building Relationships and Capacity

In addition to our teaching roles in the classroom, we also play a central role in community-based research and education. As mentioned previously, we have developed a model for our community-based research that we call *CARE: Community Action Research and Education.* This model integrates action anthropology and community-based participatory research with teaching by bringing students out of the classroom to address health disparities in their communities (Lane et al. 2017b, 2011; Rubinstein et al. 2018). The CARE model builds on "Action Anthropology," as created by Sol Tax and his collaborators (Rubinstein 1986). As they developed it, Action Anthropologists pursued research on topics of concern to the communities with which the anthropologists worked and treated community members as equals in research and problem solving processes (Rubinstein 2018; Smith 2015). Following that tradition, community members are equal partners in our research group and each CARE project is implemented at the request of community leaders. It is based upon respectful participation with community members in which students, faculty, and community members work together to conduct research and undertake interventions. Faculty, community members, and students are co-authors on publications and jointly craft grant applications. Among the CARE projects we have undertaken to date are research on: food deserts, lead poisoning in rental housing, marriage promotion policies, disproportionate incarceration as a social determinant of HIV transmission, incarceration and father involvement in child rearing, neighborhood violence, and a study of healthcare for the uninsured. The work is reciprocal and iterative in the way that it applies theory to practice and then the practical application and community involvement subsequently refines and informs new theory (e.g., Bergen-Cico et al. 2014).

In line with the principles of participatory action research, of our 16 CARE articles since 2008 there are 75 student and 22 community member co-authors.

Some of the students and community members worked with us on more than one research project and subsequent article, so this is not an unduplicated list. The student co-authors included undergraduates and graduate students in anthropology, public health, medicine, education, physician assistant, and high school. The students attended Syracuse University, Upstate Medical University, Le Moyne College, and the Skaneateles and Jamesville-DeWitt High Schools. Students become aware of our CARE research through the presentations that our group makes at the universities and in the community. Those wishing to participate, self-select and ask to be involved. They are added to a CARE research team after being oriented to the values and commitments of the model.

This research has covered a broad range of the ways in which health disparities are driven by structural inequalities, racism, disproportionate incarceration, and other social determinants of health. Our CARE research was the first to locate and link food deserts in Syracuse with poor health outcomes, like low birthweight. This led to health professional students and community members working together to redress the lack of food opportunities in poor neighborhoods of color. Recently, a new supermarket was opened in reaction to their and others' advocacy, based in part on our research. Similarly, CARE research explored the ways in which environmental racism led to disproportionately high levels of lead exposure among poor people in Syracuse and linked it to mental health and behavioral problems. Advocacy for changing lead abatement statutes for rental property is ongoing and includes health professional education students; student members of our CARE research on lead poisoning presented their findings to the Syracuse Common Council, for example. A third example is the CARE work addressing on-going trauma from gun violence and gun murders (in 2016 Syracuse had the highest per capita rate of murders of any city in New York State) and how it affects the health and well-being of community members (Jennings-Bey et al. 2015). This research has energized a number of community and medical institutional responses to mitigate the effects of this trauma. All of the results of the CARE research have been presented in various classroom, lecture, and grand rounds settings.

Social Determinants of Health: An Integrating Concept

As introduced above, for the past two decades we have worked with colleagues across several institutions of higher learning: Syracuse University (our home campus), Upstate Medical University (where Lane maintains a research professor appointment in Obstetrics and Gynecology), Le Moyne College (nursing and physician assistant programs), The Sage Colleges nursing program (where Lane has been a consultant for faculty development), and University at Buffalo (with our colleague in Social Work, Robert Keefe). These collaborations have taken many forms, including shared research and publishing, developing innovative curriculum, and guest lecturing. With the Le Moyne College physician assistant program, this collaboration resulted in a successful federal grant to develop problem-based learning modules to teach cultural competence to health professional students. At Upstate, it resulted in three elective courses that paired first and second year medical students with patients in the community, in which the medical students made home visits, shopped for food with their patients, and attended clinical appointments. These collaborations also include community stakeholders who are concerned about the health of their neighborhoods. For example, community partners in Buffalo include a network of agencies addressing perinatal depression among women of color. In Syracuse, major community partners include a free clinic for the uninsured and several groups focused on prevention of neighborhood violence and trauma, and faculty in Albany partner with a respite home for the homeless.

As anthropologists, we have also played a broader role in the national conversations about social determinants of health. In 2015–2016, Lane chaired the National Academies of Science, Engineering and Medicine's committee that wrote the *Framework for Educating Health Professionals to Address the Social Determinants of Health* (National Academies of Sciences Engineering and Medicine 2016). Lane was selected for this role because of her broad experience in Syracuse teaching health professional students and also as her work as a former Ford Foundation Program Officer, in which she supported the development of community-oriented, problem-based medical education at the University of Gezira in Sudan. The Social Determinants of Health (SDH) is an explanatory model that emerged from anthropologists' influence on public health (e.g., Foster 1977). The term social determinants of health, coined by Sir Michael Marmot (2005), encompasses the environmental, policy, political, and cultural influences on health and survival. The World Health Organization established a Global Commission on the Social Determinants of Health (2005–2008), which expanded SDH to include structural violence, health injustice, inequity and disparities, as well as traditional notions of risk factors (CSDH (Commission on Social Determinants of Health) 2008). The National Academies framework for integrating SDH into health professional education calls for equitable partnerships with communities such that community members help guide the content of the curriculum, which seeks to improve the health of community members. It advocates teaching students to take action, in partnership with communities, to address health disparities. Rather than simply passive knowledge acquisition, it emphasizes innovative teaching methods and helping students to develop competencies through active learning. Table 14.1 shows the key elements of the Framework.

Route 90 Collaborative: Moving Beyond Syracuse

The *Framework* publication led to extensive discussions among faculty in four Upstate New York institutions of higher education who formed a network called the *Route 90 Collaborative* to support and promote faculty who were interested in implementing the framework in their curricula. The *Route 90 Collaborative,* named after the throughway that connects our Upstate New York cities, includes the

Table 14.1 Key elements of *A Framework for Educating Health Professionals to Address the Social Determinants of Health*. Washington, DC: The National Academies Press

Key elements of the *Framework*
• That the *Framework* be used in teaching health professionals broadly, from community health workers to physicians, nurses, social workers, and many others, in basic education and in life-long learning.
• That the education to the extent possible should use the inter-professional education model (IPE) in which students of different health professional disciplines learn together and learn from faculty who themselves represent different disciplines.
• That the Social Determinants of Health (SDH) be the basis of teaching the health professional students to take action on health inequities. Thus, the teaching and learning focus on empowering students to work in partnership with others to take active steps to improve health, especially of vulnerable communities.
• To use transformative, active, innovative, and problem-based teaching and learning approaches, rather than the older passive teaching of lectures, followed by exams. These transformative approaches should aim to do more than impart facts; instead they should help students to understand the lived experiences of the impoverished and disadvantaged groups whose health is affected by environmental, political, social and policy factors.
• That the *Framework's* focus is global, in that it addresses the educational needs of health workers world-wide and that health professional education should address global health needs.
• That the education be planned, conducted, and evaluated as equal partners with the communities who experience health disparities, have the greatest health need, and will be the patients of many of the health professional students. Also, that the curriculum reflects the priorities of those communities.
• That this curriculum be implemented in an integrated and longitudinally-organized manner, with investment and support from governmental, professional accreditation, and institutional administration bodies. But, it is recognized that many institutions will not be able to integrate the *Framework* into all levels of coursework at once; therefore, it is recommended that institutions and faculty begin to implement the framework as they are able.

following institutions, University at Buffalo (School of Social Work), Syracuse University (Anthropology, Public Health, and Marriage and Family Therapy); Upstate Medical University (Medicine and Bioethics), Le Moyne College (Physician Assistant Program); and The Sage Colleges (Nursing program). The *Route 90 Collaborative's* objectives are to share curricula, share evaluation materials, share faculty development materials, and jointly publishing of the results of integrating SDH into curricula.

An example of a *Route 90 Collaborative* educational intervention is a course that brings together Master of Social Work and Master of Marriage and Family Therapy, as well as medical, anthropology, and public health students, to help these students understand the social determinants and lived experiences of residents of neighborhoods experiencing high levels of violence and trauma. The description below about this educational intervention is drawn from Lane et al. (2019), which details the teaching strategies and 3 years of student evaluations. The Practicum in Marriage and Family Therapy (MFT) is a core Master's level course designed to assist students in their professional development as family therapists. The course structure includes classroom content, as well as hands-on learning in the Couple and Family Therapy Center, where students provide therapy to individuals, couples, and families from the community. The course addresses the core competencies of the American Association of Marriage and Family Therapy.

The education intervention took place in two 3-hr sessions, 1 week apart. Five community members and two Syracuse University faculty (from public health and anthropology), who had conducted joint research on neighborhood trauma and violence, led the first session in a large computer-equipped classroom. Prior to the class, the students read several articles on violence in Syracuse, written by the community-university research team that led the module. The presentations featured stories of community members dealing with unremitting violence and death. Integrated with those stories were maps of gunshots and murders, data on the social determinants of the violence (e.g., lead poisoning, disproportionate incarceration, poverty, school failure, and structural racism) and analyses of the consequences of the trauma (e.g., higher failure in elementary school reading and math scores in the gunshot clusters, and elevated rates of PTSD). Session 2 involved a bus tour led by community members of the high-violence areas of Syracuse and a visit to a minority-run community center led and facilitated by the five community members and two university members of the research team. Prior to the bus tour, students received a detailed bus route with descriptions of each locale, which focused on aspects of the social determinants of violence, and electronic maps of Syracuse that spatially depicted those issues, which they could use their phones to consult during the route. At the community center, the staff of nine programs gave the students brief descriptions of how each of their programs aims to reduce violence, increase academic achievement, address the needs of individuals with disability, provide outlets for physical fitness, serve the needs of those infected with or affected by HIV/AIDS, and help youth with risk reduction. Students who wanted to know more about, or wished to volunteer for those programs gave their contact information to the program staff. At the end of the bus tour the community members, faculty and students engaged in discussion and reflection.

The majority of student responses to this course were quite positive. In each year, students asked for more time in the community center and more interaction with community members. The student feedback identified areas to improve in future training. For example, students in the first cohort expressed some discomfort with riding in an air-conditioned coach bus through neighborhoods affected by poverty; for the second and third years, a school bus was rented for the tour. A couple of students in the first cohort also pointed out that they wished there had been more application to clinical work. This feedback was taken into account for the second and third years, where there were more discussions of therapeutic interventions in the course after the tour. Likewise, the students consistently reported that they wished they had more time to have direct interaction with community members; while seeing the city increased their awareness of context, they also sought to have deeper conversations. Several students suggested that the class walk through neighborhoods; however, the community members explained that it might not be safe to walk in large groups through areas of high gunshots. The primary feedback from students in all years was that the module should be expanded for greater community engagement and inclusion of broader health professionals. To respond to the students request for more interaction with community members, we lengthened the visit to the community center each year and added more discussions with program staff. In their evaluations, students came up with many ideas for future activities, including barbeques with community members, volunteer days, attending community events, and walking tours of the city. The students seemed interested in engaging with the community beyond the scope of the two-session module. The module seemed to inspire students to be more involved in the community. Other students asked about volunteering in the area or expressed an interest in working with populations affected by community violence.

Conclusion

Finding in Syracuse established medical and allied health professional educational institutions in which anthropology played a limited role, our work opened a larger space for the engagement of anthropology by working alongside existing structures. Taking the region in which we live and the health care educational institutions as our community, we did what anthropologists always do: we built relationships with our "informants" by participating with them in engaging and working to solve their day-to-day challenges. We used our anthropological skills of interviewing, archival research, participant observation, and writing for non-professional as well as professional audiences. We had to adapt each of these techniques to conform with challenges presented by the health education setting. These included that as non-clinicians we were not able to participate completely in all of the medical and health professional students' activities. In addition, the anthropological way of framing and thinking about issues we found was often foreign to those in medical education. As a result, we have followed the advice given to us by the late anthropologist M. Margaret Clark who suggested that the most effective way to communicate anthropology in medical settings is to use analogical presentation. Reflecting on her three decades teaching at the University of San Francisco, she noted that she found it most effective to convey anthropological materials to her medical colleagues and students by explaining that material by pairing "knowledge to be achieved (the target), with pieces of information already familiar to the learner (the source)" (Pena and Andrade-Filho 2008, 609).

Some of these challenges were large questions of health equity raised by people in the city. For example, although the medical community was concerned with continuing disparities in infant mortality in Syracuse, where African American infant mortality was 30.1 per 1000 in the early 1990s, higher than in several developing countries in that era, they did not connect this to broader social determinants. It was a female community member who asked the simple question "Why is it so hard for me to find a man?", which led us to research disproportionate incarceration as a social determinant of post-neonatal mortality, HIV/AIDs, and sexually transmitted infections in pregnant women (Lane et al. 2004a, 2004b; Weisz et al. 2011). Similarly, the observation by community members that they could not buy healthy food in their neighborhoods, led to work on food insecurity, and identifying lack of access to grocery stores as a risk factor for intrauterine growth restriction (Lane et al. 2008b). Others were more practical, like providing compelling materials for Grand Rounds, and other medical settings. For example, we routinely prepare PowerPoint slide decks for our community partners to present at presentations in the college of medicine. As well, these partners present these materials at policy discussion with city, county, and state officials. These PowerPoint decks integrate epidemiological, anthropological, and clinical materials.

We have faced in this work the challenges of working within our own society identified by Ablon (1977), including negotiating value conflicts, our increased personal visibility, navigating being both part of and apart from the community. And, like Schensul (1974) we have found ourselves deeply involved in a hands-on way in the lives of community collaborators and health education institutions. Relationship-building became the foundation to help create change.

Relationships developed through the CARE model led to recognition of what anthropology can contribute and attracts further collaborations. These in turn allow us to find creative ways to institutionalize anthropology within health professional education in our region. For example, we have used the maxim that it is necessary to communicate with diverse populations in idioms and forms with which they are most comfortable. Thus, as we described above, we write for non-professional audiences, hold community meetings, and produce short videos about the work. Each of these allowed sympathetic treatment by the curricula committees responsible for heatlh professional education. To replicate elsewhere what we have done in Syracuse requires the reframing of education from a semester-based, instrumental activity, to one that focuses on building enduring relationships with members of a variety of "stakeholder" communities, and then play the convener role to bring them together to collaborate. For us, one very practical method of convening these communities is to regularly host informal dinners in our home and receptions that bring people of different backgrounds together with students.

Each collaborative effort, including the research, publications, and curriculum development, is based on bringing the methods, perspectives, and approaches of anthropology into other health related fields. The CARE approach is explicitly based on action anthropology. We share the research and teaching work we do through publication. Thus, we have produced scholarly products with community members, faculty, and students. At the start of each CARE project we discuss what the "deliverables" will be, and we establish guidelines for shared authorship. We endeavor then to place our work in venues most appropriate for those who need to know this information. We have published in anthropology journals (*Current Anthropology, Human Organization*), public health journals (*Healthcare for the Poor and Underserved*), and medical journals (*Journal of Adolescent Health, Journal of Urban Health*), among others. The CARE framework brings the critical perspective of anthropology, and the respectful partnership with the community to health professional education. The *Route 90 Collaboration* shares those lessons with an even wider group of institutions (Fig. 14.1).

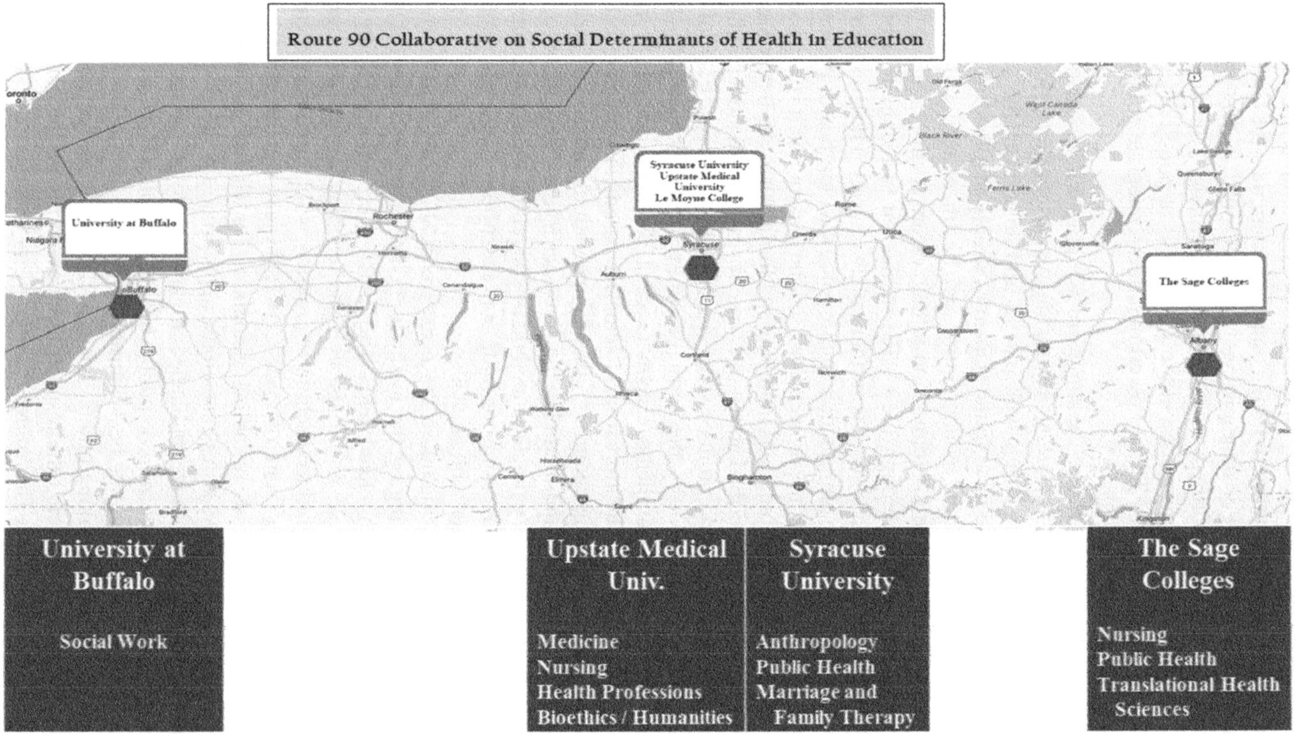

Fig. 14.1 The Route 90 Collaborative

References

Ablon, Joan. 1977. Field method in working with middle class Americans: New issues of values, personality, and reciprocity. *Human Organization* 38 (1): 69–72. http://www.jstor.org/stable/44125243.

Bergen-Cico, Dessa, Arnett Haygood-El, Timothy Jennings-Bey, and Sandra D. Lane. 2014. Street Addiction: A proposed theoretical model for understanding the draw of street life and gang activity. *Journal of Addiction Research and Theory* 22 (1): 15–26. https://doi.org/10.3109/16066359.2012.759942.

Cheng, Xin, Kenneth Ka-Ho Lee, Eric Y. Chang, and Xuesong Yang. 2017. The flipped classroom approach: Stimulating positive learning attitudes and improving mastery of histology among medical students. *Anatomy Science Education* 10 (4): 317–327. https://doi.org/10.1002/ase.1664.

Clark, M. Margaret. 1983. Cultural context of medical practice. *The Western Journal of Medicine* 139 (6): 806–810.

CSDH (Commission on Social Determinants of Health). 2008. *Closing the gap in a generation: Health equity through action on the social determinants of health. Final Report of the Commission on Social Determinants of Health*. Geneva: World Health Organization.

Daly, Robert W. 1967. Values: A view from the clinic. *Journal of Religion and Health* 6 (2): 126–136. https://doi.org/10.1007/BF01532248.

———. 1981. [The] Syracuse Consortium for the cultural foundations of medicine. In *Human values teaching program for health professionals*, ed. Thomas K. McElhinney, 117–121. New York, NY: Whitmore.

Farmer, Paul. 1999. *Infections and inequalities: The modern plagues. Updated Edition*. Berkeley, CA: University of California Press.

Foster, George M. 1977. Medical anthropology and international health planning. *Social Science and Medicine* 11 (10): 527–524. https://doi.org/10.1016/0037-7856(77)90171-8.

Goffman, Erving. 1963. *Stigma: Notes on the management of spoiled identity*. Englewood Cliffs, NJ: Prentice-Hall.

Goodenough, Ward H. 1963. *Cooperation and change*. New York, NY: The Russell Sage Foundation.

Inhorn, Marcia. 2003. Global infertility and the globalization of new reproductive technologies: Illustrations from Egypt. *Social Science and Medicine* 56 (9): 1837–1851. https://doi.org/10.1016/s0277-9536(02)00208-3.

Jennings-Bey, Timothy, Sandra D. Lane, Robert A. Rubinstein, Dessa Bergen-Cico, Arnett Haygood-El, Helen Hudson, Shaundel Sanchez, and Frank L. Fowler. 2015. The Trauma Response Team: A community intervention for gang violence. *Journal of Urban Health* 92 (5): 947–954. https://doi.org/10.1007/s11524-015-9978-8.

Lane, Sandra D. 2008. *Why are our babies dying: Pregnancy, birth, and death in America*. New York, NY: Routledge.

Lane, Sandra D., Robert A. Rubinstein, Robert H. Keefe, Noah Webster, Donald A. Cibula, Alan Rosenthal, and Jesse Dowdell. 2004a. Structural violence and racial disparity in HIV transmission. *Journal of Healthcare for the Poor and Underserved* 15 (3): 319–335. https://doi.org/10.1353/hpu.2004.0043.

Lane, Sandra D., Robert H. Keefe, Robert A. Rubinstein, Brooke A. Levandowski, Michael Freedman, Alan Rosenthal, Donald A. Cibula, and Maria Czerwinski. 2004b. Marriage promotion and missing men: African American women in a demographic double bind. *Medical Anthropology Quarterly* 18 (2): 405–428. https://doi.org/10.1525/maq.2004.18.4.405.

Lane, Sandra D., Noah Webster, Brooke A. Levandowski, Robert A. Rubinstein, Robert H. Keefe, Martha Wojtowycz, Donald A. Cibula, Joan E. Kingson, and Richard H. Aubry. 2008a. Environmental injustice: Childhood lead poisoning, teen pregnancy, and tobacco. *Journal of Adolescent Health* 42 (1): 43–49. https://doi.org/10.1016/j.jadohealth.2007.06.017.

Lane, Sandra D., Robert H. Keefe, Robert A. Rubinstein, Brooke A. Levandowski, Noah Webster, Donald A. Cibula, Adwoa K. Boahene, Olabisi Dele-Michael, Darlene Carter, Tanika Jones, Martha Wojtowycz, and Jessica Brill. 2008b. Structural violence, urban retail good markets, and low birth weight. *Health and Place* 14 (3): 415–423. https://doi.org/10.1016/j.healthplace.2007.08.008.

Lane, Sandra D., Robert A. Rubinstein, Lutchmie Narine, Inga Back, Caitlin Cornell, and Alexander Hodgens. 2011. Action Anthropology and pedagogy: University-community collaborations in setting policy. *Human Organization* 70 (3): 289–299. https://doi.org/10.17730/humo.70.3.v1hv08236w4411h6.

Lane, Sandra D., Robert A. Rubinstein, Dessa Bergen-Cico, Timothy Jennings-Bey, Linda Stone Fish, David A. Larsen, Mindy Thompson Fullilove, Tracey Reichert Schimpff, Kishi Animashaun Ducre, and Honnell Allen Robinson. 2017a. Neighborhood trauma due to violence: A multilevel analysis. *Journal of Healthcare for the Poor and Underserved* 28 (1): 446–462. https://doi.org/10.1353/hpu.2017.0033.

Lane, Sandra D., Robert A. Rubinstein, Robert H. Keefe, Lynn Beth Satterly, Tarakad Ramachandran, Sally Huntington, and Amaus Student Researchers. 2017b. Action Anthropology in a free clinic. *Human Organization* 76 (4): 336–347. https://doi.org/10.17730/0018-7259.76.4.336.

Lane, Sandra D., Robert A. Rubinstein, Tracey Reichert Schimpff, Robert H. Keefe, Timothy Jennings-Bey, Sydney Russell Leed, Brady Iles, Patricia A. Cuff, and Lynn Beth Satterly. 2019. Bringing in the community: A university-community endeavor to teach marital and family therapy students about community-based violence and trauma. *Contemporary Family Therapy* 41: 147–156. https://doi.org/10.1007/s10591-019-09488-8.

Macgregor, Gordon. 1961. Social determinants of health practices. *American Journal of Public Health* 51 (11): 1709–1714. https://doi.org/10.2105/AJPH.51.11.1709.

Marmot, Michael. 2005. Social determinants of health inequalities. *The Lancet* 365 (9464): 1099–1104. https://doi.org/10.1016/S0140-6736(05)71146-6.

National Academies of Sciences Engineering and Medicine. 2016. *A framework for educating health professionals to address the social determinants of health*. Washington, DC: The National Academies Press.

Pena, Gil Patrus, and Jose de Souza Andrade-Filho. 2008. Analogies in medicine: Valuable for learning, reasoning, remembering and naming. *Advances in Health Sciences Education Theory and Practice* 15 (4): 609–619. https://doi.org/10.1007/s10459-008-9126-2.

Rubinstein, Robert A. 1986. Reflections on Action Anthropology: Some developmental dynamics of an anthropological tradition. *Human Organization* 45 (3): 270–279. https://doi.org/10.17730/humo.45.3.j0r1w186w2162140.

———. 2018. Action Anthropology. In *Internatonal Encyclopedia of Anthropology*, ed. Hilary Callan, 21–27. London: Wiley-Blackwell.

Rubinstein, Robert A., Sandra D. Lane, Mojeed Lookman, Shaundel Sanchez, Elize Catania, Timothy Jennings-Bey, Arnett Haygood-El, and Edward Mitchell Jr. 2018. Blood in the rust belt: Mourning and memorialization in the context of community violence. *Current Anthropology* 59 (4): 439–454. https://doi.org/10.1086/698956.

Schensul, Stephen L. 1974. Skills needed in Action Anthropology: Lessons from El Centro de la Causa. *Human Organization* 33: 203–209. http://www.jstor.org/stable/44125298.

Smith, Joshua J. 2015. Standing with Sol: The spirit and intent of Action Anthropology. *Anthropologica* 57: 445–456. http://www.jstor.org/stable/26350453.

Solimeo, Samantha L., Greg L. Stewart, and Gary E. Rosenthal. 2016. The critical role of clerks in the patient-centered medical home. *Annals of Family Medicine* 14 (4): 377–379. https://doi.org/10.1370/afm.1934.

Weisz, Jessica, Sara Lozyniak, Sandra D. Lane, Robert Silverman, Emilia Koumans, Kathy DeMott, Martha Wojtowycz, and Richard H. Aubry. 2011. It takes at least two: Male partner factors, racial/ethnic disparity and Chlamydia infection and re-infection among pregnant women. *Journal of Healthcare for the Poor and Underserved* 22 (3): 871–885. https://doi.org/10.1353/hpu.2011.0086.

Robert A. Rubinstein, PhD, MsPH is a distinguished professor of anthropology and professor of international relations at the Maxwell School of Syracuse University. His medical anthropology work has focused on infectious eye disease, psychosocial epidemiology, health inequalities, and on integrating epidemiological and anthropological methods. His work has been funded by the Ford Foundation, the Edna McConnell Foundation, the US Institute of Peace, the National Science Foundation, and the Wenner-Gren Foundation, among others. He is the author or editor of 9 books and more than 100 journal articles and book chapters. He received the 2016 Victor Sidel and Barry Levy Award for Peace from the American Public Health Association, and the 2010 Robert B. Textor and Family Prize for Anticipatory Anthropology from the American Anthropological Association.

Sandra D. Lane, PhD, MPH is Laura J. and L. Douglas Meredith Professor of public health and anthropology at Syracuse University, and research professor in the Department of Obstetrics and Gynecology at Upstate Medical University. In addition to her 50 published articles and 24 book chapters, Lane authored *Why Are Our Babies Dying? Pregnancy, Birth and Death in America*; was a co-author of the CDC publication, *The Public Health Impact of Needle Exchange Programs in the United States and Abroad,* and she chaired the National Academies of Engineering, Sciences and Medicine committee that wrote, *A Framework for Educating Health Professionals to Address the Social Determinants of Health*. Her work has been funded by the CDC, EPA, HRSA, and Office of Minority Health, as well as NY State, and foundation grants. She received the 2015 Henrik L. Blum Award for Excellence in Health Policy from the American Public Health Association, and the 2019 George Foster Award for Practicing Medical Anthropology, from the Society for Medical Anthropology.

Chapter 15
Using Anthropological Perspectives to Integrate Health Equity Across a Family Medicine Residency Program in New Mexico

Mary Alice Scott, Ernesto A. Moralez, and John Andazola

Family medicine developed as a specialty in the 1960s and 1970s because of a recognition that the United States needed physicians who provide continuity of care across medical services, emphasize preventive medicine, and understand the social, emotional, and environmental factors that affect the health of patients and their families. When the specialty was formalized in 1969, the American Board of Family Practice indicated that family physicians should be trained to provide comprehensive medical care to all members of a family regardless of whether the problem facing the patient and their family is biological, behavioral, or social. They were to be advocates for patients in their communities (Gutierrez and Scheid 2002). Giving comprehensive medical care continues to be the vision of family medicine and is supported by the mission statement of the American Academy of Family Physicians (2019): "to improve the health of patients, families, and communities by serving the needs of members with professionalism and creativity."

However, the increasingly technological and bureaucratic United States health care system promotes training and practice to focus on the patient as a body and the physician as a technician who can tweak the biological and physiological make-up of the patient through medications and surgery (Wade and Halligan 2004). Thus, most residency programs focus training on intervention, testing, and procedures and only have a minimal focus on the societal components that negatively impact health. With

M. A. Scott (✉)
Department of Anthropology, New Mexico State University, Las Cruces, NM, USA
e-mail: mscott2@nmsu.edu

E. A. Moralez
Department of Public Health Sciences, New Mexico State University, Las Cruces, NM, USA

J. Andazola
Program Director, Southern New Mexico Family Medicine Residency Program, Las Cruces, NM, USA

I. L. Martinez, D. W. Wiedman (eds.), *Anthropology in Medical Education*,
https://doi.org/10.1007/978-3-030-62277-0_15

new and strengthened program requirements of the Accreditation Council for Graduate Medical Education (ACGME) for family medicine residencies to teach population health and attend to cultural and community components of health and health care (Clements 2018; Wagner et al. 2016), postgraduate medical training can serve as an opportunity to increase family physicians' capacity to return to the roots of their profession.

Medical anthropologists have long worked in clinical and medical educational settings, often focused on ethnographically-based and contextually-rich understandings of medical education and health care. These scholars (often scholar-clinicians) have made significant theoretical and methodological contributions to addressing issues that arise when attempting to address the social and cultural contexts within which health happens.

In this chapter, we describe the development and early implementation of a health equity curriculum for a family medicine residency program that uses these anthropological perspectives as its foundation. While an interdisciplinary team developed the curriculum, we focus in this chapter on the specific anthropological contributions to the curriculum. In doing so, we elevate the work of medical anthropologists in these settings whose work is sometimes not recognized as specifically anthropological and offer one example of how others may integrate anthropological perspectives into health professions curricula. In the sections that follow, we first discuss relevant frameworks from medical anthropology used to develop our curriculum. We then describe the process of curriculum development. We next describe the components of the curriculum that are grounded in anthropological foundations. We end the chapter with a discussion of the impact the curriculum has had on the residency program and the lessons we have learned in the process.

Medical Anthropology Frameworks

Psychiatrist and anthropologist Arthur Kleinman et al. (1978: 256) first articulated a clinically applied medical anthropology in the late 1970s, calling for a "clinical social science". Kleinman (1985: 70) later described clinically applied anthropologists as

> teaching and research consultants in primary care, medical specialty, public health, health policy, and research settings which can inject the 'uncomfortable science'...with our emphasis on the cultural construction and social production of sickness and clinical praxis, in the pragmatic ethos of actual health problems and programs.

Kleinman's focus was primarily on how the perspective of medical anthropology could support improved clinical encounters and teach physicians about multiple ways of understanding illness and disease. However, his framework was also broad enough to include the critical examination of the structure of biomedicine, health care, and medical education. He identified a holistic perspective, flexibility, and in-depth cultural analysis as the strengths of medical anthropologists that could be used in clinical settings.

Anthropologists have debated the value of clinically applied medical anthropology since they began working in clinical settings in the 1970s, often arguing that anthropologists have neither been able to continue to ground themselves in the values of holistic, critical praxis nor to communicate the value of anthropological perspectives to the medical community (Hemmings 2005). Yet, many have asserted that medicine needs anthropology, or at least would benefit from anthropological perspectives (Hemmings 2005; Hahn and Kleinman 1983; Konner 1991), not just in terms of recognizing the importance of patients' cultures, but also understanding and critically evaluating the culture of medicine itself (Kleinman et al. 1978; Stein 1985; Taylor 2003). Therefore, medical anthropologists can, arguably, be both critical and clinical (Morgan 1990). At the time of this debate among medical anthropologists, several issues were raised concerning integrating critical anthropology into clinical work that we also encountered (Chrisman and Maretzki 1982; Phillips 1985; Press 1990). For example, in our work in graduate medical education, it was challenging to translate theoretical concepts to practical applicability in clinical settings. We also struggled to define our role as non-reimbursable, yet critically valuable, members of a healthcare team.

Medical anthropologists have long served several roles in clinical and medical educational settings—as teachers, consultants, and researchers. All of these roles require that anthropologists immerse themselves in biomedicine in order to understand its complexity, nuances, and worldviews (Kleinman 1982; Stein 1985). Teaching has typically focused on learning cultural competency (and more recently cultural humility) and identification of patients' explanatory models while cautioning against simplistic and stereotypical uses of culture (Benbassat et al. 2003; Culhane-Pera et al. 2000; Fetters 1998; Jenks 2011; Kleinman 1982; Mull et al. 2001; Stein 1982). As consultants, anthropologists additionally have had the opportunity to highlight patient perspectives on illness and disease and expand the contexts (social, economic, political, etc) in which physicians understand illness and disease and patients experience them, thereby challenging often taken-for-granted norms and values within biomedicine (Kleinman and Benson 2006; Willen and Carpenter-Song 2013).

More recently anthropologists have contributed to medical and medical education research by introducing more robust qualitative methods into their studies. Anthropologists working in clinical settings have long paid attention to ethnography as crucial to their work in the field (Stein 1991), but in the last 20 years they have contributed more methodologically-focused works to improve clinical research and practice (see for example Borkan et al. 2001; Cohen and Crabtree 2008; Crabtree and Miller 1999; DiCicco-Bloom and Crabtree 2006; Griffiths et al. 2010; Guetterman et al. 2015; Henry and Fetters 2012; Ventres and Frankel 1996).

In all of these areas, anthropologists often exemplify the reflexive stance that has become central to critical anthropology, reminding both physicians and other anthropologists of the importance of self-reflection on one's actions, perspectives, biases, and assumptions and of considering the impact of that on one's patients, learners, and colleagues (Ventres and Fort 2014).

While there has been debate among anthropologists since the emergence of clinically applied medical anthropology about whether anthropologists working in clinical settings had been co-opted and had lost the critical perspective so central to medical anthropology, at the same time, there were calls for anthropologists to begin "studying up." In her presidential address to the Society for Medical Anthropology in 1997, Carole Browner (1999: 135) argued that while anthropologists "have much to offer to the world of biomedical research," we also run the risk of "sacrific[ing] what has made us unique." She warned about the movement towards accepting rather than critiquing biomedical categories and explanations and losing a holistic approach to analysis.

One specific framework that builds on much of the above cited work is "structural competency," a concept developed and elaborated in collaboration with medical anthropologists. Structural competency is "the trained ability to discern how a host of issues defined clinically as symptoms, attitudes, or diseases...also represent the downstream implications of a number of upstream decisions about such matters as health care and food delivery systems, zoning laws, urban and rural infrastructures, medicalization, or even about the very definitions of illness and health" (Metzl and Hansen 2014: 128). The core competencies for this type of education, as defined by Metzl and Hansen (2014: 128–131) include "(1) recognizing the structures that shape clinical interactions...(2) developing an extra-clinical language of structure...(3) rearticulating 'cultural' presentations in structural terms...(4) Observing and imagining structural intervention...moreover, (5) developing structural humility".

As noted above, anthropologists have continued to balance between critical analysis of biomedicine, biomedical practice, and health care systems and collaborative efforts to improve medicine by participating in medical education and health care systems (Martinez 2015). Unfortunately, publication of the work that medical anthropologists have done to maintain this balance is limited. Our intention in this chapter is to contribute to an ongoing conversation about how medical anthropologists can remain true to our critical foundations and also work collaboratively with our health professions colleagues. We are inspired by the work of the medical anthropologists who have come before us and have continued to exemplify the value of anthropological perspective for medicine.

Setting

The Southern New Mexico Family Medicine Residency Program (SNMFMRP) is a 3-year post-graduate program sponsored by Memorial Medical Center of Las Cruces the local health care facility located in Dona Ana County, New Mexico (which makes up part of the US/Mexico border), serving approximately 300,000 county residents. The program has 20 residents: 8 in post-graduate year 1 (PGY1), 6 in PGY2, and 6 in PGY3. The two additional residents in PGY1 go on to complete their second and third years in a rural New Mexico community. The residents are diverse regarding national origin, cultural background, gender, race/ethnicity, and age.

The SNMFMRP's mission is to eliminate health disparities in New Mexico and train family physicians who will stay in the border region after graduation. The SNMFMRP, following ACGME requirements, has long maintained a community medicine curriculum and rural health rotations that have contributed to learning about social determinants of health. However, in part due to the restrictions of the ACGME requirements, most of the curriculum has followed a traditional model of 4-week rotations that focus on clinical and hospital-based care and exposure to other medical specialties such as emergency medicine, orthopedics, and pediatrics. The residency has recently, due to the leadership of the program director (Andazola), refocused its efforts on moving more of the training outside the walls of the clinic and hospital and increasing its training in health equity, beyond simply social determinants of health.

Scott, a medical anthropologist, had previously conducted ethnographic research on teaching and learning in graduate medical education. Her work demonstrated that primary care residents often felt that their ideals were being "taught out of them" as they went through residency. Many chose a career in primary care because of their belief that the philosophy of primary care would allow them to be physician advocates creating change in their local communities. As they continued through residency, they discovered that their education included few tools or perspectives that would help them become that kind of physician. With that background, Scott and Andazola began to work together to develop a graduate medical education curriculum that would support these initial values of primary care physicians. Together, they formed an interprofessional team of experts from both academic and medical professions who collaborated to reform the medical education model in the residency program. This Health Equity Action Team (HEAT) began to create a new health equity curriculum (HEC) that would be integrated longitudinally in the 3-year family medicine residency program. In addition to the medical anthropologist, the team included academic faculty in public health (Moralez), two social workers, a psychologist, a family physician with extensive experience in health policy, family medicine residents, a member of the city fire department, and the residency program coordinator.

The initial task of HEAT was to review the medical education requirements established by the ACGME for all family medicine residency programs, identifying the competencies that were related to health equity. Each team member reviewed the program requirements and created a list of specific competencies that address health equity. The team refined the list to focus on those competencies that aligned most closely with the expertise of team members. Residency faculty then added additional components that they identified as essential to developing high-quality family physicians who could address both the medical and social needs of the community. Then the team reviewed the existing curriculum to identify which competencies were already being taught. Finally, the team revised the existing curriculum and developed new curricular components that met both the ACGME requirements and faculty-identified competencies.

Social Determinants of Health Curriculum Prior to Revisions

Before social scientists' integration into the residency, the residency had a community medicine curriculum focused on training residents in community agencies that address health at a population level (for example, with the Department of Health and school-based health centers). The goals of the curriculum included increasing understanding of the implications of patient health problems in the greater context of a community and assessing barriers to optimal health among different subpopulations within a given community.

The residency also supported a rural medicine rotation during which residents spend a month working at a rural clinic site. Some of the goals of this curriculum included training residents to develop respectful therapeutic relationships with vulnerable patients and families, implement health promotion and risk and harm reduction strategies, and apply community-oriented primary care strategies. Residents typically completed two rural medicine rotations in two different communities in southern New Mexico.

Also, the residency had been working for several years to develop an integrated behavioral health faculty and curriculum to train residents to engage in behavioral health with their patients and learn how to work on interprofessional teams. In particular, this rotation focused on understanding the interrelationships among biological, psychological, social, and cultural factors in all patients and recognizing the role of the family physician in maintaining behavioral health.

Revisions and New Components of Curriculum with Anthropological Foundations

HEAT drew from critical and clinical medical anthropological perspectives and related perspectives from other disciplines to conclude that the focus on social determinants of health alone is too often individualized in the context of medical education. For example, discussions often assume that patients *have* specific social determinants of health that physicians can address by referring them to services that will provide resources for that individual to address those social determinants. We took a broader, more comprehensive, and more critical approach which led us to develop a health equity focus for our curriculum revision.

Using the framework of structural competency, we understand health disparities to be the result of unequal distribution of wealth and power across communities. While disparities are embodied in individuals, the institutions/structures that produce them affect entire communities/populations. If we are to address health disparities and improve patient health outcomes, we must work to create a more equitable distribution of resources and power. Sometimes that means that the work our residents do may not look like health care in a traditional sense. However, it can help reconnect physicians to their ideal vision of being advocates for their patients and communities.

Community Medicine Curriculum

We began with a revision of the community medicine curriculum to include more rotation sites that did not provide direct medical care but instead moved residents into community-based sites that were addressing the contexts in which health happens. This rotation utilizes the structural competency framework to encourage residents to consider the ways that institutions such as schools and social service agencies may contribute to health equity (or inequity). They are able to experience for themselves the ways that they may, as physicians, become more integrated into their local communities. The ACGME requires a community medicine experience and additionally includes requirements to "communicate effectively with patients, families, and the public, as appropriate, across a broad range of socioeconomic and cultural backgrounds." This, among other requirements, guided our selection of specific sites to be included in the rotation.

For example, the community medicine rotation now includes two half days at a local middle school that is the first community school in our area. A community school is a publicly funded school that partners with the community to serve as both a school and a community center (Coalition for Community Schools 2019). In collaboration with the community school's coordinator in the public school district, we developed experiences in which residents do not provide medical care to the students at the community school. Instead, they talk with students about the process of becoming a doctor, help students with homework, and assist teachers in the classroom. The purpose of this experience is to expose residents to the educational environment for students in our community and to give them an opportunity to participate in one intervention that aims to improve that environment. This exposure outside of medical practice encourages residents to better understand the structures that influence their patients and that underlie much of their clinical practice whether it is immediately obvious or not.

Care of Marginalized Populations Curriculum

We have also developed a 4-week elective rotation called "Care of Marginalized Populations" which gives residents an opportunity to spend a month engaging in the health care of a particular population they are interested in caring for as a physician. The team initiated this curriculum in part because of our collaboration with a member of the fire department who runs a mobile integrated health unit, visiting people who call 911 frequently to better understand what social needs they may have that lead them to make these calls. The team recognized that this population was one of many in our community that lived in the margins and therefore was not well understood.

During the first 2 weeks of this rotation, residents visit several different agencies that work with specific populations marginalized in the context of access to health care. They then choose one agency to work with more closely during the second 2 weeks of the rotation with a focus on the way the agency works to increase access to care for the population they serve. The focus of this rotation is to engage residents in a deeper understanding and experience of the social and structural barriers that their patients may face when they are part of a marginalized community. We developed the specific experiences in this rotation to ensure that the residents can meet the ACGME requirement that residents develop a "sensitivity and responsiveness to a diverse patient population, including but not limited to diversity in gender, age, culture, race, religion, disabilities, and sexual orientation." While residents certainly cannot learn everything about the influences on a marginalized community during a 1-month rotation, this rotation does help them to develop the "structural humility" that is part of the structural competency framework. They can begin to approach patients, whether from marginalized communities or not, with the understanding that there are more influences on a patient's life and health than what is explicitly brought up in a clinic visit.

Health Policy Curriculum

Finally, we have developed a health policy elective rotation in which residents spend 4 weeks learning about how they can participate in policymaking at the local, state, and national levels. Residents are to spend their time attending legislative meetings, participating in a county-wide coalition that focuses on addressing the social determinants of health that most impact health outcomes in the county, and write op-eds, letters to legislators, and resolutions for their professional organizations. This rotation moves residents far beyond traditional medical care to engage residents in policy-making efforts that have the potential to decrease health disparities and improve health equity in the communities where residents live and work. The team developed the rotation in collaboration with a local federally qualified health center (FQHC), which will provide policy-related education regarding FQHCs as part of the rotation.

We used the ACGME requirement that residents "advocate for quality patient care and optimal patient care systems" to guide curricular development. This requirement aligns with arguably the most complex and challenging part of the structural competency framework. Policy changes are the most likely to have a broad impact on the structures that residents learn about in the previous two rotations but learning how to engage in policy as a practicing physician often feels overwhelming. This rotation provides residents with tools to engage that are manageable for a family physician.

Longitudinal Health Equity Curriculum

These rotations are part of a longitudinal health equity curriculum that will infuse a structural competency lens across all educational experiences in the residency and allow residents to engage in longer-term community-based work and deeper discussions of structural competency. This curriculum uses structural competency directly as a framework for curricular design but also draws on the ethnographic work on teaching and learning conducted by Scott. It is foundationally anthropological both in theory and in practice.

Challenges: Graduate Medical Education (GME) Structure

We have faced several challenges in our work thus far including the difficulty in changing long-standing models of residency education, a need to work within a specific set of accreditation requirements, and resistance by some residents who are concerned that this education will take away from what they need to know to be competent physicians. Our analysis of these challenges and work to address them is also influenced by specific anthropological perspectives. Scott has identified most of these challenges through participant observation, a central anthropological method, within the residency program. The discussion below reflects an anthropological analysis of the organization of residency education.

Residency education has typically been organized into 1-month block rotations to ensure that programs meet the ACGME requirements. This organization encourages thinking about medicine as distinct body systems or interventions (e.g., a neurology rotation followed by a urology rotation or a surgery rotation followed by a radiology rotation). Additionally, it makes it challenging to establish longitudinal educational experiences in which residents can make broader connections across areas of healthcare and between healthcare and the communities where their patients live.

The newest ACGME requirements do include education in social determinants of health and health equity. Since family medicine residencies are already required to include vast amounts of information and a wide range of experiences, it is challenging to add anything extra to the curriculum. The challenge is to develop curricular areas that both meet ACGME requirements and perhaps push beyond specific requirements to more fully incorporate anthropologically-based frameworks like structural competency. Additionally, there are limited ways of incorporating experts in those areas onto residency faculty particularly when the residency is community-based rather than based in an academic center. In our case, much of the work was conducted by part-time and volunteer social science faculty and physician faculty who all have to fit this work into already full schedules.

One of the primary outcomes that the ACGME measures to determine the quality of residency programs is the percentage of residents who pass the board exam near the end of their residency program. Programs receive citations from the ACGME if they do not have a high board pass rate, and residents will find it more difficult to find employment when they graduate if they have not passed the board exam. Given that orientation, residents and faculty often feel pressure to focus teaching and learning "to the test". This pressure is part of a powerful, hidden curriculum in medical education that sometimes undermines an explicit focus on community-oriented medicine by subtly supporting a more physiological and clinically-based education through focusing the majority of time in education on biology and physiology and encouraging the highest performing students to enter the most highly technical and specialized medical fields. For example, although population-based care is a section of the board exam, it accounts for only 4% of the examination. The musculoskeletal, cardiovascular, and respiratory sections, however, account for 31% of the exam (New England Journal of Medicine 2019). Tension arises between teaching skills and perspectives that will make the most substantial difference in health outcomes and teaching medical knowledge that will appear on the exam.

One example of the way this tension plays out in our daily work in the residency is in planning didactic education, which is the classroom or lecture-style educational experience as opposed to the experiential education of taking care of patients. Didactics occurs one afternoon a week for 4 h. The goal of didactics, according to the ACGME, is to provide a "forum for residents to explore and analyze evidence pertinent to the practice of family medicine." However, it is generally viewed as a time to review medical knowledge that may be on the exam. The residency has recently created a new didactics schedule organized by board exam areas with emphasis relatively equivalent to the percentage of questions on the exam that fit under that area. In this new schedule, it is difficult to include topics that may be "pertinent to the practice of family medicine" but not necessarily on the exam.

Related to the above, residency education focuses on "evidence-based medicine." While that makes sense on the face of it, it only applies to those treatments and practices that have been studied in a way that leads to the type of evidence that fits with medical training. For example, randomized control clinical trials can produce evidence that a beta blocker will likely work to control hypertension in a particular population of patients. These types of studies often drive practice in medicine. This paradigm presents a challenge to social scientists who use different types of evidence, in particular, qualitative evidence, to make arguments and propose action. For example, Scott's ethnographic research in Mexico demonstrated that women understood that drinking excessive amounts of soda was not healthy and could be contributing to their diabetes and obesity. However, their reasons for drinking soda were not always related to health. Sometimes they were more related to maintaining social and familial relationships or enjoying a small moment during a hard day. How does this type of evidence translate into the clinical practice of a physician whose goal is to get a patient's diabetes under control?

Impact

We recognize that much of the impact of our work will be seen in the practice of the residents after graduation. However, there were immediate changes made to the SNMFMRP because of the implementation of curricular changes. Our work has been informed by clinical and critical medical anthropological frameworks in shaping our role as consultants and researchers to broaden the frame of medical training using a structural competency framework. We also continue to maintain a critical perspective on the structure of medical education, challenging traditional models when they contradict the goal of curricular development. However, we maintain a collaborative approach, recognizing that the residency program is dependent on accreditation from a national body that maintains standards for the structure of residency education. Our effort is focused on practical next steps and continues to be flexible as we discuss changes with faculty, residents, and community members.

Our team has expanded the scope of the SNMFMRP to include a more tailored community-informed approach to the resident curriculum focused on encouraging residents to account for their patients' social conditions and how those conditions could be impacting health outcomes. This expansion is supported by the meaningful interprofessional collaboration between the medical teaching faculty and the social science experts. This collaboration was critical to ensuring that, along with the biomedical model emphasized by graduate medical education, every resident was given a unique opportunity to reframe their knowledge within the structural competency framework. By collaborating across professions and disciplines, we were able to create a model that fits with multiple perspectives on health, health care, and health systems. This model encourages both critique and action. We believe that the modifications to the curriculum and the added rotations gave residents a more nuanced perspective about what health equity means and the inequities facing the communities they serve.

Additionally, the SNMFMRP began to promote the HEAT on their website and recruitment materials which led to attracting applicants who had an explicit interest in health equity. Over the last several years, more residents have entered the program who are already aligned with a holistic, critical perspective and show more immediate support of the work of our team.

Finally, there has been a proposal by the SNMFMRP Program Director (Andazola) to change the name of the residency to The New Mexico Residency in Social Medicine. This along with the promotion of structural competency will be instrumental in changing the culture at the SNMFMRP and fulfilling the original vision of the program from the program director and further supporting the centrality of structural competency to resident education as well as modifying the existing post-graduate medical education paradigm with an emphasis on caring for patients not just in the context of the clinic but also in the context of their community.

Lessons Learned

In the process of collaborating to develop a health equity curriculum that places medical anthropological ideas at the center, we have learned several lessons that may be helpful to others seeking to do similar work. We quickly realized when we began the work that we needed to understand the language of both medical education and medicine in order to fully engage with our physician colleagues and to be able to translate our concepts to residents in ways that they could connect with their medical frameworks. We addressed this by learning how the residency faculty implements ACGME requirements, develops curriculum, and evaluates residents. It also included learning the language of medicine so that we could understand how residents and faculty communicate with each other and understand the trajectories of common diseases that family physicians encounter. Only by doing so could we effectively connect work on health equity to a family physician's daily practice. Our growing facility with medical language and concepts as well as with biology and physiology has also increased our credibility beyond the residency as we present our work in other medical settings.

Second, implementing a non-standard curriculum in a residency program requires creativity. Residency programs must adhere strictly to accreditation requirements that are designed to focus on the key sets of skills and knowledge needed to become family physicians. Not meeting these requirements could result in citations for the program, and if severe enough, program closure. These requirements are extensive and designed to fill 3 years of training. Any training outside of these requirements requires justification for administrators, faculty, residents, and accreditors. However, some of the requirements are written quite generally and could be fulfilled in many different ways. While some components of our curriculum clearly meet ACGME requirements (e.g., assess community, environmental and family influences on the health of patients), others need further explanation. We addressed those components that do not clearly fit with ACGME requirements in two ways. First, some of our curricula meet requirements in non-traditional ways. For example, the ACGME requires that residents "participate in identifying system errors and implementing potential systems solutions" (ACGME 2013: 7). Typically, residency programs meet this requirement by doing a root cause analysis after an unexpected bad outcome in the hospital to address hospital system errors and potential solutions. We argue that visiting legislative offices to discuss health policy bills with legislative staff also teaches residents to identify larger system errors and implement systems solutions. A second way that we address components that do not clearly meet requirements is to argue that they do support the overall goals of family medicine to improve the health of patients, families, and *communities*. This strategy requires champions. One benefit of working with this particular residency program is that most of the faculty have developed a commitment to teaching health equity regardless of whether it is explicitly stated in the ACGME requirements or not.

Third, in order to successfully work collaboratively with the residency program to develop our curriculum, we needed strong buy-in from the leadership. This was particularly essential as we were bringing in critical perspectives that sometimes challenged the traditional ways of teaching and learning that had been long established in the program. For example, as we discuss further below, we have just begun to explore the possibility of creating a different structure for the residency program so that residents can engage in more longitudinal experiences, which we see as essential to developing a sophisticated understanding of health disparities and the set of skills necessary for a physician to work towards health equity. In order to even consider such a fundamental change to the program, the program director at a minimum, and preferably the rest of the faculty had to consider this change not only possible but potentially beneficial to the program. Buy-in from the program director came as a result of applying anthropological methods and values that include establishing trust, developing a shared language and maintaining cultural relativism. In her preliminary research on teaching and learning in the residency, some of Scott's findings were critical of the standard educational methods that were also used in Andazola's program. She brought those forward first to the program director and faculty to discuss whether her interpretation made sense to them and what they would like to do next rather than immediately presenting recommendations or unproductively critiquing the residency. The program director also reviews all manuscripts for publication prior to submission to maintain transparency and ensure both the accuracy of reporting and the protection of the program's faculty and residents. Through this process, Scott and Andazola developed a shared language that Andazola was able to use to communicate to the value of the new curriculum to the residency faculty.

Finally, although medical anthropology is itself a holistic discipline, we recognized that we needed multiple other perspectives to complement that holism and provide more specific sets of expertise in our curriculum development. Although not all of the areas we would like to be represented are regularly at the table at our meetings, we have worked to include as many critical perspectives as possible. This includes not just health care professionals and social scientists, but also members of the community who do health equity-related work and can provide a more community-based perspective as we design our curriculum.

In conclusion, the perspectives of both critical and applied medical anthropology have been essential to the development of a curriculum that addresses health equity in family medicine residency. Anthropology's holistic perspective and commitment to both critique and advocacy have resulted in a productive, collaborative effort that we believe will contribute to developing family physicians who engage in health equity work in their communities moving forward. They will do so with both a commitment to improving the lives of their patients and with a critical eye towards the health care system—not just accepting that the system presents barriers but working to change it from within. Many of the gaps in graduate medical school education mentioned in this chapter were addressed by having an interprofessional team (HEAT) collaborating on changes to one residency's curriculum. For example, an important HEAT objective was to emphasize to residents the role of a patient's social context in their health outcomes and the existence of health disparities, particularly those disparities most prevalent in the region. Immediate plans include evaluating the modified curriculum and following residents after graduation to determine how they use their training in structural competency in their practices. Additionally, we also plan to train social science students to work on similar types of multi-disciplinary, interprofessional teams to build a future collaborative workforce that can balance the critical and applied perspectives in our field. It is the hope of the authors that medical anthropologists can be more involved in discussions about medical curriculum, sharing our unique perspectives to influence how graduate medical education happens in residencies.

References

Accreditation Council for Graduate Medical Education. 2013. *The Family Medicine Milestone Project. Accreditation Council for Graduate Medical Education 2013*. https://www.acgme.org/Portals/0/PDFs/Milestones/FamilyMedicineMilestones.pdf?ver=2017-01-20-103353-463. Accessed 19 Jan 2019.

American Academy of Family Physicians. 2019. *AAFP Mission Statement*. https://www.aafp.org/about/policies/all/mission.html. Accessed 19 June 2019.

Benbassat, Jochanan, Reuben Baumal, Jeffrey M. Borkan, and Rosalie Ber. 2003. Overcoming barriers to teaching the behavioral and social sciences to medical students. *Academic Medicine* 78 (4): 372–380. https://doi.org/10.1097/00001888-200304000-00009.

Borkan, Jeffrey, Schmuel Reis, and Jack Medalie. 2001. Narratives in family medicine: tales of transformation, points of breakthrough for family physicians. *Families, Systems & Health* 19 (2): 121–131. https://doi.org/10.1037/h0089536.

Browner, Carole H. 1999. On the medicalization of medical anthropology. *Medical Anthropology Quarterly* 13 (2): 135–140. https://doi.org/10.1525/maq.1999.13.2.135.

Chrisman, Noel J., and Thomas W. Maretzki. 1982. Anthropology in health science settings. In *Clinically applied anthropology: anthropologists in health science settings*, ed. Noel J. Chrisman and Thomas W. Maretzki, 1–31. Boston: D. Reidel Publishing.

Clements, Deborah S. 2018. Social determinants of health in family medicine residency education. *Annals of Family Medicine* 16 (2): 178. https://doi.org/10.1370/afm.2211.

Coalition for Community Schools. 2019. *Frequently asked questions about community schools*. http://www.communityschools.org/aboutschools/faqs.aspx. Accessed 19 June 2019.

Cohen, Deborah J., and Benjamin F. Crabtree. 2008. Evaluative criteria for qualitative research in health care: controversies and recommendations. *Annals of Family Medicine* 6 (4): 331–339. https://doi.org/10.1370/afm.818.

Crabtree, Benjamin F., and William L. Miller, eds. 1999. *Doing qualitative research*. Newbury Park, CA: SAGE Publications.

Culhane-Pera, Kathleen A., Robert C. Like, Patricia Lebensohn-Chialvo, and Ronald Loewe. 2000. Multicultural curricula in family practice residencies. *Family Medicine* 32 (3): 167–173.

DiCicco-Bloom, Barbara, and Benjamin F. Crabtree. 2006. The qualitative research interview. *Medical Education* 40: 314–321. https://doi.org/10.1111/j.1365-2929.2006.02418.x.

Fetters, Michael D. 1998. The family in medical decision making: Japanese perspectives. *The Journal of Clinical Ethics* 9 (2): 132–146.

Griffiths, Frances, Jeffrey Borkan, David Byrne, Benjamin F. Crabtree, Chris Dowrick, Jane Gunn, Renata Kokanovic, Sarah Lamb, Antje Lindenmeyer, Michael Parchman, Shmuel Reis, and Jackie Sturt. 2010. Developing evidence for how to tailor medical interventions to the individual patient. *Qualitative Health Research* 20 (12): 1629–1641. https://doi.org/10.1177/1049732310377453.

Guetterman, Timothy C., Michael D. Fetters, and John W. Creswell. 2015. Integrating quantitative and qualitative results in health science mixed methods research through joint displays. *Annals of Family Medicine* 13 (6): 554–561. https://doi.org/10.1370/afm.1865.

Gutierrez, Cecilia, and Peter Scheid. 2002. *The history of family medicine and its impact in US health care delivery*. Leawood, KS: AAFP Foundation.

Hahn, Robert A., and Arthur Kleinman. 1983. Biomedical practice and anthropological theory: frameworks and directions. *Annual Review of Anthropology* 12: 305–333.

Hemmings, Colin P. 2005. Rethinking medical anthropology: how anthropology is failing medicine. *Anthropology & Medicine* 12 (2): 91–103. https://doi.org/10.1080/13648470500139841.

Henry, Stephen G., and Michael D. Fetters. 2012. Video elicitation interviews: a qualitative research method for investigating physician-patient interactions. *Annals of Family Medicine* 10 (2): 118–125. https://doi.org/10.1370/afm.1339.

Jenks, Angela C. 2011. From "lists of traits" to "open-mindedness": emerging issues in cultural competence education. *Culture, Medicine, and Psychiatry* 35: 209–235. https://doi.org/10.1007/s11013-011-9212-4.

Kleinman, Arthur. 1982. The teaching of clinically applied medical anthropology on a psychiatric consultation-liaison service. In *Clinically Applied Anthropology: anthropologists in health science settings*, ed. Noel J. Chrisman and Thomas W. Maretzki, 83–115. Boston: D. Reidel Publishing.

———. 1985. Interpreting illness experience and clinical meanings: how I see clinically applied anthropology. *Medical Anthropology Quarterly* 16 (3): 69–71.

Kleinman, Arthur, and Peter Benson. 2006. Anthropology in the clinic: the problem of cultural competency and how to fix it. *PLoS Medicine* 3 (10): e294. https://doi.org/10.1371/journal.pmed.0030294.

Kleinman, Arthur, Leon Eisenberg, and Byron Good. 1978. Culture, illness, and care: clinical lessons from anthropologic and cross-cultural research. *Annals of Internal Medicine* 88 (2): 251–258. https://doi.org/10.7326/0003-4819-88-2-251.

Konner, Melvin. 1991. The promise of medical anthropology: an invited commentary. *Medical Anthropology Quarterly* 5 (1): 78–82.

Martinez, Iveris L. 2015. Integrating anthropology in medical education: opportunities, challenges, and lessons. *Practicing Anthropology* 37 (1): 35–39.

Metzl, Jonathan M., and Helena Hansen. 2014. Theorizing a new medical engagement with stigma and inequality. *Social Science & Medicine* 103: 126–133. https://doi.org/10.1016/j.socscimed.2013.06.032.

Morgan, Lynn M. 1990. The medicalization of anthropology: a critical perspective on the critical-clinical debate. *Social Science & Medicine* 30 (9): 945–950. https://doi.org/10.1016/0277-9536(90)90141-E.

Mull, Dorothy S., Nghia Nguyen, and Dennis J. Mull. 2001. Vietnamese diabetic patients and their physicians: what ethnography can teach us. *Western Journal of Medicine* 175: 307–311. https://doi.org/10.1136/ewjm.175.5.307.

New England Journal of Medicine: Knowledge +. 2019. *ABFM Family Medicine Blueprint*. https://knowledgeplus.nejm.org/products/abfm-family-medicine-blueprint/. Accessed 19 June 2019.

Phillips, Michael R. 1985. Can "clinically applied anthropology" survive in medical care settings? *Medical Anthropology Quarterly* 16 (2): 31–36. https://doi.org/10.1111/j.1937-6219.1985.tb00964.x.

Press, Irwin. 1990. Levels of explanation and cautions for a critical clinical anthropology. *Social Science & Medicine* 30 (9): 1001–1009. https://doi.org/10.1016/0277-9536(90)90146-J.

Stein, Howard F. 1982. The ethnographic mode of teaching clinical behavioral science. In *Clinically Applied Anthropology: anthropologists in health science settings*, ed. Noel J. Chrisman and Thomas W. Maretzki, 61–82. Boston: D. Reidel Publishing.

———. 1985. Principles of style: a medical anthropologist as clinical teacher. *Medical Anthropology Quarterly* 16 (3): 64–67. https://doi.org/10.1111/j.1937-6219.1985.tb00983.x.

———. 1991. The role of some nonbiomedical parameters in clinical decision making: an ethnographic approach. *Qualitative Health Research* 1 (1): 6–26. https://doi.org/10.1177/104973239100100102.

Taylor, Janelle S. 2003. Confronting "culture" in medicine's "culture of no culture". *Academic Medicine* 78 (6): 555–559.

Ventres, William B., and Meredith P. Fort. 2014. Eyes wide open: an essay on developing an engaged awareness in global medicine. *BMC International Health and Human Rights* 14: 29. http://www.biomedcentral.com/1472-698X/14/29.

Ventres, William B., and Richard M. Frankel. 1996. Ethnography: a stepwise approach for primary care researchers. *Family Medicine* 28: 52–56.

Wade, Derick T., and Peter W. Halligan. 2004. Do biomedical models of illness make for good healthcare systems? *BMJ* 329: 1398–1401. https://doi.org/10.1136/bmj.329.7479.1398.

Wagner, Robin, Nancy J. Koh, Carl Patow, Robin Newton, Baretta R. Casey, Kevin B. Weiss, and CLER Program. 2016. Detailed findings from the CLER National Report of Findings 2016. *Journal of Graduate Medical Education* Supplement, May: 35–54. https://doi.org/10.4300/1949-8349.8.2s1.35.

Willen, Sarah S., and Elizabeth Carpenter-Song. 2013. Cultural competence in action: "Lifting the hood" on four case studies in medical education. *Culture, Medicine, and Psychiatry* 37: 241–252. https://doi.org/10.1007/s11013-013-9319-x.

Mary Alice Scott, PhD is Associate Professor of Anthropology and graduate faculty in the integrated Behavioral Health Program at New Mexico State University. She is also adjunct research faculty at the Southern New Mexico Family Medicine Residency Program. She received her B.A. in Women's Studies from Duke University and her M.A. and Ph.D. in Anthropology from the University of Kentucky. Her current research is part of an academic-community collaboration with a team of NMSU students and faculty and the residency program. The team documents cultures of medicine, focusing on the professional development of new physicians. The objectives of the research are (1) to develop innovative educational systems that better prepare physicians to deliver high quality health care in increasingly complex social and cultural environments and (2) to challenge traditional cultures of medicine that have led to harm to physician well-being, patient safety, and community health outcomes. She has expertise in community-based participatory research and has served as a qualitative research design consultant on two NIH-funded grants that have used mixed-methods strategies for data collection. Her research has been funded by the National Science Foundation, a Fulbright-García Robles grant, the University of Kentucky Graduate School, Elon University, the New Mexico State University College of Arts & Sciences, the Southwest and Border Cultures Institute, the New Mexico Humanities Council, and the National Institutes of Health.

Ernesto A. Moralez, is an Assistant Professor of Public Health and Co-Coordinator of the Public Health Minor at St. Lawrence University in Canton, New York. He received his Master's of Public Health from New Mexico State University and his Ph.D. in Health and Behavioral Sciences from the University of Colorado Denver. His graduate research focused on the impact of chronic illness on depression treatment in primary care among low-income patient populations. His clinical research experience has focused on training family medicine residents in communication strategies to discuss pain symptoms and treatment management. He has also served as a program evaluator for clinic-based interventions aimed at tobacco cessation among pregnant women and the use of community health workers in hospital settings.Currently, he is exploring the roles of community health workers and their capacity to address cancer health disparities in rural communities. He has published in the Journal of Cancer Prevention, the Journal of Education and Health Promotion, the Journal of Consulting and Clinical Psychology, and the Journal of the American Board of Family Medicine. He has taught both undergraduate and graduate courses in public health, integrative health practices, health and wellness coaching, and health psychology.

John Andazola, MD, FAAFP is the Program Director of the Southern New Mexico Family Medicine Residency Program in Las Cruces, New Mexico. He received his MD from the University of New Mexico School of Medicine. He completed his Family Medicine residency at the Southern New Mexico Family Medicine Residency Program in Las Cruces, New Mexico. He also completed fellowships in Advanced Hospital Training for Family Physicians and in Faculty Development in Phoenix, Arizona and the University of Arizona. Dr. Andazola has been involved in academic medicine his entire career and has presented at numerous local, state, and national conferences. He has authored several book chapters and peer-reviewed publications. He is President of the Board for the New Mexico Primary Care Training Consortium, Past President of the New Mexico Academy of Family Physicians, and a board member of the Center for Health Innovation (New Mexico's Public Health Institute). He is also an inaugural member of the National Physician Advisory Board for LifePoint Health. His interests include health equity, inter-professional training, and social accountability in medical education. Dr. Andazola has numerous state and national awards that recognize his contributions to public service and to the community.

Part V
Conclusion

Chapter 16
Contributions, Constraints, and Facilitations for Sustained Engagement of Anthropology in Medical Education

Dennis W. Wiedman and Iveris L. Martinez

Introduction

The chapters in this book present a broad historical and global perspective of the many roles anthropologists have had in medical education, medical schools, and the training of physicians. While anthropologists have engaged in medical education for over 100 years, their roles and opportunities in medical schools has significantly expanded since the early 1980s with the community health movement, deinstitutionalization of mental hospitals, grass-roots political movements calling for more equitable and accessible care of minorities, health management organizations, and national policies, priorities and funding for patient-centered and socially responsible health care. These political and economic structural factors empowered applied and practicing anthropologists to address a wide array of human concerns, among which is the medical school training of physicians. The years from the late 1980s to the present will be looked back upon as a time of shifting priorities and transformational responses to medicine and medical care (Chap. 2).

Anthropologists are being called upon to join medical school initiatives to reconfigure a more humanistic curriculum, to refocus on clinical patient care, on patient life situations in the family and community, health inequalities, distribution of health services, and caring for culturally diverse patients, as well as government

---

Dennis W. Wiedman and Iveris L. Martinez contributed equally to the thinking, writing, and production of this chapter.

D. W. Wiedman (✉)
Department Global and Sociocultural Studies, School of International and Public Affairs, Florida International University, Miami, FL, USA
e-mail: wiedmand@fiu.edu

I. L. Martinez
Center for Successful Aging, College of Health and Human Services, California State University - Long Beach, Long Beach, CA, USA

I. L. Martinez, D. W. Wiedman (eds.), *Anthropology in Medical Education*,
https://doi.org/10.1007/978-3-030-62277-0_16

policies. Many chapter author's reflections on their individual experiences reveal the personal and professional tensions these new roles generated, the awkwardness, and the status differences. Stepping back from these personal reflections, we see that these tensions stem from a commonality of being enmeshed in shifting health care priorities, structural reorganizations, and transformational responses of the time. The most recent generation of anthropologists in medical education often find themselves in newly created, named and contested departments within the very traditional hierarchical social structure of biomedicine. Anthropologists are not specifically trained to teach social, cultural, and humanistic principles to biological science and clinical based medical students. Numerous authors reflect on this feeling of professional inadequacy working on issues that had not been published in the journal literature, or being so busy, they did not have time to review. This is a generation of innovators, creating things as they encountered new situations in their medical school careers.

It is from the experiences of this generation of anthropologists in medical schools in the last 25 years that we assemble the major contributions, constraints, and ways to facilitate anthropology's impact and influence on the future training of anthropologists, physicians, and health professionals for better health care for all. We begin with contributions, or the various ways that anthropology contributed to the planning, curriculum, management, and evaluation of medical schools. Constraints are those aspects of medical education, the culture of medicine or anthropology, institutional structures, policies, and other factors that restrict anthropologists successful engagement in medical education. Facilitations are actions that would facilitate, or make easier anthropological engagement in medical school teaching, research and successful careers.

Many of these constraints are not new. In fact, Thomas Weaver succinctly identified many of these in the late 1960s:

> These problems have involved difficulties in accommodating his materials and teaching methods to medical curriculum requirements, in resolving methodological and conceptual differences between himself and the medical field, in adjusting to a different social and academic environment, and in compensating for the inadequate development of his own science. (Thomas Weaver 1968, 6)

The aim of this chapter is to summarize what anthropologists, as well as the field of medical education, can do better to ensure more successful and sustained engagement of anthropologists in medical education. Applied medical anthropologists primarily emphasize improving health outcomes for populations, including changing health care delivery for the better. Strategically, one of the key ways to do this is to influence the training of physicians.

Methods

Given the richness of the chapter information in this volume, and the array of topics covered, we implemented an analytical method to prioritize the contributions, constraints, and facilitations to highlight in this chapter. We analyzed the "data" from each chapter by assigning topical key phrases and words, aggregating these into major topics, searching for patterns and importance. From this process emerged a narrative weaving together the most salient points emerging from the chapters in this volume. Special attention was placed on issues recurrently reported on by authors or issues that the editors considered critical to the future engagement and influence of anthropologists. Hopefully, this chapter stimulates readers to return to the original chapters.

Contributions

Contributions of anthropology to medical education and medical research over the last century are numerous. Some notable contributions are in the areas of comparative anatomy, human evolution, forensic pathology, pediatric growth and development, nutrition, doctor-patient communication, health disparities, ethnomedicine, culture-bound syndromes, and more recently patient-centered medicine. Of critical importance are political and economic forces, including the exercise of power, in shaping wellness, disease, illness experience, and healthcare. Anthropologists have the knowledge and ability to teach medical students to consider these factors, including the ethnocentric tendency for biomedicine to summarily dismiss ancient and "alternative" treatments and local community healers, as quackery or worse, unsafe (Chap. 12). These contributions are not always encompassed within a specific course, but are often incorporated into existing courses.

Below we highlight anthropology's four core contributions to medical education: 1) ethnography, 2) community engagement and understanding the socio-cultural context of health, 3) communication and collaborative skills, as well as 4) organizational development and management.

Ethnography

Among anthropological contributions to medical education, ethnography has been paramount. Employed in numerous ways, ethnography is frequently used as a tool for understanding medical school culture, and a method for sensitizing students to socio-cultural issues. For example, Dikomitis (Chap. 5) carried out participant observation, the principal method of ethnographic research, both inside and outside the classroom, including labs, clinical settings, lectures, and during informal contacts with students. Rushing and McMullin implemented ethnographic methods in the development of an interdisciplinary humanities curriculum at a community-based medical school (Chap. 10). Wiedman used ethnography for building a consensus among faculty, administrators, and community representatives on the university strategic plan that included a vision for a new medical school (Chap. 6).

The importance of ethnography to address community health issues in the process of educating students is highlighted throughout many chapters in this book. For example, Chileshe (Chap. 7) incorporates ethnography to engage Zambian students in local resource-poor communities. Using participant observations they take part in the family activities from morning till late afternoon with instructions to observe the social and economic situation and the cultural practices of the family. The idea behind the community home visits is to learn a holistic approach to health, as well as stimulating students to think about how best they can use local networks and resources to address local health needs in communities.

Likewise, McKellin (Chap. 8) integrated home interviews for first and second year medical students. Pairs of students were matched with people who had genetic conditions or chronic illness, observing the physical accommodations they made to their apartments and houses, and how their conditions shaped individuals' decisions about accessing medical, social, and educational services. Students were often surprised to learn that patients and families' experiences were often more profoundly affected by the barriers they encountered and the support they received in the community than by their interactions with health professionals in clinics.

These are only a few examples of how the primary method of anthropological enquiry, ethnography, can contribute to medical education.

Community Engagement and Understanding the Socio-cultural Context of Health

Anthropologists are often in the role of medical school experts in community health beliefs and practices, and as facilitators of medical school's engagement with the surrounding community, bridging the gaps between clinical medicine and community healthcare needs, and placement of medical students in community-based training experiences. Research and action programs in community-based health care systems, giving accessibility to the economically and socially marginal, and noting economic and political power hierarchies are other key roles for anthropologists in medical education. They may also serve as external evaluators of these community programs. The demand for community-engaging skills were facilitated by the community health movements of the 1960s and 1970s (Chap. 2). For example, in developing their "*CARE: Community Action Research and Education,*" to respond to social determinants of health in Upstate New York, Rubinstein and Lane (Chap. 14) saw themselves as long-term fieldworkers maintaining relationships with community partners, medical learning activities and research that benefit both the students, the community and the health care agencies.

Several medical schools have recently foregone an affiliation with one hospital and instead adopted a community-based teaching model, in which there is no primary teaching hospital, but rather students train in a network of local community health clinics, hospitals, and medical practices. This approach positions schools of medicine to meet a mission of social accountability and serve the medically underserved. Florida International University's Wertheim College of Medicine, and the University of California, Riverside School of Medicine, are two such examples highlighted in this volume (Chaps. 6, 10, and 13). The community-based medical education approach prioritizes immersing students in communities to learn about and address social determinants of health disparities. It also offers students the opportunity to observe and reflect on the complexities of health beyond the clinical setting.

Outside the United States, community-engaged approaches to medical education have a long and established history. For example, Maya and Vega detail how health care at the community level was at the foundation of training physicians in Mexico since the 1930s. Anthropologists began as faculty in the 1960s. All students in the last stage of the Medical Surgery Career Study Plan have the obligation to provide their medical services for 1 year free of charge in a rural community. According to Maya and Vega, "their social service is designed as a sustained experiential learning experience so that they may not only witness, but also contend, with how social determinants of health—specifically, gender inequality, poverty, political disempowerment, isolation in rural environments, lack of education, and racial discrimination—determine health outcomes, including who lives and who dies." (Chap. 9). This approach also aims to resist assumptions that the "indigenous worldviews" are opposed to the logic of biomedical knowledge, while developing cultural competencies for future physicians to provide culturally competent care in community clinic settings ensuring health care access, particularly for the indigenous population in Mexico.

Anthropologists are uniquely equipped to develop learning opportunities in community contexts, and especially in building medical school relationships with communities of diverse cultural groups.

Communication and Collaboration Skills

One of the key contributions of the field of anthropology to medical education is our cross-cultural collaboration skills. Anthropology is unique among academic disciplines for its dominant perspective of "holism," the perspective that the mind, body, individuals, society, and the environment are integral to understanding the whole of the human condition. Encompassing past, present, and future with biology, society and culture, anthropology transects the full range of academic inquiry from the hard sciences to the humanities. Anthropology holism tries to integrate all that is known about human beings and their activities. The way anthropology defines, describes, and evaluates a problem is holistic, seeing the tensions and gaps between the individual, the system, and institutional elements. Anthropologists strive to translate the languages used by the different peoples and disciplines into something an ordinary person can understand, and attempt to correct misunderstandings and contradictions in values, meanings and procedures.

Hence, anthropologists can be effective communicators and collaborators, not only with local communities, but also across academic disciplines that medicine intersects with in practice. Understanding the language and communication styles of medicine and medical education in order to effectively engage physician colleagues is similar to learning a second language when anthropologists do fieldwork abroad. Collaboration and good communication skills are key to buy-in from leadership, other faculty, and community. Scott and Moralez (Chap. 15) attribute their success in integrating anthropological perspectives into a family medicine residency program on their being effective collaborators and not only critical of the prior curricular content and structure.

Furthermore, anthropologists can help medical students become better communicators and collaborators. As Iida and Nishigori (Chap. 4) note, anthropology can provide the viewpoints and frameworks that allow practitioners to verbalize their uncertain feelings and consider the issues in the social and cultural contexts in which they occur. Their approach in clinical case conferences is to illustrate that apparently irrational narratives and behaviors have meanings in the context of patients' lives and social relations. While similar at first glance, the collaborative clinical case conference approach is distinct from a narrative-based approach that has been popularized in medicine in the last twenty years, as they introduce anthropological theoretical concepts throughout the process.

Another area where anthropologists enhance communication and collaboration is facilitating communication among medical disciplines in order to provide interdisciplinary teamwork so critical in the clinical setting. Martinez (Chap. 13) demonstrates the effectiveness of teaching students to communicate and function as part of an interprofessional team, a skill that is now referred to as IPE or IPP, interprofessional teamwork education and practice. Margaret Read (1970) alluded to the usefulness of anthropology in interprofessional experiences as far back as the early 1970s. The role of anthropology in interprofessional education goes hand in hand with our role in highlighting and addressing health disparities. Medical students and physicians are often overwhelmed by the health disparities and social issues that impact their patient's health, and therefore become frustrated by the presentation of information that they feel they cannot do anything about. Anthropologists can play an important role in teaching them to communicate and function as part of an interprofessional team to address these concerns by recognizing when issues exist and learning to refer patients to other professions, such as social work, dietetics, psychologists, and community support resources (Chap. 14). Barriers to health is an area that anthropologists have and can contribute to as they function as cultural brokers between disciplines that often miscommunicate with each other.

Organizational Development and Management

Anthropologists serve in roles and functions that contribute to making medical schools more effective. Teaching courses and conducting research are the expected indicators of academic productivity, however, service to departments and universities may be even more important for the anthropological profession to influence positive changes while supporting the organization's mission and goals. As a profession, anthropology has over a hundred years of research on social group formation, social structures and culture change processes. Many chapters provide examples of anthropologists working to develop new programs, organizing faculty, and managing administrative units, while communicating anthropological perspectives. These provide examples of how anthropologists purposefully and consciously direct their time and efforts to influencing the structures of medicine.

For example, Rushing and McMullin (Chap. 10) led a work group of interdisciplinary faculty in developing an innovative health humanities program at the University of California-Riverside Medical School merging health training with academic anthropological theory to develop a curriculum while creating an organizational structure for the humanities program. Translation among divergent paradigms and pedagogy of the humanities, arts and social sciences demonstrates their knowledge of sociocultural and organizational change processes to actually implement these in the management of the organizations. Bridging organizational cultures within the health sciences is a skill that promotes the career long success of anthropologists in medical schools.

Likewise, Iveris Martinez (Chap. 13) played several influential administrative roles during her tenure at the newly formed Wertheim College of Medicine at Florida International University. As the founding Chief of the Division of Medicine & Society in the Department of Health and Humanities, she developed the original vision, created policies to ensure equity among the faculty, and played a key role in establishing an interprofessional household visiting program. Both her background in anthropology and community-based participatory research developed and implemented this innovative program. As an anthropologist, her ability of working across professional cultures led to her establishing and chairing an interprofessional education committee that organized a yearly workshop with approximately 500 students across nine health professions. She also chaired the college of Medicine's admissions committee, helping establish processes for diversifying the pool of admitted students as part of the college's mission to recruit students that represented the diversity of the local community.

Dennis Wiedman (Chap. 6) served as Director of an out-patient community mental health clinic of the Department of Psychiatry, University of Miami Miller School of Medicine. This administrative role implemented the concept of "culture broker" theorized by anthropologist Hazel Weidman as a professional role for clinical anthropologist managers who could liaison between biomedical culture and the local community to provide culturally sensitive health care. This prepared him to work in the Provost Office of Florida International University contributing to policy development, planning, accreditation, and program evaluations establishing institutional structures that continue long into the future such as the planning and conceptualization of the Wertheim College of Medicine. Over the years, he published on these practicing anthropology roles from the perspective of directing organizational culture change.

Robert Rubenstein and Sandra Lane (Chap. 14) effectively established a consortium across health and education institutions in upstate New York to address community health concerns. They collaboratively brought together faculty and students from the Upstate Medical University, Medicine and Bioethics programs; University at Buffalo School of Social Work; Syracuse University programs in Anthropology, Public Health, Marriage and Family Therapy; Le Moyne College Physician Assistant Program; and the Nursing program at Sage Colleges to share curriculum, evaluation materials, faculty development materials, and jointly publish results of integrating the curricula. Sandra Lane was also pivotal at the national level chairing the National Academies of Science, Engineering, and Medicine Committee that authored the Framework for Educating Health Professionals to Address the Social Determinants of Health (2016). This framework for integrating the social determinants of health into health professional education, is being used nationally to guide the development and implementation of curriculum across the health professions.

Contributions of anthropologists to program development, policies, and management are important ways for anthropologists to influence organizational structures and future behaviors.

Constraints

Science, Humanism, and What Counts as Evidence

Despite changes in requirements for entry into medical school, the majority of medical students come from a physical or biological science background. While social sciences has increasingly become a component of medical education, social science knowledge is often still considered peripheral learning content by medical students. Clinical and basic science faculty tend to reinforce these misunderstandings and misconceptions of the social sciences and anthropology contributions to medical education (see Chap. 5). Socio-cultural information is often deemed "common sense," "fluff," or non-science, and therefore not critically assessed or integrated into clinical thinking.

In general, "science" as recognized by biomedicine is a reductionist process where exceedingly complex phenomena are reduced to the smallest unit and some type of formula is presented to resolve the problem. Scientific reductionism versus narrative explanations of phenomena is a major challenge for anthropologists and humanists teaching in medicine. Medical students expect teachers to reduce knowledge down to the simplest, easiest memorizable formula. Reading and preparing for tests (which in turn impacts class rank) in medical school traditionally entails memorization of "facts" especially in the first 2 years of study. Studying social science and humanism, requires a different type of skills, including reflection, abstraction and critical analysis. Therefore, it is not uncommon to have medical students who may not have been exposed to social science and humanism to underline and highlight their reading materials in search of "facts" to memorize. This was noted by more than one medical teacher in this volume (see Chaps. 3 and 5, for example). This is one of the greatest challenges faced by anthropologists for success in medical education, particularly since anthropologists tend to express themselves in abstract theory and principles primarily in narrative and story form, instead of brief, succinct factual statements.

Within humanities faculties, anthropologists may face challenges based on moral medical practices and teaching pedagogies built upon the western philosophy of the individual and self. Allopathic medicine is focused on the body, diseased part, diseases and the individual patient's responsibility to follow the doctor's regimen. As Rushing and McMullin (Chap. 10) explain, at the foundation of Medicine is the central humanist model of the autonomous self, a coherent, bounded individual with intentional thought, action, and belief. This emphasis on the individual becomes problematic for anthropologists entering a medical humanities program who question the hegemony of the humanist tradition that transforms differences in patients, communities and cultures, into familiar western epistemologies and ontologies. Anthropologists find themselves in a tense but fundamental role to problematize the cultural specificity of the Western ideal of the self and related values of individualism. It becomes the role of anthropologists to draw upon the cross-cultural ethnographic evidence on cultural variations of 'personhood,' integrating into medical education the biological, social, cultural, historical, political, economic, technological and environmental conditions that make possible the selves of patients, doctors, as well as the broader constructions of the Western self.

This science-humanism constraint exists within the discipline of anthropology itself. Anthropology institutional structures continue to constrain anthropologists since the culture wars that occurred in anthropology with the ascendency of postmodernism's denial of scientific validity. During the 2000–2010s, many Departments of Anthropology fractioned into the humanists versus the scientific. This ideological conflict affected the editors of the flagship journal the "American Anthropologist," as well as the premier professional organization, the American Anthropological Association (AAA). Founded in 1902, the AAA is the largest professional organization for anthropologists in the world. It was founded as a scientific society and is today considered both a science and a humanities. By 2004 however, an influential portion of AAA membership rejected the idea that anthropology can be or should be a science. This science v. humanism ideological and structural conflict within the discipline of anthropology continues to impact the effectiveness of students we train who want to join medical school faculty. Anthropologists working with biomedical scientists in medical schools must be able to rationally argue with each other to find the best approach. Medical schools are not the ideal employment for anthropologists who think science itself is the problem. Anthropology is arguably both a science and a humanity.

Clinical Relevance

Similarly, anthropologists are challenged to be succinct and demonstrate the relevance and applicability of anthropological knowledge in clinical discussions, such as ground rounds and in patient care settings. Grand rounds are a methodology of medical education that consists of presenting medical problems and treatment of a particular patient to an audience of attending physicians, residents, and students. Anthropologists are challenged to succinctly answer questions about a patient in grand rounds, often giving an example through a story. However, depending on the nature of this story and how it is framed, they may or may not be effective with the majority of medical students.

Funding and Research Constraints

Non-clinician anthropologists are not able to participate completely in all of the medical and health professional students' activities. This distinction is reinforced with research funding and criteria for promotion. Clinical and basic research with scientific based controlled laboratory studies are preferred. Especially in the US, financial pressures that academic health centers face have bolstered the expectation that all medical school faculty participate in grant and contract revenues to generate a portion of their salaries. Conducting extramurally funded research provides salary reimbursement, benefits, and institutional overhead. This usually involves securing highly competitive National Institute of Health grants to fund "science-based" medical research on topics of programmatic interest to the funding agency. Clinical research brings in much larger amounts of dollars from national foundations and government agency grants and contracts.

These aspects of biomedical academic life can devalue the types of research anthropologists do. Rigorously conducting clinical research in assessing the safety and efficacy of novel pharmaceutical drugs, medical devices, and procedures, are costly, impersonal, and narrowly focused on random controlled tests (RCT). These are the gold standard that treatments must undergo to be considered "evidence-based." Anthropologist's research and teaching on traditional healing and medicines used in the community are less valued. Centuries of historical use and experimentation are not recognized as high quality evidence in the evidence-based model (EBM) of medicine today (see Chap. 12). Furthermore, clinical faculty may question anthropological methods of ethnography, interviewing, archival research, and participant observation.

Publishing in medical fields usually presents highly technical journal articles with multiple faculty listed as authors. This is in contrast to anthropology where sole author journal articles are the ideal and most rewarded. These discipline distinctions and cultural values affect teamwork versus individual researcher dynamics within the everyday life in the department influencing social interactions, support networks, and academic promotions over one's career. Even the kinds of research questions and methodological designs influence how anthropologists are integrated into the medical school culture. While anthropologists are generally good at developing relationships with communities, they are generally trained to be lone scholars and teachers, which can be challenging in integrating into medical education and research.

Status Gap

Anthropology faculty are usually associated with "lower grade" subjects (Read 1970) such as prevention, community, family medicine, and psychiatry. Anthropologists find themselves at the bottom of the hierarchy in the medical setting under other basic science Ph.D. faculty that teach foundational courses in biochemistry, anatomy and physiology, etc. who are themselves under clinician faculty (MDs). Physician salaries are significantly greater than those offered Ph.D.s, and females continue to have pay inequalities. These powerful social structural constraints with resulting status and income inequalities, may go counter to the values that bring persons into anthropology in the first place and make it difficult for them to function. This "status" gap is also reflected in the time allocated to social science and humanities topics in the curriculum. Finding "time" in the curriculum to effectively teach this material is a major challenge. Medical schools and residencies are nationally rated and ranked according to student performance on standardized tests. "Teaching to the test" and the "hidden curriculum" structurally dominates decisions for what is allowed in the curriculum and the time spent on each topic. Numerous instances in these chapters tell of the struggles to place the social sciences and humanities in the curriculum, then the gradual reduction over time of these topics.

Hidden Curriculum

Anthropology is among the subjects that while not explicitly stated as such is associated with learning of less importance. Several chapter authors noted the "hidden curriculum" is just as important in enculturating students to the culture of medicine and the medical school. The "hidden curriculum" resides outside the formal curriculum and reflects what students learn implicitly by example as they learn to become physicians. The hidden curriculum consists of "positive and negative lessons, which are embedded in organizational structure and culture, are the hidden curricula conveyed in medical schools, residency programs, hospitals, and clinics." (Lehman et al. 2018). This is often contradictory to what is explicitly taught in teaching settings. This moral economy of values, ritual behaviors, beliefs and ethical assumptions are important as much, if not more, than medical knowledge and technical skills. Dikomitis (Chap. 5) explores how the hidden curriculum is a cultural process through which students learn what is and what should be valued in clinical practice. Physicians-in-training learn to subjectively define patients in ways that guide their interactions and influence decisions about the patient's medical care. Higashi et al. (2013) argue that providing the 'best care possible' becomes a highly qualified, subjective endeavor, and strategies for accomplishing this are learned through the medical school "hidden curriculum."

Medical Teacher Credentialing

Accreditation requirements, at least in the United States, specify that teachers have degrees in the field they are teaching, or a certain number of graduate credits on the topic. Although Ph.D. anthropologists are employed in medical schools, it is the M.D. faculty that have the accreditation legitimacy to teach the courses and to serve in authoritative administrative positions. This segregation pertains to all the behavioral, humanities, and social sciences Ph.D. faculty in medical schools marginalizing their direct training of future physicians. Often team teaching resolves this issue with an M.D. faculty as the lead teacher, the instructor of record who is responsible for the course content and assigning grades. Furthermore, disciplinary investments, individual personalities, and institutional expectations often thwart attempts to include anything new into medical education, particularly courses that are not taught by MDs and raises concerns among some physicians who believe that students' professional socialization by physicians is diluted by non-physician teachers. Although the anthropologist may be the primary developer of the course content, we see a tendency over time for an M.D. to take over the course encouraging the anthropologist to move along to other endeavors, overlooking the unique contributions of anthropological frameworks and a loss of interest in anthropology. While social science principles are increasingly recognized as important to understanding of health and disease by accrediting bodies (AAMC 2011; General Medical Council 2018), sociology and psychology are often mentioned, with anthropology yet to be explicitly recognized as a contributing discipline. On one hand accreditation calls for more behavioral science, on the other hand criteria constrain the recognition of anthropology in medical school curriculum and training of physicians.

Identity Loss and Isolation

Anthropologists employed in medical schools often assimilate to the culture of biomedicine taking on the role expected of them while losing the identity and core values of anthropology. Chapter authors often expressed their experiences in awkward social roles, feeling caught between differing worldviews, and identity loss. This is perhaps most clearly illustrated by Crowder and McDonald (Chap. 11) in their chapter on implementing a medical humanities program at the University of Texas. By constructing and redefining their own individual and professional identities in this process, they found themselves "wearing a cloak and many hats." This loss of identity and the subsequent sense of isolation was highlighted by various authors. In fact, as early as 1968, Weaver noted the predominant "utilitarian case study approach" of medical education and research, focusing on specific individuals or diseases, results in "philosophical isolation" of anthropologists (Weaver 1968: 6).

Isolation is also from one's own field of anthropology. Anthropologists who practice in medicine are seen by fellow anthropologists as at risk of losing the critical perspective central to medical anthropology and as being "co-opted" by medicine. Furthermore, it is hard to find the anthropologists and the anthropological contributions in medicine because the task of teaching and publishing in medical education can be all-absorbing. They may be required to publish mainly in recognized medical journals, instead of anthropological ones. They may attend medical education conferences, instead of anthropology conferences. Moreover, they may have little time or opportunity to engage in anthropological scholarship.

Lack of Adequate Preparation for Roles in Medicine

Anthropologists often enter medical education by chance, or when an unexpected opportunity presents itself. A career in medical education does not appear to be an expected or planned career option for anthropologists. It almost appears serendipitous by being in the right place at the right time, meeting those who are open to the skills and knowledge base of anthropologists, rather than a systematic area of study and career track. Barriers to practice in medical education also stem from within anthropology itself as a field, and the training anthropologists receive. There is a general lack of understanding into the process of medical education and culture of biomedicine, as well as a lack of empathy for the enculturation process through which medical students are put through to turn them into physicians. Leze is a prime example of what can be a shocking experience at first for anthropologists teaching in medicine (Chap. 3).

Diverse four-field training of anthropologists in biological, archaeological, linguistic and cultural anthropology is a strength of anthropology's holism setting it off from the other academic disciplines. When anthropologists join a medical school faculty each bring their distinct anthropology training theories, methods, and data.

There is no one "Anthropology." This makes it difficult for medical school deans and faculty to understand how anthropologists can contribute. The wide variety of roles and programs contained in these chapters, is evidence of this diversity.

Anthropology has been very adept at criticizing biomedical culture and the process of enculturation of medical students, rarely have these critiques been of a constructive nature. Furthermore, knowledge of these critiques within biomedicine can create resistance and skepticism about anthropologist's motives (Johnson 1991, p.127). The dominant political-economy theory of "Critical Medical Anthropology," often has harsh words for allopathic physicians, their hegemony in the health care system, and the biomedical model of disease. We now have 20 years of training medical anthropology students from the critical anthropology perspective making it the most pervasive perspective in the field. "Structural violence," "Biomedical Domination," are recurrent phrases that portray the cultural themes in our narratives and publications. These same phrases and theoretical positions create responses from physicians and biomedical scientists that further marginalize anthropologists from the core of medical education, creating resistance and skepticism about anthropologist's motives. To be effective in medical education, anthropologists must be trained to purposefully deconstruct their own positions, theoretical foundations, and professional institutional structures in order to facilitate their career success in medical schools.

Facilitating Sustained Engagement and Impact

Are anthropologists employed in medical schools a sustainable trend or passing fancy? This book brings to light and discusses many critical issues about anthropology's role in medical schools. How effectively has anthropology been integrated into medical school education? What is anthropology's role and magnitude of influence? Beyond the individual, what are the institutional commitments or structures that would facilitate sustained engagement? What are some potential models or strategies for sustained engagement? How do we better prepare anthropology students to fulfill emerging roles in medical education?

> The anthropologist cannot make a real contribution. . .if he simply acquires the jargon of the science, and is content for the rest to "trot out" his little ethnographic museum of esoteric curios. He can make a real contribution...only if he remains an anthropologist, a student of culture, defined as a patterned way of experiencing both extra-social and social reality. George Devereux (1956: 47)

While there is a recognition of the value of anthropology to medical education for several decades and calls for their integration, the engagement of anthropologists with medical educators has been inconsistent at best. Throughout the decades of anthropologists teaching in medical schools, concrete recommendations have been made for success in these roles. However, many of these recommendations are buried in the literature, many of which are not readily available. Moreover, given the changing nature of medical practice and education, these challenges need to be revisited and expanded upon to be useful to anthropologists today. By way of concluding this volume, we offer several ways that anthropological engagement in medical education can be improved and sustained moving forward.

Maintaining Anthropological Identity

One of the professional challenges that anthropologists in medical schools often suffer from like others in applied or practice settings, is a loss of identity as an anthropologist and isolation from the very field and paradigms that makes them valuable. While anthropologists may be tempted to hide their identification as an anthropologist in a "stealth" mode, by doing so we miss the opportunity to have others understand the importance of the specific contributions of anthropology as a field compared to other disciplines. This includes ensuring the understanding and buy-in of key stakeholders, including medical students, medical educators, clinicians and administrators, as well as providing them with practical and specific ways that can facilitate the integration of anthropology into medical education.

While anthropologists often find themselves "hiding" their anthropological identities in order to integrate into roles in medical education, ironically, maintaining an identity as an anthropologist is perhaps one of the key facilitators to being more effective as medical educators. As chapter author Mutale Chileshe succinctly expressed:

> I had suspended the 'anthropological identity' in order for me to fully integrate with the medical school. I had abandoned the anthropological tools, perspectives, methods and way of doing things. This approach, however, did not work. Looking back I came to understand that at a medical school the anthropologist assumes no fixed participation but is constantly moving through the different categories of participation. What was important for me then was to keep the 'anthropological identity' in every role. I had to keep and use all the properties—methods, perspectives—of anthropologists which are unique such as fieldwork, participatory approaches which make anthropologists distinct from other disciplines. (see Chap. 7)

Strategies identified by chapter authors that can facilitate anthropologists to maintain their professional identity include repeatedly emphasizing anthropological areas of expertise, always introducing oneself as an anthropologist, being active in professional anthropological associations by presenting papers, serving on committees, editorial and governance boards.

Making Anthropological Perspectives Palatable

Anthropologists teaching in medicine must be able to modify their teaching activities to fit with medical approaches and demonstrate clinical relevance of material, while at the same time trying to communicate the complexities and nuances of anthropological perspectives. Blonder (Chap. 12) notes that the role of anthropologists is not simply to impart relevant information, but to inspire learners to identify prejudices in science-based medicine that may prevent them from investigating traditions and modalities that would otherwise be of value in practice. The chapters in this volume demonstrate diverse strategies to successfully integrate anthropological perspectives to improve the understanding of medical students on the complexities of socio-cultural context and experiences of health and illness, cross-cultural communication, managing uncertainty, valuing integrative medicine, to name a few.

Anthropologists need to be better at expressing theory in short, understandable ways. We need to utilize authoritative scientific journal articles where anthropologists present both grand theories and specific ways in which these affect an individual's biology to demonstrate theoretical constructs in tangible ways. Finding examples within themselves and their daily lives is a powerful teaching tool for medical students. It is also a means of humanizing and countering the process of detachment of themselves as social, cultural and spiritual beings that is prevalent in the enculturation to the culture of medicine. Chapters in this volume provide numerous examples of how this can be done. One format of conveying relevant information that medical students become familiar with and may be helpful to anthropologists "telling stories" is the "clinical pearl." Clinical pearls are best defined as small bits of free standing, clinically relevant information often presented by medical teachers based on their clinical experience or observation. They are part of the vast domain of experience-based medicine and can be helpful in dealing with clinical problems for which controlled data do not exist (Lorin et al. 2008). Moreover, Johnson (1991: 140–141) and Howard Stein (1990) suggest participating actively in attending rounds with physicians and students at the patient's bedside to seize "teaching moments" thereby encouraging students to incorporate anthropology data in their presentation and progress notes. Scott, Moralez, and Andazola recommend that anthropologists can work effectively within the medical education accreditation standards by linking curriculum to required competencies (see Chap. 15). Integrating anthropological content requires flexibility and creativity within a strict structure, as well as using it as a guiding framework.

Changing the Culture of Anthropology: Training Anthropologists for Medical School Careers

For anthropologists to have a greater impact in medical education, they need to be trained specifically on how to do so, by understanding the process of medical education, the culture of biomedicine, and engaging in a process of constructive criticism when necessary without alienating one's students and employers. Four-field graduate programs in anthropology provide a strong foundation for many academic, applied, and practicing careers. Over the past 25 years, M.A. and Ph.D.

granting departments have specialized in training focused on specific applied and practicing career tracks that do not lead to a professorial role in Departments of Anthropology (Nolan 2013). From the chapters in this book, we can discern common career trajectories, necessary skills, and perspectives, that if taught more systematically in graduate schools, their graduates would more likely succeed in medical school roles.

Several important skills and knowledge a graduate school curriculum training anthropologists for roles in medical education should strive for include :

1) Culture, language, and history of biomedicine, faculty and student expectations.
2) Basic comprehension of biological terminology and disease categorizations of biomedicine.
3) Translating major anthropological theories with practical clinical implications.
4) Community studies approaches integrating medical schools, clinics and hospitals.
5) Ethnography with mixed methods approaches combining quantitative and qualitative methods.
6) Teamwork and interprofessionalism.
7) Organizational culture change, planning, policy development, program evaluation, administration and management.
8) Negotiating one's role and compensation within medical education.

Future anthropologists in medical education should be able to differentiate themselves from other discipline, including:

1) Comparative health care systems.
2) Cultural relativity of knowledge and truth, ethnomedical perspective.
3) Holistic perspectives broadening from the biological and anatomical view of disease, methods for understanding views, values, and perceptions of people, both in the community and in the various health professions.
4) Grand time depth of human adaptations resulting in diversity in phenotypes, languages, cultures and health care traditions.

Training programs should include field experiences in hospitals, clinics, neighborhood homes, and alternative health care systems. Dual degree training in M.D./Anthropology Ph.D., public health, and clinically oriented disciplines is another effective way for anthropologists to have a life-long successful health career.

Academic anthropologists often ascribe lower status to applied and practicing anthropologists. An often-heard phrase is that being a university administrator is joining the "dark side," reflecting the worker–employer tension in the social hierarchy of power relationships. Physicians and medical schools are one of the most elite careers and professions with great power and authority. Anthropologists employed in medical schools and anthropology graduate students should be trained to be conscious organizational change agents in order to confidently take on administrative roles that empower them to direct organizational culture change (Wiedman 2013; McCabe and Briody 2018).

Our own professional associations, journals, and funding agencies must recognize and support this influential employment category. Professional organizations need to be more welcoming and supportive of anthropologist careers in medical schools. The Anthropology of Higher Education Interest Group of the Society for Applied Anthropology (SfAA) formed only a half dozen years ago. Their organized sessions provided a forum for the session that brought together the anthropologists for this book, as did a session sponsored by the Society for Medical Anthropology (SMA) at an American Anthropological Association (AAA) conference. The National Association for the Practice of Anthropology (NAPA) and the Council on Anthropology and of Education (CAE) could also strengthen their efforts. A unique organization for medical school anthropologists, or anthropologist-physicians is yet to form. Hopefully, this volume stimulates medical school anthropologists to volunteer on committees and executive boards of these organizations where they can be spokespersons for this important career track.

Furthermore, there is room in the engagement of anthropologists in medical education to emphasize less what is wrong with medical education to focus more on the changes that anthropology as a field can make to be more effective in medicine (see Chap. 7). Very often anthropologists and anthropology as a field has been resistant to this change or perceive it as a negative one. Anthropology as a field should move beyond its "purist" stance and create a "New Anthropology" (Chap. 4), and explore how collaborations with medicine can reshape anthropology in a positive way, shifting from the "anthropology of medicine" to "anthropology with medicine."

Institutional Supports

Finally, for anthropologists to be effective in integrating theories, methods, and perspectives in medical schools, they need to be courageous as applied culture change agents. Teaching courses and conducting research are the expected indicators of academic productivity, however, service to the Department and University may be even more important for the anthropological profession to influence positive changes while supporting the organization's mission and goals. Many chapters provide examples of anthropologists innovatively inserting topics and agendas into medicine and training of future health care providers. A goal of this book is to urge anthropologists to purposefully and consciously direct their time and efforts to influencing the culture of medicine. Facilitating anthropological engagement in medical education goes, however, beyond individual efforts and skills. It requires institutional support both within the field of medicine and anthropology at various levels and involving diverse potential change agents. This includes accrediting bodies, challenging hierarchies within medical school culture, better training anthropologists for success in roles in medical education, and ultimately conversations between professional bodies in both disciplines.

Accreditation Association Policies Accreditation policies can facilitate the integration of anthropologists in medical education. Anthropologists in medical schools need to work to refine professional, accreditation, and national policies specifying behavioral and social science competency. Each country has its own standards for who can practice medicine, their level of training, curriculum content, and years of study. The call for social science, behavioral, and humanistic curriculum in allopathic medical schools has occurred at various times in the countries represented in this book.

At the National Autonomous University of Mexico Medical School, elective subjects related to anthropology have been offered since the mid-1960s. It was in 1985 that the course "History and Philosophy of Medicine" was included as a required course (see Chap. 9). For the United Kingdom, the General Medical Council (GMC) included the social and behavioral sciences as core and vital areas of medical education in 1993 (see Chap. 5). In France (see Chap. 3), a 1995 Ministerial Order required humanities and social sciences in the first year of undergraduate medical studies. The reform of 2009 required Health, Society, and Humanity provide "culture of health" first year core coursework to all the health professions with a common culture and ethics: medicine, pharmacy, odontology, maieutics, and physiotherapy. Meanwhile, in Canada, where both healthcare and medical education are publicly funded, the medical curriculum renewals in the 1990s and 2000s, shifted undergraduate medical education programs to focus on their social responsibilities to their communities and patients (see Chap. 8). Similar efforts came at a later date in the United States (see Chap. 13) and Japan. In 2011, the American Association of Medical Colleges (AAMC) outlined core behavioral and social science competencies for future physicians, noting the contribution of Anthropology to medical education is to: "Accurately describe the influence and potential implications of culture and community context on health behaviors, beliefs and outcomes, as well as how physicians should appropriately integrate this knowledge into patient care." As of 2018, the Liaison Committee on Medical Education, the accrediting body for allopathic medical schools in the United States and Canada, published "Cultural Competence and Health Care Disparities," highlighting the need to address gender and cultural biases and recommending content on "the manner in which people of diverse cultures and belief systems perceive health and illness and respond to various symptoms, diseases, and treatment," as well as health disparities and professional attributes needed for effective care for a diverse society (AAMC, March 2018).

Anthropology and sociology were first incorporated into the model core curriculum of Japanese medical education in 2017. The Educational Commission for Foreign Medical Graduates (ECFMG), announced in 2010 that starting in 2023 physicians applying for ECFMG Certification will be required to graduate from a medical school that has been appropriately accredited through a formal process using accepted criteria, such as those developed by the World Federation for Medical Education that incorporate the social sciences, including medical anthropology (Chap. 4). Therefore, anthropologists need to take an active role in influencing accrediting bodies and their policies to facilitate the integration of anthropology in medical education.

Reducing the Status Gap With the incorporation of psychology, behavioral, social, and cultural in the curriculum, medical school administrators are challenged in creating workable administrative structures to organize social science faculty within traditional medical school departments. Since the early 2000s, new departments with names such as medical humanities and bioethics have formed. From within these institutional structures, anthropologists are taking major roles in curriculum design, course content for training physicians, and research on different aspects of medical education. Some have taken department leadership positions where they have significant power and authority to design new programs, implement budgets, and institutionalize policies and procedures, but often without explicit recognition of the role of anthropological perspectives in these contributions. Dikomitis (Chap. 5) suggests integrating anthropologists as permanent staff members fully into all aspects of the medical education process curriculum development, educational delivery, and assessments, as well as training other faculty to prioritize and integrate social science content.

Dialogue between Medicine and Anthropology at Higher Levels While progress has been made in integrating social science principles in medical education, the role and contributions of anthropology have yet to be explicitly recognized. This will require higher level engagement between professional bodies of medicine and anthropology. Issues of what is recognized as scholarship, job security, and status need to be addressed at the highest levels. The research questions asked and methods used by anthropologists affect obtaining tenure or subsequent promotions, especially if their work does not obviously and significantly contribute to their field. Anthropological contributions addressing health inequalities, how to collaborate, and understand diverse communities is highly valued. Transforming these into the teaching needs of a professional medical school is optimal but raises questions about how to situate the resulting knowledge within disciplinary fields of medicine and anthropology. Disciplinary boundaries are difficult to cross, or blend, leading to the question of how anthropological work in medicine can lead to tenure and promotion if the work does not obviously fit into the field of medicine or anthropology.

Power and authority to be organizational change agents resides much more clearly in administrative positions. Department Chairs, Deans, Presidents, division directors and support roles are opportunities for anthropologists to use our theory, methods, and perspectives to make lasting structural, policy and academic cultural changes. University contracts with medical school faculty frequently differ from regular tenure earning faculty in academic departments. Term limited 1-year, or multiple term contracts, are often the medical school professional relationship with faculty. Since practicing physicians can more easily obtain employment outside of the medical schools, this is the norm at many medical schools. Whereas, life-long tenured contracts are the typical relationship in Departments of Anthropology. This leads to professional mental and economic strains on anthropologists as they uneasily move through their careers and changing roles within the medical school. Once an anthropologist takes a practicing role such as this in a medical school, it is difficult for them to later move to tenure-track positions in traditional anthropology departments. Anthropology departments that desire to train graduate students to teach in a medical school must consider hiring anthropologists with practicing experience in medical schools.

In conclusion, as this volume and chapter demonstrates, anthropologists have made substantial contributions to medical education and to the practice of medicine throughout the last century. The recent call for expanding physician learning to include behavioral and social sciences competencies has widened the space for greater contributions. With the highlighted facilitations in place, including institutional support both within anthropology and medicine, anthropologists employed in medical schools should be better poised to contribute to the field of medical education and play a greater role in improving health outcomes for all.

References

Association of American Medical Colleges (AAMC). 2011. *Behavioral and social science foundations for future physicians*. Washington, DC: Association of American Medical Colleges.

Devereux, George. 1956. Normal and abnormal: the key problem of psychiatric anthropology. In *Some uses of anthropology: theoretical and applied*, ed. Joseph B. Casagrande and Thomas Gladwin. Brooklyn: Theo. Gaus' Sons.

General Medical Council. 2018. Outcome for graduates. https://www.gmc-uk.org/education/standards-guidance-and-curricula/standards-and-outcomes/outcomesfor-graduates. Accessed 26 Aug 2019

Higashi, Robin T., Allison Tillack, Michael A. Steinman, C. Bree Johnston, and G. Michael Harper. 2013. The 'worthy' patient: rethinking the 'hidden curriculum' in medical education. *Anthropology & Medicine* 20 (1): 13–23.

Johnson, Thomas M. 1991. Anthropologists in medical education: ethnographic prescriptions. In *Training manual in applied medical anthropology*, ed. C.E. Hill. Washington, DC: American Anthropological Association.

Lehmann, Lisa Soleymani, Lois Snyder Sulmasy, and Sanjay Desai. 2018. Hidden curricula, ethics, and professionalism: Optimizing clinical learning environments in becoming and being a physician: a position paper of the American College of Physicians. *Annals of internal medicine* 168 (7): 506–508.

Lorin, Martin I., Debra L. Palazzi, Teri L. Turner, and Mark A. Ward. 2008. What is a clinical pearl and what is its role in medical education? *Medical Teacher* 30 (9-10): 870–874.

McCabe, Maryann, and Elizabeth Briody, eds. 2018. *Cultural change from a business anthropology perspective*. Lanham, MD: Lexington Books.

Nolan, Riall W. 2013. *The handbook of practicing anthropology*. Hoboken, NJ: Wiley Blackwell.

Read, Margaret. 1970. Some problems in teaching medical anthropology. *Social Science & Medicine*. 4 (1): 163–167.

Stein, Howard. 1990. *American medicine as culture*. Boulder: Westview Press.

Weaver, Thomas. 1968. *Medical anthropology: trends in research and medical education. Essays on Medical Anthropology*, 1–12. Athens: University of Georgia Press.

Wiedman, Dennis. 2013. Anthropologists working in higher education. In *Handbook of practicing anthropology*, ed. Riall Nolan, 184–195. Hoboken, NJ: Wiley/Blackwell.

Dennis W. Wiedman, PhD, is Professor of Anthropology, Department of Global and Sociocultural Studies. Florida International University. Miami, Florida. He received his Ph.D. in Anthropology from the University of Oklahoma in 1979 where he trained in medical anthropology at the University of Oklahoma College of Medicine. Employment in the Department of Psychiatry at the University of Miami School of Medicine in the Office of Transcultural Education and Research grounded him in clinical anthropology as Director of a Department of Psychiatry community mental health unit. He is the Founding Director of the FIU Global Indigenous Forum with the mission to bring the Indigenous voice to FIU, South Florida, and the world. His research interests include Native American health, Type II diabetes, organizational culture, applying anthropology, and directing culture change. He specializes in social and cultural factors for the global pandemic of Type II diabetes and metabolic syndrome. He teaches courses in medical anthropology, anthropological theory, and ethnohistorical research methods. During more than a decade in the FIU Provost Office he was the Assistant to the Provost, University Accreditation Officer and first Director of Program Review. As lead strategic planner for the university's first major strategic plan he had a key role in planning and envisioning the new FIU Medical school incorporating medical anthropology principles and a community focus. He served on the Executive Board of the American Anthropological Association (AAA) in the practicing/professional seat, and was President of the National Association for the Practice of Anthropology (NAPA). Throughout these academic, applied, and practicing leadership experiences, he consistently published on organizational culture theory and analysis in leading journals and book chapters.

Iveris L. Martinez, PhD is Professor, Archstone Foundation Endowed Chair in Gerontology, and Director of the Center for Successful Aging at California State University, Long Beach. She was a founding faculty member of the Herbert Wertheim College of Medicine (HWCOM) at Florida International University where she served as chief of the Division of Medicine & Society and chaired the admissions committee for the college for 5 years. Between 2007 and 2018, she taught the first year introductory course and other course content on health disparities, cultural competency, and social determinants of health at HWCOM, as well as led an annual interprofessional clinical workshop across the health sciences. An applied anthropologist, she has received funding from the National Institutes of Health, the Macarthur Foundation, and others for her community-based research on social and cultural factors influencing health, with an emphasis in aging, Latinos, and minority populations. Her current research interests include improving services for caregivers of persons with Alzheimer's, reducing social isolation in aging, as well as interprofessional efforts to create age-friendly communities. She previously served as the Chair of the Board of the Alliance for Aging, Inc., the local area agency on aging for Miami-Dade and Monroe Counties, and President of the Association for Anthropology, Gerontology, and the Life Course. She holds a joint Ph.D. in Anthropology and Population & Family Health Sciences (Public Health) from Johns Hopkins University.

Index

I. L. Martinez, D. W. Wiedman (eds.), *Anthropology in Medical Education*,
https://doi.org/10.1007/978-3-030-62277-0

F

G

H

I

N

O